The S∧GES Manual

The SAGES Manual

Volume 2 Advanced Laparoscopy and Endoscopy

Third Edition

Ninh T. Nguyen, MD
University of California Irvine Medical Center,
Orange, CA, USA

and

Carol E.H. Scott-Conner, MD, PhD, MBA
University of Iowa Hospitals and Clinics,
Iowa City, IA, USA

Editors

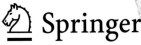

Springer

Editors
Ninh T. Nguyen
Department of Surgery
Division of Gastrointestinal Surgery
University of California Irvine
Medical Center
Orange, CA, USA

Carol E.H. Scott-Conner
Department of Surgery
University of Iowa Hospitals
and Clinics
Iowa City, IA, USA

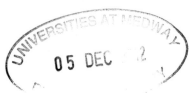

ISBN 978-1-4614-2346-1   e-ISBN 978-1-4614-2347-8
DOI 10.1007/978-1-4614-2347-8
Springer New York Dordrecht Heidelberg London

Library of Congress Control Number: 2012932411

Springer is part of Springer Science+Business Media (www.springer.com)

Foreword

As the Society of American Gastrointestinal and Endoscopic Surgeons complete its 30th year, our commitment to education burns as brightly as ever. The first SAGES manual was published in 1998. Since then it has continued to be a well-organized, clear, and to the point reference in minimally invasive surgery written by experts in the field and aimed at the surgical resident. That said, it will also be useful to students and attending surgeons alike. This third addition of the SAGES manual reflects the best of what has been a leading reference in minimally invasive surgery yet at the same time incorporating many new concepts that have evolved since the second addition. This is mirrored by the tireless efforts of Carol E.H Scott Connor, MD who has overseen this project since its inception and the addition of Ninh T. Nguyen, MD and Nathanial (Nat) Soper, MD as editors of the 3rd edition. Together this team has organized this brilliant reference in the field of minimally invasive surgery.

Surgical residents and practicing surgeons will find this addition completely reorganized as the field of minimally invasive surgery continues to grow. Dividing the manual into 2 volumes allows for a convenient method of keeping it handy as well as reorganizing this book into basic (volume 1) and advance procedures (volume 2). Students of history, who recall that SAGES' roots grew out of flexible endoscopy, will also no doubt notice the increasing prominence of flexible endoscopy in this manual. This reflects the rise in interest of *surgeon* performed endoscopy as a therapeutic tool complementing other MIS techniques. Surgical residents interested in a career in gastrointestinal surgery should pay close attention to the increasing role that the endoscope will play in their future. While the first 2 chapters of this edition of the SAGES manual highlight the roles of the Fundamentals of Laparoscopic Surgery (FLS) and Maintenance of Certification (MOC) play in the educational process, future editions will clearly also include information on the Fundamentals of Endoscopic Surgery (FES) and other key offerings as well.

Even as this book comes to press, controversies concerning optimal treatment strategies continue to swirl as issues of endoluminal therapies, surgical robotics, and natural orifice translumenal endoscopic surgery

(NOTES) are debated around the world. Even the issue concerning the optimal number and size(s) of trocars in our bread and butter commodity procedure, such as laparoscopic cholecystectomy, remains unsettled. Clearly, we should get working on the fourth edition.

I was recently asked if medical texts are destined for the same desolate fate as ice boxes, typewriters, and mimeographs in the annals of history, all supplanted by newer technologies. Clearly, the organization of medical information is evolving rapidly with so much information now available at our fingertips in digital form. The available "infostream" is coming at us like water spouting wildly from a fire hose, but amidst all that data, where do we find truly useful information concisely organized? I suspect it will be in places like the SAGES Manual, and yes, this reference too will be available in a digital format for those who wish to abandon paper altogether.

Whether on paper or in a digital format, I am sure you will enjoy using this reference (at least until the next edition comes out).

Steven D. Schwaitzberg, MD
SAGES President 2011–2012
Cambridge, MA, USA

Preface

In creating this third edition of *The SAGES Manual* we have completely restructured, reorganized, and revised the entire manual. Rather than put the manual on a diet, we have separated it into two volumes for better portability. Volume I covers the fundamentals and procedures performed during surgical residency. We anticipate that Volume I will be the first volume used by students, residents, and allied healthcare professional trainees. Do not be deceived; however, we have added material to these fundamentals and procedures that should also be of interest to experienced surgeons. Volume II covers more advanced procedures, generally taught during fellowship. If you own an old, dog-eared copy of the second edition, you will find much that is new in both volumes.

All of the sections have been reorganized with a critical eye to the needs of the modern minimal access surgeon. Two new editors have been added. Although many chapters have new authors, many stalwart authors have continued to contribute. We have also added color photographs.

As before, the manual strives to strike a balance between completeness and conciseness. Significant additional information, including videos, is available from the SAGES Web site (see Appendix, at the end of Volume I). But, as always, we want you to think of this manual as a way to take SAGES experts along with you throughout your surgical journey.

Nathaniel J. Soper
Saint Louis, MO, USA
Ninh T. Nguyen
Orange, CA, USA
Carol E.H. Scott-Conner
Iowa City, IA, USA

Contents

Part I Laparoscopic Bariatric Surgery

Part II   Benign and Malignant Esophageal Disease

Part III   Laparoscopic Gastric Surgery: Advanced Procedures

Part VI   Other Adjunct Minimally Invasive Procedures for Gastrointestinal Surgeons

Contributors

John N. Afthinos, MD
Department of Surgery, St. Luke's-Roosevelt Hospital Center,
New York, NY, USA

Brian Bello, MD
Department of Surgery, University of Chicago Pritzker
School of Medicine, Chicago, IL, USA

Noelle L. Bertelson, MD, FACS
Division of Colon & Rectal Surgery, Mayo Clinic,
Scotsdale, Phoenix, AZ, USA

Marylise Boutros, MD
Department of Colorectal Surgery, Cleveland Clinic Florida,
Weston, FL, USA

Stacy A. Brethauer, MD
Bariatric and Metabolic Institute, Cleveland Clinic,
Cleveland, OH, USA

Joseph C. Carmichael, MD
Assistant Clinical Professsor, Department of Colon & Rectal Surgery,
University of California Irvine Medical Center, Orange, CA, USA

Alfred Cuschieri, MD, DSc, FRCS, FACS, FRS, FMedSC
Institute for Medical Science & Technology,
University of Dundee, Dundee, Scotland, UK

Anthony P. D'Andrea, MS
Research Associate, Department of Colorectal Surgery,
Lankenau Medical Center & Institute for Medical Research,
Wynnewood, PA, USA

Conor P. Delaney, MD, PhD
Department of Surgery, Division of Colorectal Surgery,
University Hospitals Case Medical Center, Cleveland, OH, USA

James A. Dickerson II, MD
Department of Surgery, Duke University Medical Center,
Durham, NC, USA

Robert B. Dorman, MD, PhD
Department of Surgery, University of Minnesota,
Minneapolis, MN, USA

Brian J. Dunkin, MD, FACS
Section of Endoscopic Surgery,
The Methodist Hospital, Houston, TX, USA

Joanne Favuzza, DO
Department of Surgery, Division of Colorectal Surgery,
University Hospitals Case Medical Center, Cleveland,
OH, USA

Joseph L. Frenkel, MD
Department of Colorectal Surgery, Lankenau Medical Center &
Institute for Medical Research, Wynnewood, PA, USA

Michel Gagner, MD, FRCSC, FACS, FASMBS, FICS, AFC(Hon.)
Professor of Surgery, Department of Surgery, Hôpital du Sacré Coeur,
Montreal, QC, Canada

Erin W. Gilbert, MD
Department of Surgery, Oregon Health & Science University,
Portland, OR, USA

Jayleen Grams, MD, PhD
Assistant Professor, Department of Surgery, Division of Gastrointestinal
Surgery, University of Alabama at Birmingham, Birmingham,
AL, USA

Roberto Gullo, MD
Fellow, Department of Surgery, University of Chicago
Pritzker School of Medicine, Chicago, IL, USA

Paul D. Hansen, MD
Program Director, Department of Surgical Oncology,
Portland Providence Cancer Center, Portland, OR, USA

Helen M. Heneghan, MD
Bariatric and Metabolic Institute, Cleveland Clinic,
Cleveland, OH, USA

John G. Hunter, MD
Department of Surgery, Oregon Health and Sciences University,
Portland, OR, USA

Matthew M. Hutter, MD, MPH, FACS
Department of Surgery, Massachusetts General Hospital,
Boston, MA, USA

William B. Inabnet, MD
Department of Surgery, Mount Sinai Hospital,
New York, NY, USA

Sayeed Ikramuddin, MD
Department of Surgery, University of Minnesota,
Minneapolis, MN, USA

Timothy D. Jackson, MD, MPH, FRCSC
Department of Surgery, Division of General Surgery,
University Health Network - Toronto Western Hospital,
Toronto, ON, Canada

Garth R. Jacobsen, MD
Department of Surgery, University of California, San Diego, CA, USA

Gregg H. Jossart, MD, FACS
Department of Surgery, California Pacific Medical Center,
San Francisco, CA, USA

Namir Katkhouda, MD, FACS
Department of Surgery, University of Southern California,
Los Angeles, CA, USA

Kent W. Kercher, MD, FACS
Department of General Surgery, Carolinas Medical Center,
Charlotte, NC, USA

Abraham Krikhely, MD
Resident, Department of Surgery, New York University Medical Center,
New York, NY, USA

Marina Kurian, MD
Assistant Professor, Department of Surgery,
New York University Medical Center, New York, NY, USA

John G. Lee, M.D.
Professor, Department of Medicine, Division of Gastroenterology,
UC Irvine Medical Center, Orange, CA, USA

Catherine A. Madorin, MD
Department of Surgery, Mount Sinai Hospital, New York, NY, USA

Jeffrey M. Marks, MD, FACS
Director, Department of General Surgery, Case Western Reserve
Medical Center, University Hospitals of Cleveland, Cleveland,
OH, USA

John H. Marks, MD
Department of Colorectal Surgery, Lankenau Medical Center
& Institute for Medical Research, Wynnewood, PA, USA

Brendan Marr, MD
Department of Minimally Invasive Surgery,
Ohio State University Medical Center, Columbus, OH, USA

W. Scott Melvin, MD
Department of Surgery, Division of General and GI Surgery,
Ohio State University Hospital, Columbus, OH, USA

Shai Meron-Eldar, MD
Bariatric and Metabolic Institute, Cleveland Clinic,
Cleveland, OH, USA

Marc P. Michalsky, MD
Department of Pediatric Surgery, National Children's Hospital,
Columbus, OH, USA

Pippa Newell, MD
Department of Surgical Oncology,
Portland Providence Cancer Center, Portland, OR, USA

Allan K. Nguyen, BS
Research Fellow, Department of Surgery,
Division of Gastrointestinal Surgery, University of California Irvine
Medical Center, Orange, CA, USA

Ninh T. Nguyen, MD
Department of Surgery, Division of Gastrointestinal Surgery,
University of California Irvine Medical Center, Orange, CA, USA

Richard Novack Jr., MD
Department of Surgery, New York University Medical Center,
New York, NY, USA

Christopher R. Oxner, MD
Department of General and Oncological Surgery,
City of City Hospital, Duarte, CA, USA

Chan W. Park, MD
Department of Surgery, Duke University Medical Center,
Durham, NC, USA

Marco G. Patti, MD
Department of Surgery, University of Chicago Pritzker
School of Medicine, Chicago, IL, USA

Jeffrey H. Peters, MD, FACS
Department of Surgery, University of Rochester School of Medicine,
Rochester, NY, USA

Melissa S. Phillips, MD
Department of Surgery, University Hospitals Case Medical Center,
Cleveland, OH, USA

Alessio Pigazzi, MD, PhD
Department of Surgery, Division of Colon and Rectal Surgery,
University of California, Irvine, Orange, CA, USA

Aurora D. Pryor, MD
Department of Surgery, Duke University Medical Center,
Durham, NC, USA

Assar A. Rather, MD
Department of Colorectal Surgery,
Cleveland Clinic Florida, Weston, FL, USA

Kevin M. Reavis, MD, FACS
Department of Surgery, Division of Gastrointestinal Surgery,
University of California Irvine Medical Center, Orange, CA, USA

Jason F. Richardson, MD
Department of Surgery, University of California Irvine Medical Center,
Orange, CA, USA

Barry Salky, MD
Department of Surgery, Division of Laparoscopic Surgery,
Mount Sinai School of Medicine, New York, NY, USA

Philip R. Schauer, MD
Bariatric and Metabolic Institute, Cleveland Clinic,
Cleveland, OH, USA

Bruce David Schirmer, MD, FACS
Department of Surgery, University of Virginia,
Charlottesville, VA, USA

Brian R. Smith, MD, FACS
Department of Gastrointestinal Surgery, University of California
Irvine Medical Center, Orange, CA, USA

Nathaniel J. Soper, MD
Loyal and Edith Davis Professor and Chair,
Department of Surgery, Northwestern University Feinberg
School of Medicine, Chicago, IL, USA

Michael J. Stamos, MD
Department of Surgery, University of California Irvine Medical Center,
Orange, CA, USA

Vivian E. Strong, MD
Department of Surgery/Gastric Mixed Tumor Service,
Memorial Sloan-Kettering Cancer Center, New York, NY, USA

Lee L. Swanstrom, MD, FACS
Department of Surgery, Orgeon Health Sciences University,
Portland, OR, USA

Mark A. Talamini, MD
Department of Surgery, University of California, San Diego, CA, USA

Steven Teich, MD
Department of Pediatric Surgery,
National Children's Hospital, Columbus, OH, USA

Julio A. Teixeira, MD, FACS
Department of Surgery,
St. Luke's-Roosevelt Hospital Center, New York, NY, USA

Christopher C. Thompson, MD, MSc, FACG, FASGE
Division of Gastroenterology, Brigham and Women's Hospital, Boston,
MA, USA

Elsa B. Valsdottir, MD
Department of General Surgery,
University Hospital of Iceland, Reykjavik, Iceland

Esteban Varela, MD
Department of Surgery, Division of General Surgery,
Section of Minimally Invasive Surgery,
Washington University in St. Louis School of Medicine,
St. Louis, MO, USA

Rabindra R. Watson, MD
Department of Medicine, University of California, Los Angeles,
Los Angeles, CA, USA

Eric G. Weiss, MD
Department of Colorectal Surgery, Cleveland Clinic Florida,
Weston, FL, USA

Steven D. Wexner, MD
Department of Colorectal Surgery, Cleveland Clinic Florida,
Weston, FL, USA

Tonia M. Young-Fadok, MD, MS, FACS, FASCRS
Division of Colon and Rectal Surgery, Mayo Clinic, Scotsdale,
Phoenix, AZ, USA

Part I
Laparoscopic Bariatric Surgery

1. Laparoscopic Bariatric Surgery: Principles of Patient Selection and Choice of Operation

Richard Novack, Jr., M.D.
Abraham Krikhely, M.D.
Marina Kurian, M.D.

A. Indications

Obesity is a worldwide epidemic and efforts to decrease the rising rates have not been effective. In the USA, obesity currently affects 36% of the population. Obesity has been classified in different ways but mostly based upon the body mass index (BMI). Class I obesity is a BMI between 30 and 34.9, class II is between 35 and 39.9, and class III is over 40. Class III obesity is also considered morbid obesity. Surgically treatable obesity is considered severe obesity, and generally implies that the patient has approximately 100 lbs to lose. Approximately 6.2% of the US population is considered morbidly obese, which represented over 18 million people in 2011. In 1991, an NIH consensus panel was convened to look at effective treatments for morbid obesity. The NIH has examined surgery for morbid obesity several times since then, most recently in 2004, but the 1991 guidelines remain applicable. Obesity-related deaths are estimated to be over 300,000 per year. Combined deaths from colon, breast, and lung cancer are 248,000 in 2010. Obesity is the number two preventable cause of death, with smoking being number one. Treating morbid obesity improves a variety of comorbid conditions, including cardiovascular disease, hypertension, diabetes, sleep apnea, and joint disease to name a few.

N.T. Nguyen and C.E.H. Scott-Conner (eds.), *The SAGES Manual: Volume 2 Advanced Laparoscopy and Endoscopy*, DOI 10.1007/978-1-4614-2347-8_1, © Springer Science+Business Media, LLC 2012

B. Patient Selection

Patients with morbid or severe obesity are at least 100 lbs above their ideal body weight, which is determined based on their height and body shape based on the 1984 Metropolitan Life Tables. This extra 100 lbs or more is considered the **excess weight** that the patient has to lose. Not all severely obese patients are candidates for weight loss surgery. Patients must have a BMI of 35–39.9 with a severe comorbid condition or a BMI≥40 with or without a comorbidity. In addition, they must have failed nonsurgical management of their morbid obesity (including diet, exercise, medications, and behavior modification). The patient has to understand the risks of surgery and commit to the aftercare and necessary behavior modifications.

C. Preoperative and Postoperative Care

Prior to weight loss surgery, the patient is screened by a multidisciplinary team, which includes a dietitian, clinical psychologist, and the surgeon. Most insurance companies require documentation of prior weight loss history and may have other requirements as well. The psychological and dietary evaluations help assess and prepare the patient for the postoperative changes expected after the different weight loss procedures. The patient is guided as to the preoperative and postoperative diets as well as necessary behavioral changes. The detailed history and physical in the surgeon's office helps to fully evaluate the patient's physical preparedness for weight loss surgery. Some patients may need to be further optimized for surgery by a cardiologist, pulmonologist, or endocrinologist in addition to their primary care physician. Patients need a risk assessment before this elective surgery as many morbidly obese patients have some degree of underlying cardiovascular risk. A cardiologist may need to assess and optimize the patient's cardiac risk. A pulmonologist may need to assess the patient for sleep apnea and determine the need for preoperative CPAP. Asthma, obesity hypoventilation syndrome, or narcolepsy with pulmonary hypertension is also assessed by the pulmonologist. A hematology evaluation may be necessary in patients with a history of DVT/PE and/or hypercoagualable disorder. An individual patient's medical history will guide the necessary preoperative evaluations. Patients considered high risk, with a history of DVT, PE, venous stasis disease, or super morbid hormone produced mainly by P/D1 cells lining the fundus of the human stomach and epsilon cells of the pancreas. It stimulates hunger. Numerous studies indicate that sharp declines in fasting and postprandial levels of this orexigenic hormone following LSG cause a long-term reduction in hunger feeling, which significantly reduces oral intake.

2. **Efficacy**: The early results seem to quite promising, with weight loss that approaches other well-established procedures. The postoperative percent excess weight loss (%EWL) is 49.9% ($n=159$), 64.2% ($n=138$), 67.9% ($n=77$), 62.4% ($n=34$), and 62.2% ($n=9$) at 3, 6, 12, 24, and 36 months, respectively. In addition, resolution of comorbidities, including diabetes, hypertension, hyperlipidemia, and sleep apnea, has been reported in many patients 12–24 months after LSG. These results are comparable to those of other restrictive procedures. Long-term data (>5 years) for weight loss and comorbidity resolution are just being obtained for LSG.

3. **Complications**: The two most common operative complications after LSG are staple-line bleeding and anastomotic leaks. These complications can be life-threatening. Published complication rates range from 0 to 24%, with an overall reported mortality rate of 0.39%. The postoperative staple-line bleeding rate can be as high as 7.3%. In early experience, sleeve gastrectomy had an early complication rate equivalent to that of LRYGB, BPD-DS, and LAGB, without the late complications of marginal ulcerations, internal hernias, malabsorption issues, adjustments, or foreign body complications. LSG is also an effective and generally safe operation as a first-stage procedure for high-risk surgical patients who are undergoing bariatric surgery. There is increasing evidence that it also serves as a definitive weight loss operation for many patients. LSG is a restrictive rather than a malabsorptive procedure, thereby minimizing nutritional concerns compared with other procedures.

I. Emerging Technology

Application of newer techniques, such as NOTES and single incision laparoscopy, has not been widely adopted to date. These procedures further reduce scar compared to standard laparoscopy and provide a cosmetic benefit to the patient. New endoscopic procedures for weight loss include endoluminal stapling to create a narrow pouch (TOGA), endoscopic plications to create an endoscopic sleeve (POSE trial by USGI) as well as procedures to place various stents to create the effect of an intestinal bypass (Endobarrier). The field of bariatric surgery is an exciting one, full of innovation at this time.

Selected References

Buchwald H, Avidor Y, Braunwald E, et al. Bariatric surgery: a systematic review and meta-analysis. JAMA. 2004;292:1724–8.

Farrell TM, Haggerty SP, Overby DW, Kohn GP, Richardson WS, Fanelli RD. Clinical application of laparoscopic bariatric surgery: an evidence-based review. Surg Endosc. 2009a;23:930–49.

Farrell T, Haggerty S, Overby W, et al. Clinical application of laparoscopic bariatric surgery: an evidence-based review. Surg Endosc. 2009b;23:930–49.

Fielding G, Ren C. Laparoscopic adjustable gastric band. Surg Clin North Am. 2005;85:129–40.

Fuks D, Verhaeghe P, Brehant O, Sabbagh C, Dumont F, Delcenserie R. Results of laparoscopic sleeve gastrectomy: a prospective study in 135 patients with morbid obesity. Surgery. 2009;145(1):106–13.

Gluck B, Movitz B, Jansma S, Gluck J, Laskowski K. Laparoscopic sleeve gastrectomy is a safe and effective bariatric procedure for the lower BMI (35.0–43.0 kg/m2) population. Obes Surg. 2010;21:1168–71.

Gulkarov I, Wetterau M, Ren CJ, Fielding GA. Hiatal hernia repair at the initial laparoscopic adjustable gastric band operation reduces the need for reoperation. Surg Endosc. 2008;22(4):1035–41.

Kinzl JF, Schrattenecker M, Traweger C, et al. Psychosocial predictors of weight loss after bariatric surgery. Obes Surg. 2006;16(12):1609–14.

Lalor P, Tucker O, Szomstein S, Rosenthal R. Complications after laparoscopic sleeve gastrectomy. Surg Obes Relat Dis. 2008;4:33–8.

Moy J, Pomp A, Dakins G, Parikh M, Gagner M. Laparoscopic sleeve gastrectomy for morbid obesity. Am J Surg. 2008;196(5):56–9.

Parikh M, Fielding G, Ren C, et al. U.S. experience with 749 laparoscopic adjustable gastric bands. Surg Endosc. 2005;19:1631–5.

Parikh M, Laker S, Weiner M, Hajiseyedjavadi O, Ren C. Objective comparison of complications resulting from laparoscopic bariatric procedures. J Am Coll Surg. 2006;202(2):252–61.

Parikh M, Ayoung-Chee P, Romanos E, Lewis N, Pachter HL, Fielding G, et al. Comparison of rates of resolution of diabetes mellitus after gastric banding, gastric bypass, and biliopancreatic diversion. J Am Coll Surg. 2007;205(5):631–5.

SAGES Guidelines Committee. SAGES guideline for clinical application of laparoscopic bariatric surgery. Surg Endosc. 2008;22:2281–300.

Silecchia G, Boru C, Pecchia A, Rizzello M, Casella G, Leonetti F, et al. Effectiveness of laparoscopic sleeve gastrectomy (first stage of biliopancreatic diversion with duodenal switch) on co-morbidities in super-obese high risk patients. Obes Surg. 2006;16: 1138–44.

2. Laparoscopic Roux-en-Y Gastric Bypass: Techniques and Outcomes

Robert B. Dorman, M.D., Ph.D.
Sayeed Ikramuddin, M.D.

A. Introduction

The Roux-en-Y gastric bypass (RYGB) is the "gold standard" bariatric surgical procedure. According to the American Society for Metabolic and Bariatric Surgery, the RYGB is currently the most common bariatric procedure performed in the USA. The RYGB has both restrictive and malabsorptive properties due to the combination of a small gastric pouch and total bypass of the duodenum and the proximal jejunum. Today, over 90% of RYGB are performed laparoscopically. In this chapter, we highlight the history of the RYGB, operative indications, operative techniques, postoperative management, common complications and outcomes.

The RYGB has evolved significantly over the previous decades. Edward Mason was the first to describe the gastric bypass operation in 1967 as a treatment for morbid obesity. The stomach was divided creating a 100 mL horizontal, proximal gastric pouch to which a loop gastrojejunostomy was constructed. Later, Mason and colleagues reduced the pouch size to <50 mL to increase weight loss and reduce the frequency of anastomotic ulcer formation. Later in 1977, a horizontal stapled, undivided pouch was introduced by John Alden which was followed by the introduction of the Roux-en-Y reconstruction by Ward Griffen. This served to prevent alkaline reflux into the gastric pouch. The stomach was later divided from the pouch to reduce the incidence of gastrogastric fistula. Torres and Oca modified the Roux limb by lengthening it, a technique that was later popularized by Brolin and colleagues to augment weight loss. In 1994, Wittgrove and colleagues described the first laparoscopic RYGB with an end-to-end stapler technique. In 1999, Kelvin Higa described the first laparoscopic RYGB with a hand-sewn gastrojejunostomy.

N.T. Nguyen and C.E.H. Scott-Conner (eds.), *The SAGES Manual: Volume 2 Advanced Laparoscopy and Endoscopy*, DOI 10.1007/978-1-4614-2347-8_2, © Springer Science+Business Media, LLC 2012

B. Indications

1. Per the criteria set forth by the 1994 National Institute of Health Consensus Statement, bariatric surgery is indicated for patients with a body mass index (BMI) greater than or equal to 40 kg/m^2 or with a BMI greater than or equal to 35 kg/m^2 if one additional major comorbidity is present.
   a. A major comorbidity could include type 2 diabetes, obstructive sleep apnea, or hypertension.
   b. Since this statement was released, the profound effect of bariatric surgery on metabolic disease, particularly type 2 diabetes, has been thoroughly documented. Studies are currently underway to investigate the effect of the RYGB on patients with type 2 diabetes who have a BMI less than 35 kg/m^2.

C. Preoperative Evaluation

Preoperative planning includes evaluations by the patient's primary care physician, a mental health professional, and a nutritionist. Commitment of the patient to attend several preoperative appointments serves as a litmus test for their ability to follow-up after surgery as well. In our practice, all patients are followed for a minimum of 3 months after referral before undergoing their procedure. At least 6 months of preparation with lifestyle and dietary modification is preferred.

1. A letter provided by the primary care physician upon referral should include previous weight loss strategies, such as exercise and dietary regimens as well as any previously attempted medical weight loss treatments. Also, a chronologic history of the patient's weight should be documented. Ultimately, surgery is only a tool and the long-term success of the operation is often determined by adherence to a diet and exercise plan postoperatively.
2. Polysomnography should be obtained when sleep apnea is suspected based on history, with the implementation of a continuous positive airway pressure (CPAP) device if warranted.
3. Referral to a cardiologist is recommended for patients over the age of 45 years with a diagnosis of type 2 diabetes or any patient older than 50 years with concomitant risk factors, such as a history of smoking, dyslipidemia, or hypertension. An echocardiogram

is recommended for patients with a history of fluramine and phentermine (Fen-Phen) use of 6 months duration.

4. A history of deep venous thrombosis or other clotting abnormality with unknown etiology triggers a hematology consultation.

5. The presence of severe pulmonary hypertension should prompt preoperative placement of a temporary inferior vena cava filter as a pulmonary embolism would be poorly tolerated in this patient population.

6. Physical medicine and rehabilitation is consulted if a patient has limited exercise ability due to neurologic, muscle, or joint disorders.

7. All patients should be screened for deficiencies in iron, vitamin B12, thiamine (B1), folate (B9), 25-hydroxy-vitamin D and calcium preoperatively.

8. Preoperative weight loss is a core component of preparation. The ability to accomplish this solidifies a patient's commitment to the weight loss process.

9. Documented smoking cessation is required for patients who smoke.

10. Exclusion criteria for RYGB include inflammatory bowel disease, ulcer diathesis, and those who are dependent on nonsteroidal anti-inflammatory medications.

11. A relative contraindication for a laparoscopic procedure includes a history of one or multiple previous intra-abdominal surgeries, where evaluation of the small bowel due to adhesions may be suboptimal. A previous colectomy may serve as a relative contraindication to a laparoscopic RYGB because distal adhesions may precipitate early postoperative bowel obstruction and increase the likelihood of an anastomotic leak. Thought should also be given to patients at increased risk for gastric cancer who would require frequent surveillance of their gastric remnant.

12. The use of esophagogastroduodenoscopy with *Helicobacter pylori* testing preoperatively remains controversial.

D. Operative Technique

In the preoperative area, all patients receive subcutaneous low-molecular weight heparin and sequential compression devices are applied as prophylaxis against deep venous thrombosis. Antibiotics (e.g. cefoxitin 2 g) are administered within 30 minutes of incision.

Ideally, the room should be equipped with an operating table capable of holding 1,000 pounds and providing at least 45° of reverse Trendelenburg position. The table should also have the ability to be fitted with extenders for length and width. A footboard is essential to prevent patient movement during manipulation of the operating table. Extra-long instruments may be necessary and should include toothed and atraumatic graspers, ultrasonic scissors, endoscopic staplers, liver retractors, and suction aspirators.

1. Position the patient supine position with arms out to the side and padding under both knees. Place a Foley catheter and secure the feet with tape and padding to the footboard. Place a safety strap just above the patient's knees.

2. The surgeon stands on the patient's right side with the assistant on the left. We operate with four ceiling-mounted monitors placed at shoulder level of both the surgeon and the assistant.

3. Establish pneumoperitoneum through a 15 cm Veress needle in the left upper quadrant at the junction of the mid-clavicular line just beneath the costal margin if no previous midline or left-sided incisions are present. Once pneumoperitoneum is established, place a 5-mm trocar at this site. Routinely, a total of five extra-long trocars are placed across the upper abdomen. An 11-mm trocar is placed approximately 15 cm below the xiphoid just to the left of midline under direct vision. A 10 mm, 45° laparoscope is then placed through the 11 mm port and the patient is placed in steep reverse Trendelenburg. Two ports are then placed along the patient's right side; one subcostal at the mid-clavicular line (5 mm) and the second (12 mm) is placed medial to the midclavicular line and just rostral to the camera port. A 5 mm trocar is placed in the right flank for liver retraction, and a sixth 5 mm working port can be placed in the patient's left flank for retraction when necessary (Fig. 2.1).

4. To create the gastric pouch, first divide the lesser omentum with a Harmonic scalpel. The left gastric artery should be easy to identify. Take care to avoid dividing a replaced or accessory left hepatic artery, if present.

5. Transect the neurovascular fat bundle along the lesser curve using a 6 cm linear endostapler with a vascular staple cartridge. Bovine pericardium or other staple-line reinforcement product reduces bleeding from staple lines.

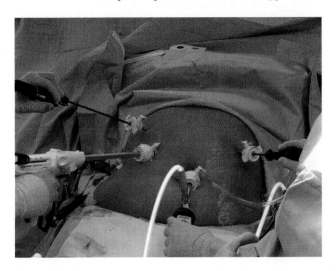

Fig. 2.1. Port placement. Five ports are routinely placed across the upper abdomen for maximum maneuverability and optimal exposure.

6.   Next, orient the endostapler transversely 2–3 cm distal to the gastroesophageal junction and just distal to the left gastric artery; and fire it to complete the transection of the neurovascular pedicle.

7.   Create a 20–30 mL vertically oriented gastric pouch with the endostapler using 3.5 mm staples or a "blue" staple load. Sizing of the pouch with a balloon has proven not to be necessary. First, perform a transverse application of the stapler, with subsequent applications oriented toward the angle of His parallel to the lesser curve (Fig. 2.2). Apply Surgicel® as a topical hemostatic agent to control any oozing. Take care to avoid any incorporation of gastric fundus in the pouch. Repair any staple line defects in the pouch or gastric remnant with endo-suturing techniques. Alternative techniques include formation of the gastric pouch with the use of ring reinforcement and the micro-pouch technique.

8.   We perform an antecolic, antegastric anastomosis. If a retrogastric anastomosis is planned or necessary due to a foreshortened mesentery, adhesions posterior to the remnant must be divided. Divide the greater omentum to improve reach of the Roux limb.

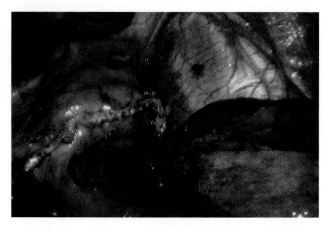

Fig. 2.2. Gastric pouch. The gastric pouch (*left*) following transection from gastric remnant (*right*).

9.   Next, perform the gastrojejunostomy. Return the table to a neutral position and then identify the ligament of Treitz by lifting the transverse mesocolon rostrally. Measure out 100 cm of jejunum from the ligament of Treitz and a small defect is created in the mesentery. Pass a Penrose drain through. Rotate the proximal bowel one-half turn clockwise and bring the loop of jejunum up to the gastric pouch in an antecolic, antegastric fashion. At this time, the proximal Roux limb is to the patient's right and the biliopancreatic limb is to the patient's left.

10. Return the table to reverse Trendelenberg. Form the back row of the gastrojejunostomy anastomosis using an Endostitch™ (Covidien) with a 3–0 braided nylon running seromuscular suture beginning at the angle of His at the rostral aspect of the gastric pouch staple line. On the Roux limb, start the back row suture close to the mesentery.

11. At the right inferior portion of the pouch, create a gastrotomy with the Harmonic® scalpel (Ethicon Endo-Surgery). Similarly, create an enterotomy at a corresponding point on the Roux limb. Insert a blue staple load into the pouch and Roux limb to no more than 2.0 cm and fire it to create the gastrojejunostomy (Fig. 2.3).

12. Pass a 30-Fr endoscope through the mouth, into the pouch, through the anastomosis and into the Roux limb. Use an Endostitch™ to close the defect over the endoscope in two layers. Next, use a white load cartridge to divide the jejunum just

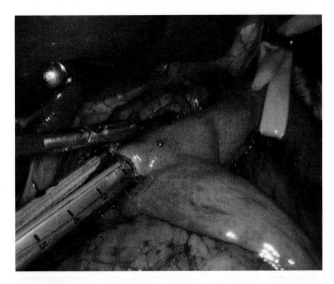

Fig. 2.3. Gastrojejunostomy. Following suturing of the back wall of the anastomosis a blue load endostapler is used to create the gastrojejunostomy. The Penrose drain in the background marks 100 cm from the ligament of Treitz and is the future site of division of the jejunum.

to the left of the gastrojejunal anastomosis. If the small bowel is unusually thick, consider a blue load to divide the small bowel. Remove the Penrose drain from the abdomen.

13. To test the anastomosis, place a bowel clamp 5 cm distal to the gastrojejunostomy and submerge the site of anastomosis in saline irrigation. Insufflate air through the endoscope with monitoring for bubbles. Oversew any areas suspected of leaking and then repeat the insufflation process. Drains at the site of the gastrojejunostomy are rarely used.

14. A 150 cm Roux limb is standard. It is measured from the gastrojejunostomy.

15. Sew the distal biliopancreatic limb, the stapled end created in step 11 above, to the Roux limb at their antimesenteric borders in preparation for a functional side-to-side stapled anastomosis. Take extra care to be certain that the mesenteries are properly aligned and no twists are present.

16. Make enterotomies in the Roux limb and biliopancreatic limb with a Harmonic® scalpel. Insert a 6 cm white cartridge load to its full length in each limb to create the anastomosis. Place a single suture to secure the heel of the anastomosis (Fig. 2.4a).

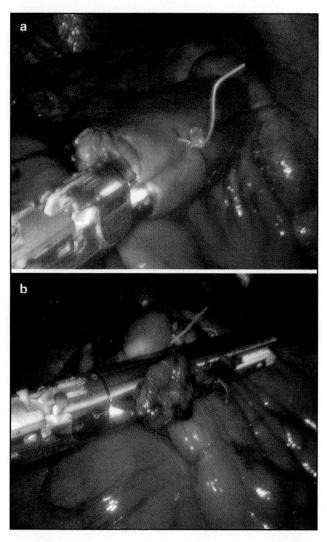

Fig. 2.4. Jejunojejunostomy. A side-to-side functional anastomosis is formed between the two enterotomies with an endostapler (**a**) and the common enterotomy is closed with an endostapler as well (**b**). An anti-obstruction stitch is placed to aid in preventing future kinking of the anastomosis (**c**). (Part **c** Reprinted with permission has been granted from J Gastrointest Surg. 2007;11:217–28, for Fig. 2.4).

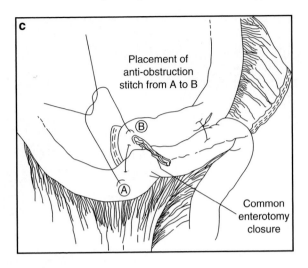

Fig. 2.4.   (continued)

17. Approximate the edges of the common enterotomy with an Endostitch™, and close the enterotomy with an additional firing of a white load with the 6 cm endostapler (Fig. 2.4b). Approximate any areas of separated serosa with Lembert sutures.

18. Place an "anti-obstruction stitch" from the Roux limb to the biliopancreatic limb to prevent kinking (Fig. 2.4c). Close the small mesenteric defect with a running suture (Fig. 2.5). Apply fibrin glue to the staple line to reduce adhesions and bleeding.

19. Close Peterson's defect with a purse-string suture (Fig. 2.6).

20. Remove trocars and close all skin incisions with staples. These can be removed and replaced with Steri-Strips™ (3M Corporation) on postoperative day 2.

E. Postoperative Management

Postoperative management is directed toward avoidance and early detection of complications. Nasogastric tubes are not routinely left in place. On postoperative day 1 an upper gastrointestinal contrast study is obtained to look for evidence of an anastomotic leak or a Roux limb

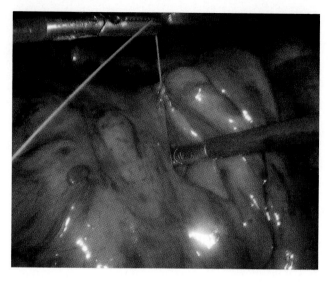

Fig. 2.5. Mesenteric defect. A short running suture is used to close the short mesenteric defect after creation of the jejunojejunostomy.

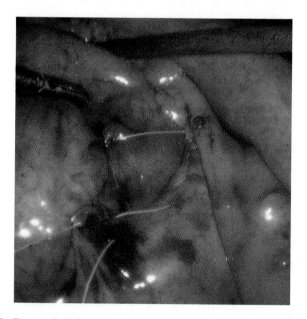

Fig. 2.6. Peterson's defect. Peterson's defect is closed with a purse string suture to reduce the likelihood of future internal hernia formation.

obstruction. If negative, patients are started on clear liquids that morning. Typically, patients are discharged home on postoperative day 2 with follow-up in bariatric surgery clinic at 1 week and at 1, 3, 6, 9, and 12 months.

F. Complications

Complications can be divided into two groups: non-technical and technical.

Non-technical complications include nausea and vomiting, deep venous thrombosis, and pulmonary embolism. Technical complications include anastomotic leak, stricture, bowel obstruction, and hemorrhage.

1. A leak rate of <1% is anticipated.
2. A rate of deep venous thrombosis of <1% is expected.
3. A stricture rate of 5–8% is appropriate.
4. The rate of internal hernias is between 1 and 3%.
5. Marginal ulcer rate is anywhere from 1 to 10%.
6. An overall 30-day mortality rate of 0.2% has been reported.

G. Outcomes of RYGB

1. In a study published by Adams et al., with a mean follow-up of 7.1 years, the mortality rate for patients who underwent RYGB was 2.7% versus 4.1% in BMI-matched controls. Disease-specific mortality was reduced by 56%, 92%, and 60% for coronary artery disease, diabetes, and cancer, respectively.
2. Major adverse events are predicted by a history of deep venous thrombosis or pulmonary embolism, a history of obstructive sleep apnea and impaired functional status. Major complications have also been shown to be predicted by male gender, higher BMI, advancing age and preoperative presence of bleeding disorders.
3. 90-day readmission rate following laparoscopic gastric bypass is between 6 and 7% with the most common complications resulting in readmission being nausea/vomiting/dehydration and stricture.

4. Weight loss at 1 year on average equals 70% of excess weight.
5. Twenty to thirty percent total weight loss at 10 years has been reported.
6. Failure rate, defined as a follow-up BMI ≥35 kg/m² for morbidly obese or ≥40 kg/m² for super obese, is 35% at 10 years overall with 58% failure rate among the super obese.
7. The effect of RYGB on comorbid illnesses is profound. A large meta-analysis by Buchwald et al. demonstrated that RYGB resulted in 84% resolution of type 2 diabetes, 94% of patients experienced improvement in hyperlipidemia, and 75% demonstrated resolution of their hypertension.

H. Summary

1. The laparoscopic RYGB is the most commonly performed bariatric procedure in the USA today.
2. Preoperative evaluation and appropriate patient selection are key factors for a successful weight loss operation.
3. The effect of the RYGB on metabolic disease is profound, and studies are currently underway to explore the utility of the RYGB outside the current BMI guidelines making the RYGB a metabolic operation as well as a weight loss operation.

Selected References

Adams TD, Gress RE, Smith SC, Halverson RC, Simper SC, Rosamond WD, LaMonte MJ, Stroup AM, Hunt SC. Long-term mortality after gastric bypass surgery. N Engl J Med. 2007;357:753–61.

Brolin RE. The antiobstruction stitch in Roux en Y enteroenterostomy. Am J Surg. 1995;3:355–7.

Buchwald H. Overview of bariatric surgery. J Am Coll Surg. 2002;194(3):367–75.

Buchwald H, Buchwald JN. Evolution of operative procedures for the management of morbid obesity 1950–2000. Obes Surg. 2002;12:705–17.

Buchwald H, Avidor Y, Braunwald E, Jensen MD, Pories W, Fahrbach K, Schoelles K. Bariatric surgery: a systematic review and meta-analysis. JAMA. 2004;292(14):1724–37.

Christou NV, Look D, MacLean LD. Weight gain after short- and long-limb gastric bypass in patients followed for longer than 10 years. Ann Surg. 2006;244(5):734–40.

Cohen R, Pinheiro JS, Correa JL, Schiavon CA. Laparoscopic Roux-en-Y gastric bypass for BMI <35 kg/m^2: a tailored approach. Surg Obes Relat Dis. 2006;2(3):401–4.

Fobi MAL. Placement of the GaBP ring system in the banded gastric bypass operation. Obes Surg. 2005;15:1196–201.

Ikramuddin S, Kendrick ML, Kellogg TA, Sarr MG. Open and laparoscopic Roux-en-Y gastric bypass: our techniques. J Gastrointest Surg. 2007;11(2):217–28.

Lancaster RT, Hutter MM. Bands and bypasses: 30-day morbidity and mortality of bariatric surgical procedures as assessed by prospective, multi-center, risk-adjusted ACS-NSQIP data. Surg Endosc. 2008;22:2254–63.

le Roux CW, Aylwin SJ, Batterham RL, Borg CM, Coyle F, Prasad V, Shurey S, Ghatei MA, Patel AG, Bloom SR. Gut hormone profiles following bariatric surgery favor an anorectic state, facilitate weight loss, and improve metabolic parameters. Ann Surg. 2006;243(1):108–14.

Livingston EH, Huerta S, Arthur D, Lee S, De Shields S, Heber D. Male gender is a predictor of morbidity and age a predictor of mortality for patients undergoing gastric bypass surgery. Ann Surg. 2002;236(5):576–82.

The Longitudinal Assessment of Bariatric Surgery (LABS) Consortium. Perioperative safety in the longitudinal assessment of bariatric surgery. N Engl J Med. 2009; 361(5):445–54.

Rubino F, Moo TA, Rosen DJ, Dakin GF, Pomp A. Diabetes surgery: a new approach to an old disease. Diabetes Care. 2009;32(2):S368–72.

Sapala JA, Wood MH, Sapala MA, Schuhknecht MP, Flake TM. The micropouch gastric bypass: technical considerations in primary and revisionary operations. Obes Surg. 2001;11:3–17.

Schneider BE, Villegas L, Blackburn GL, Mun EC, Critchlow JF, Jones DB. Laparoscopic gastric bypass surgery: outcomes. J Laparoendosc Adv Surg Tech A. 2003;13(4): 247–55.

Sjöström L, Lindroos A-K, Peltonen M, Torgerson J, Bouchard C, Carlsson B, Dahlgren S, Larsson B, Narbro K, Sjöström CD, Sullivan M, Wedel H. Lifestyle, diabetes, and cardiovascular risk factors 10 years after bariatric surgery. N Engl J Med. 2004; 351(26):2683–93.

3. Laparoscopic Gastric Banding[*]

Jason F. Richardson, M.D.
Brian R. Smith, M.D., F.A.C.S.

A. Introduction

Adjustable gastric banding is a restrictive bariatric procedure during which a fluid-filled silicone band is wrapped around the gastric cardia. The volume of fluid within the band may be adjusted through percutaneous access to a subcutaneous port that is connected to the band by flexible tubing and attached to the anterior abdominal fascia. Increasing band fluid volume results in greater extrinsic compression and more limited flow of luminal contents through the gastric cardia.

B. Indications

The 1991 National Institutes of Health Consensus Development Conference recommended that bariatric surgery could be considered in well-informed and motivated patients with body mass indexes (BMI) >40 kg/m^2 (or >35 kg/m^2 with at least one high-risk, obesity-related comorbid condition) who have failed established weight control programs and who have been determined to have acceptable operative risks after being evaluated by a multidisciplinary team. Obesity-related comorbid conditions include cardiomyopathy, coronary artery disease, dyslipidemia, gastroesophageal reflux, hypertension, infertility, obstructive sleep apnea, osteoarthritis, pseudotumor cerebri, type-2 diabetes, urinary stress incontinence, and venous stasis, to name some. In February 2011, The Food and Drug Administration (FDA) expanded the approved use of

---

[*]This chapter was contributed by Todd A Kellogg, M.D. and Sayeed Ikramuddin M.D. in the previous edition.

N.T. Nguyen and C.E.H. Scott-Conner (eds.), *The SAGES Manual: Volume 2 Advanced Laparoscopy and Endoscopy*, DOI 10.1007/978-1-4614-2347-8_3, © Springer Science+Business Media, LLC 2012

laparoscopic adjustable gastric banding (LAGB), to include adults who have a BMI ≥30 and at least one obesity-related comorbid condition.

In the arsenal of bariatric surgical operations currently performed, certain procedures may be more appropriate for specific patients. The choice of operation should be based primarily on the patient's BMI and comorbid conditions. When compared to LAGB, laparoscopic Roux-en-Y gastric bypass (GBP) has been shown to be more effective at achieving long-term weight loss and reducing obesity-related comorbid conditions, but carries a higher mortality rate. Average 30-day mortality rates for GBP and LAGB are 0.16% and 0.06%, respectively.

One prospective randomized trial involving LAGB found excess body weight loss (EBWL) to be a 37% at 1 year and 42% after 3 years. Other studies have found EBWL to be around 50% after 1 year. Two prospective randomized trials have suggested that LAGB patients with relatively lower preoperative BMI have greater EBWL over time. The cutoff in one study was a preoperative BMI <50 kg/m^2, whereas the other study used a preoperative excess body weight <50 kg. Regarding long-term reoperations, 23% of LAGB patients either required conversion to another procedure or experienced <20% EBWL at 4 years. Male sex has been found to be a significant predictor of poor weight loss after LAGB. Many studies demonstrate a 60–72% improvement in obesity-related comorbid conditions after LAGB. Although this is similar to LGBP, such improvements are typically less pronounced and take longer to occur after LAGB (are weight-loss related).

Considering the above findings, LAGB may be better suited for patients who are:

- Older or have more severe comorbidities.
- Starting with a lower BMI (≤50).
- Female.
- Non-diabetic.

Independent predictors of surgical morbidity and mortality after LAGB include age ≥45 years, BMI ≥50 kg/m^2, cigarette smoking, hypertension, and male gender. Relative contraindications are the same as bariatric surgery in general, and include:

- High cardiopulmonary risk.
- End-stage liver disease.
- Uncontrolled severe psychiatric disorders.
- Alcohol or drug dependence.
- Tobacco smoking.
- Inability to comprehend or adopt postoperative lifestyle changes.

C. Preoperative Management

1. Weeks Prior to Surgery:
   a. **Workup**—Patients preparing for LAGB require preoperative medical evaluation and optimization. Work-up should include a 12-lead EKG, chest radiograph, lipid profile, nutritional panel, and blood chemistries. A history of dysphagia or gastroesophageal reflux may warrant additional evaluations, such as contrast fluoroscopy, endoscopy, and manometry.
   b. **Diet**—Some surgeons recommend a low fat, low carbohydrate, and high protein liquid diet for 2 weeks prior to bariatric surgery. Patients who were able to attain ≥5% EBWL prior to surgery were found prospectively to have a lower BMI and higher EBWL 1 year after surgery. Therefore, success with preoperative weight loss may identify patients with the discipline necessary to achieve sustained weight loss after surgery. Weight loss prior to surgery also decreases the volume of a fatty liver and may facilitate intraoperative retraction of the left lobe and access to the angle of His while decreasing the likelihood of liver injury during retraction.
   c. **Medication Adjustments**—Diabetic patients should be counseled to reduce their dose of oral hypoglycemic agents and long-acting insulin preparations for the day prior to surgery. A frequently successful practice is to halve the long-acting insulin dose and eliminate any afternoon oral hypoglycemics.
2. Immediately Prior to Surgery
   a. **Deep venous thrombosis (DVT) prophylaxis**—Most patients for whom bariatric surgery is indicated fall into a high-risk category for VTE. Consequently, the use of pneumatic compression devices is mandatory and chemoprophylaxis preoperatively is strongly encouraged.
   b. **Infection avoidance**—Since LAGB involves the insertion of an implantable device, sterile technique must be closely followed to avoid contamination. Without entry into the gastrointestinal tract, the surgical technique described in this chapter would be classified as a clean procedure under

the Centers for Disease Control and Prevention (CDC) wound classification system. Routine preoperative antibiotic prophylaxis is indicated, should be directed at common skin bacteria, and be dosed prior to incision according to patient weight. Alternative antibiotics may be necessary if the patient is known to be colonized by resistant microorganisms.

c. **Equipment**—Flush the gastric band and port with saline prior to insertion to evaluate for device leaks. As with any surgery, it is important to verify the presence and functionality of all the required equipment prior to surgery. This includes the availability of an additional band and port to be utilized as a backup in the event that the first one is damaged or contaminated during surgery. Some surgeons choose to have an orogastric balloon catheter available for calibrating the gastric pouch size during band placement.

d. **Monitoring**—Routine cardiac noninvasive monitoring is essential. Arterial, central venous, and urinary catheters are only indicated when additional monitoring is necessary based on patient comorbidities. An orogastric tube for decompression is optional.

e. **Patient positioning**—Some surgeons prefer the lithotomy position with the surgeon located between the patient's legs since it allows for an optimized operative posture and orientation of the laparoscopic instruments, thereby minimizing shoulder fatigue. It has the disadvantage of increasing the risk of common peroneal nerve injury if the patient is not positioned properly. An alternative and arguably easier position is supine with arms abducted bilaterally and secured to arm-boards. A footboard and upper thigh belt minimizes patient slippage during reverse intraoperative positioning. In this position, the surgeon stands on the right side of the patient, and the assistant on the left.

D. Operative Technique

1. Port placement varies greatly among surgeons and usually involves either four or five trocars ranging from 5 to 15 mm. Our approach has an advantageous balance between ideal liver

retraction, surgeon ergonomics, and near universal utility between various patients and foregut procedures. Place a Veress needle through a left supraumbilical incision and insufflate the abdominal cavity to 15 mmHg prior to exchanging the needle for a 12-mm trochar (camera port). Introduce an angled laparoscope and use it to evaluate for any inadvertent bowel injury during entry. Place three 5-mm trochars under laparoscopic visualization in the far right subcostal margin (liver retractor), right upper quadrant (surgeon's left hand), and far left subcostal margin (assistant's right hand). Place a 15-mm trochar in the right hypogastric region (surgeon's right hand).

2. Place the patient in a steep reverse Trendelenburg position, and position a liver retractor to elevate the left lobe of the liver (Fig. 3.1). Use a blunt grasper to introduce the gastric band through the 15-mm trocar and place it away from the operative field. Evaluate the diaphragm for large defects and herniation, and repair these before band placement.

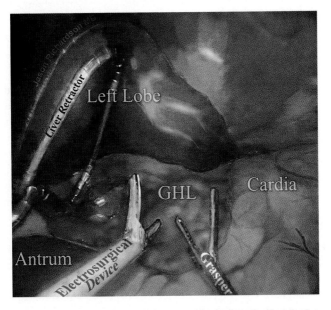

Fig. 3.1. Configuration of instruments in preparation for band placement. Gastrohepatic ligament (GHL), gastric cardia, gastric antrum, serpentine liver retractor lifting left lobe of liver.

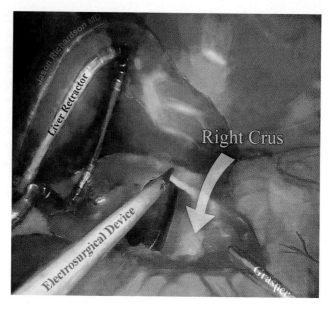

Fig. 3.2. Opening the gastrohepatic ligament with electrosurgical device, exposing right crura of diaphragm.

3. We advocate the pars flaccida approach because it minimizes the risk of postoperative posterior band slippage compared to the perigastric technique. To begin, divide the gastrohepatic ligament using a thermal energy device (Fig. 3.2). Initiate a retrogastric dissection by dividing the peritoneum at the posterior confluence of the diaphragmatic crura directly anterior to the right crus (Fig. 3.3). Use two closed blunt instruments to gradually develop the retrogastric space through this window while avoiding entry into the lesser sac or injury to the esophagus, stomach, or spleen.

4. Once the window is created, replace the blunt instruments with a single articulating blunt dissecting instrument, and pass this with minimal pressure cephalad and anterolateral toward the angle of His (Fig. 3.4). Once this is properly positioned, divide the peritoneum overlying its tip.

5. Feed the leading edge of the gastric band onto the exposed tip of the articulating instrument and pull it into the retrogastric

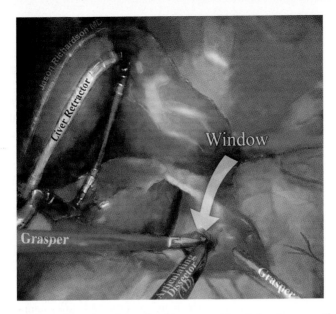

Fig. 3.3. Blunt dissection of pars flaccida retrogastric window in preparation of placement of an articulating esophageal dissector (AD).

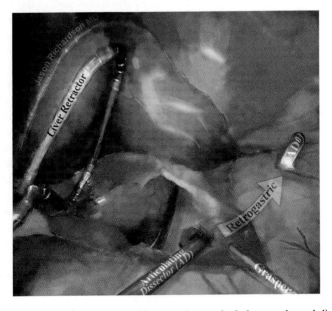

Fig. 3.4. Once retrogastric tunnel is created, an articulating esophageal dissector (AD) is inserted and articulated adjacent to angle of His in preparation for attachment of gastric band.

space, as the dissector is withdrawn. Free the band from the articulating instrument and allow it to rest around the posterior stomach.

6. Use two blunt instruments to buckle the band over the gastric cardia in the fashion recommended by the specific band manufacturer. In an attempt to secure the band in a 45° angle and reduce postoperative anterior band slippage, use several interrupted nonabsorbable sutures to wrap the stomach over the band by plicating the gastric body to the gastric cardia anterior to effectively covering the band on its anterior aspect.

7. To minimize the risk of contaminating the band during the following few steps, it is important to avoid patient abdominal skin contact with the port and tubing. Extract the end of the band tubing through the 15-mm trocar, and completely remove the trochar. Cut the tubing to a length that avoids redundancy, flush the system, and then connect the tubing to the port.

8. Sharply widen the skin incision sufficiently to accommodate the port. Bluntly develop a subcutaneous pocket over the fascia. Techniques vary among surgeons as to how best to close the 15 mm fascial defect and secure the access port to the fascia. Our preference is to close the defect using a suture-passing instrument and a single nonabsorbable suture. One of the free tails of the tied fascial suture is passed through the eyelet of the port that is opposite from the port-tubing connection. This suture is then tied to the tail of the remaining free suture, thereby securing the port to the fascia at one point.

9. Ensure that there are no sharp angles along the band tubing, which may increase the risk of future tube breakage or kinking. A second nonabsorbable suture is passed through the fascia directly to each side of the port-tubing connection with the use of a suture-passing instrument. The port is then secured to the fascia at a second point.

10. Remove all instruments and trochars. Cover the port with interrupted absorbable suture to reapproximate subcutaneous adipose tissue prior to skin closure. Use a running stitch to seal the band port incision tightly. Close the remaining skin incisions at the dermal level with absorbable suture. Apply adhesive strips over the closed skin incisions.

As the band typically provides restriction immediately upon placement, saline instillation in the postoperative period is unnecessary, and it is left unfilled until at least 4 weeks after surgery.

E. Postoperative Management

1. **Monitoring**—Patients who experience any intraoperative cardiopulmonary problems or have a history of obstructive sleep apnea or other severe cardiopulmonary condition should remain overnight in a unit with continuous cardiac monitoring and pulse oximetry. Other patients should be able to be transferred to a ward bed. Some surgeons perform LAGB as an outpatient procedure.

2. **Activity**—Patients are encouraged to ambulate the evening of surgery, and pneumatic compression devices and DVT chemoprophylaxis are continued until discharge. Routine physical exercise is essential for optimal long-term weight loss, and a progressive exercise routine is recommended for patients to continue at home.

3. **Medication Adjustments**—Additional adjustments are necessary to the medication regimens of diabetic patients. It is frequently possible to continue half of the preoperative regimen of long-acting insulin dose and oral hypoglycemic agents. Postoperative episodes of hyperglycemia can usually be controlled using an insulin sliding scale.

4. **Nutrition**—An upper gastrointestinal fluoroscopy study to evaluate for leak, obstruction, and band position is optional on the first postoperative morning prior to starting a sugar-free clear liquid diet. If tolerated, the patient is advanced to a full liquid diet and discharged home that afternoon. Commercial supplements are used to ensure that the full liquid diet is high in protein and low in fat, sugars, and total calories. Each 2 weeks, patients are transitioned to the next dietary stage. This equates to 2 weeks on each of the following: full liquids, pureed foods, and soft foods. Finally, patients transition to a modified regular diet that they maintain thereafter. The modified regular diet comprises three small slowly consumed high-protein meals daily with occasional inter-meal snacks as needed. Patients are counseled to stop eating the moment they first feel full, to consume 64 oz of water daily, and to avoid consuming fluids within 30 min of meals due to the risk of accelerating food transit through the gastric band. They are educated that consumption of liquid foods mostly comprises fat or carbohydrates will greatly limit any weight loss. Daily multivitamin intake is

recommended to avoid deficiencies in vitamins A, B_1, B_{12}, D_{25}, calcium, folate, and iron[13].

5. **Follow-up**—Outpatient follow-up office visits are scheduled for postoperative week 1, month 1, and then every 2–3 months thereafter. These visits provide the surgeon with an opportunity to provide behavioral and dietary counseling, to monitor for complications and nutritional deficiencies, and to provide gastric band fluid adjustments as needed.

6. **Band Adjustments**—The majority of healing and resolution of edema has occurred by the time of the second office visit (1 month after surgery) and the patient has usually lost sufficient weight to benefit from additional band restriction at that time. A ≥22 G noncoring deflected-point needle (Huber) ≥2 in long is attached to a 10–20 ml syringe. After standard skin prep and draping, the needle is used to access the subcutaneous port and aspirate all of the saline. The needle is left embedded in the port as the syringe is disconnected, evacuated of its contents, and refilled with fresh saline. The amount of fresh saline should be between 0.25 and 1 ml greater than the quantity previously removed from the port. Older bands with smaller reservoirs may require adjusted volumes. The syringe is reconnected to the needle and the fresh saline instilled prior to removal of the needle from the port. The patient is then provided with a small glass of room-temperature water to drink. Severe dysphagia or regurgitation may necessitate immediate readjustment. Some surgeons selectively perform fluoroscopy during adjustments to tailor the rate of oral contrast passage through the band.

7. **Support Groups**—It has been demonstrated that patient participation in regular bariatric support group meetings can result in significantly improved and sustained weight loss. It is recommended that all patients routinely attend such a group function on a monthly basis.

F. Complications

1. **Perioperative complications**—Early complications after LAGB are often related to performing surgery on obese patients rather than issues specific to the band itself. Pulmonary complications, DVT, hemorrhage, wound infections, and band

leak each have a rate less than 1%, which results in a total perioperative complication rate between 2.3 and 2.8% and a mortality rate of 0.06%.

2. **Late complications**—Late complications include port or tubing problems (up to 4% at 5 years), band slippage (approximately 3%), and band erosion (1–2%). Flipped ports that impair needle access can be repositioned as outpatient procedures. Although the band slippage rate has decreased with adoption of the pars flaccida approach and anterior gastrogastric plication, this complication can result in extrinsic compression of the left gastric artery, consequent gastric ischemia, necrosis, and eventual free perforation if left unidentified. Some surgeons perform routine surveillance radiographs to evaluate for changes in the 45° band angle that suggest slippage. If a slipped band is discovered, the band should be immediately deflated and the patient scheduled for a laparoscopic band repositioning (or removal) with gastrogastric plication over the band. If the band is found to be in the perigastric position, replacement via the pars flaccida technique should be considered. Due to the scarring associated with the gradual nature of band erosion through the wall of the stomach, free intraperitoneal perforation rarely occurs. Instead, a patient with band erosion may present with a delayed port site infection after intraluminal bacteria have traveled from the band to the port along the tubing. Upper endoscopy is indicated and may reveal an intraluminal segment of the band. If discovered, an eroded band should be removed promptly and the gastrotomy repaired.

3. **Band Removal**—In one prospective multicenter trial, band removal rates totaled 18% of the patients within 5 years. Indications for band removal included erosion, inadequate weight loss, obstruction, pouch dilation, and slippage. Band removal rates in other studies range from 1.4% to 5.8%.

G. Conclusions

LAGB demonstrates the lowest rate of complications and least weight loss of the mainstream bariatric operations. Although, perhaps better suited for less obese patients who are older or have more severe comorbidities, it may be the most accessible procedure due to the approved use expansion by the FDA in early 2011. Optimal results are achieved through appropriate patient selection, proper positioning technique, and patient participation with diet and exercise regimens and support group meetings.

References

Belachew M, Belva PH, Desaive C. Long-term results of laparoscopic adjustable gastric banding for the treatment of morbid obesity. Obes Surg. 2002;12(4):564–8.

Buchwald H, Estok R, Fahrbach K, et al. Trends in mortality in bariatric surgery: a systematic review and meta-analysis. Surgery. 2007;142:621–32.

Favretti F, Cadiere GB, Segato G, et al. Laparoscopic banding: selection and technique in 830 patients. Obes Surg. 2002;12(3):385–90.

Greenstein RJ, Martin L, MacDonald K, et al. The Lap-Band® system as surgical therapy for morbid obesity: intermediate results of the USA, multicenter, prospective study. Surg Endosc. 1999;13:S1–18.

Mechanick JI, Kushner RF, Sugerman JH, et al. American Association of Clinical Endocrinologists, the Obesity Society, and American Society for Metabolic & Bariatric Surgery medical guidelines for clinical practice for the perioperative nutritional, metabolic, and nonsurgical support of the bariatric surgery patient. Endocr Pract. 2008;14:1–83.

Nguyen NT, Slone JA, Nguyen XT, et al. A prospective randomized trial of laparoscopic gastric bypass versus laparoscopic adjustable gastric banding for the treatment of morbid obesity; outcomes, quality of life, and costs. Ann Surg. 2009;250:631–41.

O'Brien PE, Brown A, Smith PJ, et al. Prospective study of a laparoscopically placed, adjustable gastric band in the treatment of morbid obesity. Br J Surg. 1999; 85:113–8.

Ren CJ, Fielding GA. Lapasroscopic adjustable gastric banding: surgical technique. J Laparoendosc Adv Surg Tech. 2003;13(4):257–63.

Zinzindohoue F, Chevallier JM, Douard R, et al. Laparoscopic gastric banding: a minimally invasive surgical treatment for morbid obesity: prospective study of 500 consecutive patients. Ann Surg. 2003;237(1):1–9.

4. Laparoscopic Sleeve Gastrectomy

Gregg H. Jossart, M.D., F.A.C.S.

A. Introduction

Laparoscopic sleeve gastrectomy has emerged as an acceptable surgical option for the treatment of morbid obesity. The earliest experience with this operation dates back to the development of the duodenal switch procedure. The laparoscopic approach was first introduced in 1999 after completion of a porcine feasibility study. It was initially used on higher risk, higher BMI patients as a first stage of a duodenal switch procedure. Currently, it is also offered to lower BMI patients as an alternative to adjustable gastric banding and gastric bypass.

The apparent technical simplicity of this procedure is appealing. There is no foreign body, no anastomoses and no intestinal bypass. The long-term risk profile is appealing as the risk of foreign body and intestinal bypass complications is eliminated. The preservation of the pylorus and resection of most of the stomach may also offer hormonal and motility benefits that are not yet well understood.

The seeming lack of technical difficulties of this procedure can be misleading. The gastric staple line is the longest of all the procedures. Brethauer et al. (2009), in a systematic review, cited staple line dehiscence at rates ranging from 0.3 to 5%. The procedure is not well standardized and controversy exists over bougie size and pouch calibration; extent of antral resection; management of reflux and hiatal hernias; and the use of buttress materials and staple line suturing methods. Moreover, postoperative problems from a suboptimal technique may not present for months or years after surgery, and thus it is difficult to evaluate differing technical preferences.

N.T. Nguyen and C.E.H. Scott-Conner (eds.), *The SAGES Manual: Volume 2 Advanced Laparoscopy and Endoscopy*, DOI 10.1007/978-1-4614-2347-8_4, © Springer Science+Business Media, LLC 2012

B. Indications for Surgery

The primary indication for sleeve gastrectomy is generally the same as for any bariatric procedure—morbid obesity. However, this procedure can be offered to many morbidly obese individuals who are otherwise not candidates for gastric banding or intestinal bypass procedures. It is worthwhile to consider for patients with inflammatory bowel disease, organ transplantation, ulcer history, and those who need anticoagulation. The lower BMI group benefit from weight loss equal or superior to adjustable gastric banding and gastric bypass without the inherent long-term risks of those procedures. The higher BMI group may benefit from the fact that it is technically easier to perform than the intestinal bypass procedures and a staged approach may offer a desirable risk reduction.

C. Preoperative Evaluation

Preoperative evaluation includes consultations with a registered dietitian and mental health professionals. Chest X-ray, 12 lead ECG, and comprehensive lab testing are also routine. Upper gastrointestinal series and/or endoscopy can be done depending on age, symptoms, risk factors, and surgeon preference. Patients over age 40 with significant reflux and risk factors for esophageal or gastric cancer should undergo an endoscopy. While the presence of a hiatal hernia is not an absolute contraindication for sleeve gastrectomy, patients should be consented for simultaneous repair and advised that the definitive antireflux procedure for them could be a Roux-en-Y gastric bypass. Reflux and hiatal hernia can be a source of complaints and may be present in up to 40% of patients, as noted by Himpens et al. (2010) and Munoz et al. (2009). Any appearance of Barrett's esophagus or the diagnosis of dysplasia on biopsy, may prove to be a relative contraindication to the procedure. Those patients with dysplasia could progress and may require an esophagectomy. The sleeve gastrectomy eliminates the gastric blood supply from the right gastric artery and makes it impossible to divide the left gastric artery and use the remaining sleeve as conduit due to inadequate blood supply.

D. Patient Position and Port Placement

1. The operating room personnel and equipment are arranged with the surgeon on the patient's right and the assistant on the left. Alternatively, the surgeon can be between the patient's legs, the assistant surgeon on the patient's right, and the camera holder to the left.

2. Place video monitors at either side of the head of the table. These should be viewed easily by all members of the operating team.

3. Instrumentation includes graspers, cautery, scissors, curved dissectors, clip appliers, liver retractor, 5-mm needle holders, linear stapler, and an energy source.

4. Ports are all at the level of the umbilicus and above. The initial and main working port can be a 12 or 15 mm port placed at the umbilicus or within a rectangular region extending as much as 5 cm superior and to the right of the umbilicus. This is often dependent on the size of the pannus and displacement of the umbilicus. Frequently, there is an umbilical hernia that allows open placement of a 12 or 15 mm port for stapling.

5. Liver retraction can be done with a sub-xiphoid Nathanson liver retractor or with a flexible retractor place through a 5 mm right anterior axillary line port.

6. The camera port is located in the left upper paramedian location. This port can range in size from 5 to 12 mm depending on the surgeon's preference for scope size and the need for a larger port in this location to possibly staple from.

7. Assisting ports can be a 5 mm right upper paramedian port for the surgeon's left hand and a 5 mm left anterior axillary line port for the assistant's right hand.

E. Diagnostic Laparoscopy

This will allow the surgeon to assess the need for a liver biopsy in the event a fatty or fibrotic liver is encountered. The presence of a hiatal hernia can be determined, although this can be very difficult in the higher BMI patient group. The gallbladder can be examined and a survey for abdominal wall hernias can also be completed.

F. Gastric Mobilization

1. **Identify the pylorus** and mark it with a suture, clip, or ink. During the dissection of the short gastric vessels, the antrum can develop spasms and make it slightly more difficult to locate the pylorus. A suture can be placed on the greater curvature 3–6 cm proximal to the pylorus to mark the site of the first stapling. This suture is also useful for retraction during stapling and for extracting the gastric specimen at the end of the procedure.

2. **Mobilization of the fundus**. Using cautery or the energy source, make a window into the omental bursa between the gastric wall and the gastroepiploic artery. Proceeding superiorly, seal and divide the short gastric vessels directly on the serosa of the stomach. Since this part of the stomach is part of the specimen, there is no concern for thermal injury. This approach also reduces the chance of deviating toward the spleen and creating a small splenic infarction or tearing of short gastric vessels that can be difficult to control. Once the fundus is mobilized, the choice to continue toward the cardia or reverse direction and proceed toward the antrum may be surgeon preference but the level of exposure may play a significant role. In the larger patients with a higher degree of visceral obesity, mobilization of the antrum next may allow for better exposure while dissecting the cardia.

3. **Mobilization of the antrum (Fig.** 4.1). Once the fundus has been mobilized, the surgeon can reverse direction on the greater

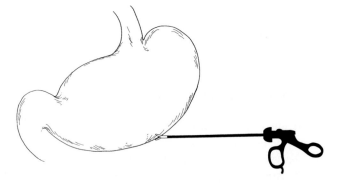

Fig. 4.1. Stomach with mid section of omentum already divided and the energy source tip dividing short gastric toward the direction of the antrum and pylorus.

curvature and proceed toward the pylorus. In this region, the omental bursa is obliterated and the posterior antrum tends to be adherent to the pancreas. As the pylorus is approached, be aware of the gastro-duodenal and right gastric artery becoming the gastroepiploic artery. Usually, stopping the dissection about 2 cm proximal to the pylorus will prevent injuring one of these vessels and preserve perfusion of the distal antrum and pylorus. Any attachments of the anterior pyloric region to the falciform, liver, or gallbladder should be divided to allow for optimal retraction during stapling.

4. **Mobilization of the Cardia**. Once the antrum has been mobilized, it will be easier to retract the stomach toward the patients right and inferiorly thus allowing better exposure of the cardia, spleen, and left crus. This is the area where any element of haphazard dissection or exposure may result in the disruption of a short gastric vessel that may subsequently retract and become difficult to control. If the angle of view of the short gastric vessels becomes difficult, it is useful to lift the stomach anteriorly and roll it over toward the right thereby placing tension on the gastric tissues and vessels that travel adjacent to the left crus. The splenic artery and the lymph node tissue adjacent to the left gastric artery can often be seen at this point and it is always wise to deviate away from these structures. The final posterior short gastric can be divided along the left crus. The anterior fat pad is often enlarged and obstructs the view of the medial cardia and the distal esophagus. Mobilize this to provide adequate exposure of this area for optimal stapling and placement of sutures.

G. Assessment and Repair of a Hiatal Hernia

1. Preoperative studies and or symptoms may have already diagnosed the presence of a hiatal hernia but a negative preoperative study does not preclude the presence of a hernia. The anterior hiatus can quickly be examined and anterior fat pad can be displaced with a grasper to determine the presence of a hiatal defect. The appropriate management of a slight indentation or laxity in the anterior hiatal membrane is unclear. Certainly, in

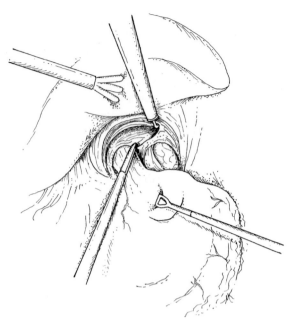

Fig. 4.2. Dissection of hiatus.

the higher BMI patient where the operation is already quite challenging, it is probably reasonable to avoid further dissection in this region. In lower BMI patients with reflux symptoms, it is reasonable to probe the posterior hiatus from the left crus and if laxity or an enlarged posterior hiatus is noted, it is reasonable to proceed with a hiatal hernia dissection and repair of the hiatus with cardiopexy (if desired).

2. **Hiatal Dissection (Fig.** 4.2). Dissect the hiatus as for any hiatal hernia repair. Once the mediastinal attachments are separated and the distal esophagus resides within the abdomen, perform crural closure. This repair is strictly a hiatal closure and can be described as an Allison repair. This approach is similar to what has been used in adjustable gastric banding to reduce the reoperative rate in patients with hiatal hernias.

3. **Posterior Closure (Fig.** 4.3). Close the right and left crura, beginning posteriorly and working anteriorly. We currently use an O-braided, permanent suture for closure and try to incorporate the endoabdominal fascia to minimize tearing of the crural

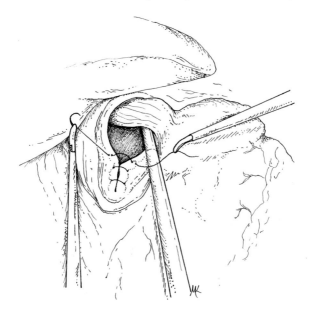

Fig. 4.3. Suture closure of hiatus.

muscle. The use of Teflon pledgets is surgeon dependent. The hiatus can be closed prior to gastric stapling or after the gastrectomy has been completed. The usual sequence is to dissect the hiatus, place the bougie, perform the gastrectomy, and then close the hiatus around the bougie. The hiatal closure can be done prior to stapling. The key point is to dissect the hiatus and reduce the stomach prior to stapling. Failure to do so may yield a gastric pouch with a proximal diverticulum of retained cardia/ fundus. These patients tend to have ongoing reflux, nausea, and globus symptoms that may require reoperation.

4. **Anterior Closure**. The anterior hiatal peritoneal covering spans a separation between the anterior right and left crus. If only a posterior closure is performed, the patient may develop an early recurrence due to the laxity in this membrane and subsequent dilation of the anterior hiatus. Usually, a single suture can be placed to approximate the anterior crus. The closure should still be slightly loose around the bougie, which is usually between 32 and 40 French.

5. **Cardiopexy**. Once the stapling phase of the sleeve gastrectomy has been completed (see next section), the cardia may be anchored to the left crus at the point of insertion of the divided phrenoesophageal ligament. This option serves to recreate the angle of His and may reduce the incidence of hiatal hernia recurrence.

H. Gastrectomy

1. **Bougie size and placement**. To date, pouch size has not been standardized. Bougie size may range from 32 up to 64 French. Placement of the stapler against the bougie and staple line suturing can also affect the volume of the pouch. Generally, a smaller pouch will lead to more durable weight loss but it may also increase complications, such as staple line bleeding, dehiscence, and stenosis. The bougie can be placed prior to stapling or the antrum can be stapled first and then the bougie be placed (Fig. 4.4). The author strongly recommends using a smaller bougie (32–38 French), placing it right against the pylorus prior to stapling and stapling directly adjacent to the bougie without stretching the gastric wall. This technique is reproducible and tends to avoid pouch malformations.

2. **The antrum is stapled first** starting at 2–3 cm proximal to the pylorus. Preserving the antrum may reduce distal gastric obstruction, but the antrum tends to enlarge and the increased volume may contribute to weight regain. Stapling within 2–3 cm of the pylorus resects part of the antrum and may contribute to better weight loss. However, the antrum is extremely thick in this location and seromuscular disruption with stapling may increase the incidence of staple line leaks. This area should be suture inverted. The choice of staple cartridge for the antrum should be green, purple, or black. Blue cartridges are contraindicated on gastric tissue. Buttress material is used selectively in this location. These materials can occupy up to 40% of the closed staple line height and may actually contribute to staple line disruption. If buttress materials are going to be used, a cartridge with greater staple line height should be selected (black or green). We use mostly black, purple, or green cartridges for

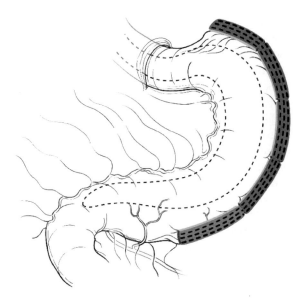

Fig. 4.4. Laparoscopic sleeve gastrectomy: creation of sleeve (Reprinted with permission from Singh K. Sleeve gastrectomy. In: DeMaria EJ, Nguyen NT, Ikramuddin S, Hutter MM, editors. The sages manual: a practical guide to bariatric surgery. New York: Springer; 2008).

the first two staplings and avoid buttress materials. By staying within 2–3 cm of the pylorus, enough antrum is resected to hopefully minimize future dilation. It is important to verify the proximity of the stapler to the bougie both anteriorly and posteriorly with each cartridge application. Failure to do this may result in an irregular outpouching that will increase the overall volume of the pouch. Since seromuscular disruption on the antrum is possible, we tend to leave just enough space between the bougie and stapler to allow for inverting (Lembert) sutures along the antral staple line.

3. **Body/Fundus stapling**. Once the antrum is stapled and the angularis is approached (usually the third cartridge), it is critical to avoid creating a relatively stenotic segment at the angularis. Functional obstruction at this level is not well described but it may contribute to an increase in the incidence of proximal staple line dehiscence, persistent vomiting, and proximal gastric

dilation. The remaining stomach can usually be stapled with purple or green cartridges. Blue cartridges may seem satisfactory but the gastric tissue thickness is probably too great and a slightly higher leak rate may occur. Stapling in this region tends to be directly on or adjacent to the lesser curvature vessels. Staple line bleeding may be increased in this region and additional sutures to control bleeding may create segmental narrowing and obstruction. Stapling slowly and the use of buttress materials may help reduce staple line bleeding in this region without narrowing the lumen.

4. **Cardia**. Placement of the last two cartridges at the top of the stomach can be the most difficult for proper calibration. There tends to be more posterior stomach that is tethered to the left gastric artery and the left crus. With an anterior view, the cartridge can be closed adjacent to the bougie quite easily, but a posterior view will expose redundant stomach in between the cartridge and the bougie. Stapling without correcting this will result in a retained proximal fundus which can lead to a need for reoperation later. It is important to rotate the stomach and the stapler anteriorly to carefully examine and retract the posterior gastric wall through the cartridge prior to closing it. The tendency to allow the stapler to deviate off the bougie with the hope that a staple line disruption will be avoided is a noble endeavor but again, it may lead to retention of a significant amount of fundus that would require a possibly riskier reoperation. The final cartridge should be placed at least 1 or 2 cm from the GE junction to allow for suture reinforcement of the cardia. This area tends to be at risk for leaks and the author routinely suture inverts (Lembert technique) this area. Once the stapling is completed, the bougie can be removed and a leak test may be performed. Staple line bleeding sites may be sutured as well. The entire staple line may be sutured to hopefully reduce the incidence of leaks and hemorrhage. This can be problematic however, as the staple line is usually on or adjacent to the lesser curvature vessels and staple line suturing can lead to additional bleeding near the left gastric artery and subserosal hematomas may also develop. Another alternative is to apply a fibrin sealant to the staple line to reduce the incidence of delayed staple line hemorrhage.

I. Omentopexy and Gastric Extraction

1. Suspending the omentum to the staple line can provide an additional modality for hemostasis and may stabilize the position of the stomach in a way that will reduce the risk for postoperative gastric volvulus or coiling. This is particularly important at the level of the angularis and below, where the stomach tends to migrate medial to the pancreas and create a relative obstruction at the angularis. Identify the divided edge of the omentum and elevate it superiorly. A suture can be placed medial to the gastroepiploic and then directly into the staple line, preferable at an intersection of staple lines as the pouch tends to have slightly more tissue in these regions.

2. The stomach can be extracted with a plastic bag or without. It is usually easiest to grab the antral part of the staple line and extract it from the largest port site after gently dilating the fascia. This fascia should be closed to avoid a port site hernia. Ports can be removed and the wounds closed per standard technique.

J. Postoperative Care

1. Nasogastric tubes and drains are only considered if there was a staple line disruption that required suturing.

2. Narcotics, antacids, and antiemetics are administered on a prn basis. Anticholinergics (Hyosamine) can be useful to reduce or treat early cardiospasm. These patients tend to have chest tightness and difficulty drinking liquids in the first 24 h. Anticholinergics can relieve this.

3. Clear liquids are given the morning of the first postoperative day. If tolerated and the patient has good pain control, they may be discharged. Higher risk patients may need an additional day of hospitalization. Upper GI studies can be done selectively or routinely. Patients are asked to remain on a liquid diet for 2 weeks to allow for complete healing of the very long staple line. Thicker foods are usually not well tolerated in the first 2 weeks and may lead to intractable vomiting and staple line disruption.

K. Early Complications

1. **Bleeding**. Postoperative bleeding after sleeve gastrectomy is rare. There is no anastomosis and no gastric remnant staple line. Intra-luminal bleeding is extremely rare. The usual sites of hemorrhage would be intra-abdominal and would include the long gastric staple line, divided short gastric vessels, and the port sites. All of these can be self-limiting or may require reoperation to control.

2. **Staple line disruption**. This can occur in the first few days and would usually require an early reoperation. After 1 week, presentation is variable and treatment options may include percutaneous drainage, reoperations, gastric decompression, or stenting.

3. **Aspiration**. This can occur at any point in the first week, especially if the patient develops cardiospasm or edema along the pouch. They may retain some fluid in the esophagus prior to laying down and may aspirate in their sleep. It is important they avoid liquids just before lying down and use the anticholinergic and antiemetic agents if necessary.

4. **Dehydration**. Consumption of liquids in the first week or two can be quite limited by the size of the pouch and spasms. Some patients will need to obtain additional intravenous fluids for dehydration even if they have not had vomiting issue.

5. **Deep Vein Thrombosis/Pulmonary Embolus**. The risks are the same as for any bariatric procedure. Theoretically, the simplicity and reduced operative time of the procedure may reduce the risk in the higher BMI patients.

Acknowledgment

The author gratefully acknowledge support from: Sutter Pacific Medical Foundation.

Selected References

Brethauer SA, Hammel JP, Schaure PR. Systematic review of sleeve gastrectomy as staging and primary bariatric procedure. Surg Obes Relat Dis. 2009;5(4):469–75.

De Csepel J, Burpee S, Jossart G, Andrei V, Murakami Y, Benavides S, Gagner M. Laparoscopic biliopancreatic diversion with a duodenal switch for morbid obesity: a feasibility study in pigs. J Laparoendosc Adv Surg Tech A. 2001;11(2):79–83.

Gulkarov I, Wetterau M, Ren CJ, Fielding GA. Hiatal hernia repair at the initial laparoscopic adjustable gastric band operation reduces the need for reoperation. Surg Endosc. 2008;22(4):1035–41.

Hess DS, Hess DW. Biliopancreatic diversion with a duodenal switch. Obes Surg. 1998; 8(3):267–82.

Himpens J, Dobbeleir J, Peeters G. Long-term results of laparoscopic sleeve gastrectomy for obesity. Ann Surg. 2010;252(2):319–24.

Marceau P, Biron S, Bourque RA, Potvin M, Hould FS, Simard S. Biliopancreatic diversion with a new type of gastrectomy. Obes Surg. 1993;3(1):29–35.

Munoz R, Ibanez L, et al. Importance of routine preoperative upper GI endoscopy: why all patients should be evaluated. Obes Surg. 2009;19(4):427–31.

Read RC. The contribution of Allison and Nissen to the evolution of hiatus herniorrhaphy. Hernia. 2001;5(4):200–3.

Ren CJ, Patterson E, Gagner M. Early results of laparoscopic biliopancreatic diversion with a duodenal switch: a case series of 40 consecutive patients. Obes Surg. 2000;10(6):514–23.

Santoro S. Technical aspects in sleeve gastrectomy. Obes Surg. 2007;17(11):1534–5.

5. Metabolic Effects of Bariatric Surgery

Helen M. Heneghan, M.D.
Shai Meron-Eldar, M.D.
Stacy A. Brethauer, M.D.
Philip R. Schauer, M.D.

A. Introduction

Obesity is associated with a constellation of weight-related comorbidities, the most prevalent of which are the conditions that comprise the metabolic syndrome, diabetes mellitus, and cardiovascular diseases (CVDs). The pathophysiological mechanisms underlying the development of these diseases are multifactorial and incompletely understood. These mechanisms include the endocrine functions of adipose tissue, the proinflammatory state induced by obesity, and the mass effect of central adiposity leading to an increase in intra-abdominal pressure (IAP). Bariatric surgery has been performed for the treatment of obesity since 1953, when Dr. Richard Varco (Minnesota) performed the first jejunoileal bypass specifically to induce weight loss from malabsorption. Although fraught with nutritional complications, this procedure was noted to induce marked weight reduction. It had a remarkable effect on circulating lipid levels in severely hyperlipidemic patients with a 90% decrease in plasma cholesterol and an even greater (96%) reduction in plasma triglycerides. In the following decades, the jejunoileal bypass was modified and refined to reduce the severity of the malabsorptive nutritional complications while retaining its weight loss and lipid-lowering benefits. This was followed by procedures, such as the biliopancreatic diversion (Scopinaro) and duodenal switch (Marceau), followed by limited bypass or restrictive procedures, such as the roux-en-Y gastric bypass (RYGB) and vertical banded gastroplasty. Indeed, as the field of bariatric surgery has evolved

N.T. Nguyen and C.E.H. Scott-Conner (eds.), *The SAGES Manual: Volume 2 Advanced Laparoscopy and Endoscopy*, DOI 10.1007/978-1-4614-2347-8_5,
© Springer Science+Business Media, LLC 2012

over the past 50 years, weight loss has almost been overshadowed by the extraordinary effects on all obesity-related comorbidities. In particular, the dramatic and prompt remission of type 2 diabetes mellitus (T2DM) has stimulated researchers to investigate the exact mechanisms responsible for this phenomenon.

B. Weight Loss: Its Role in the Metabolic Effects of Bariatric Surgery

Multiple factors are thought to contribute to the dramatic effect of bariatric surgery on glucose homeostasis. These include: decreased caloric intake secondary to restriction of the stomach, weight loss leading to increased sensitivity of peripheral insulin receptors to circulating insulin, and alterations in the release of gut hormone which stimulate pancreatic beta cells to produce insulin. The contribution of weight loss to the metabolic benefits of bariatric surgery is critical. Observations supporting this statement include the fact that restrictive procedures, such as gastric banding and sleeve gastrectomy can achieve significant metabolic benefits, which correlate directly with the amount of weight loss achieved. Buchwald's meta-analysis examining weight loss and diabetes resolution outcomes after bariatric surgery showed that DM resolution rates were proportional to the degree of weight loss; they observed remission rates as high as 95% following biliopancreatic diversion with duodenal switch, 80% for gastric bypass, and nearly 57% for gastric banding. In this analysis of 621 studies, including over 135,000 patients, the overall T2DM resolution rate after all bariatric procedures was 78%. Among studies reporting the longest follow-up at that time, resolution was sustained for at least 2 years in 74% of diabetic patients. It has also been observed that weight gain after bariatric surgery is associated with recurrence of metabolic comorbidities, including T2DM.

A **reduction in the volume of adipose tissue**, especially central adiposity, is proposed to play an important role in mediating the metabolic effects which follow weight loss surgery. Adipose tissue is not only specialized in the storage and mobilization of lipids, but it also functions as an active endocrine organ releasing numerous hormones and cytokines, including proinflammatory molecules, such as interleukin-6 (IL-6) and TNF-alpha (Table 5.1). The increased secretion of inflammatory markers observed with accumulating adipose tissue mass has been shown to occur in concert with a decrease in the production of adipokines with

Table 5.1. Summary of the proposed metabolic effects and mechanisms of various bariatric operations.

	Proximal bowel exclusion	Increased nutrient transport	Ghrelin secretion	Weight loss independent metabolic effects
LAGB	No	No	↑	No
LSG	No	Yes	↓↓	Undetermined
RYGB	Yes	Yes ++	↓	Yes
BPD-DS	Yes	Yes ++	↔	Yes

LAGB laparoscopic adjustable gastric banding, *LSG* laparoscopic sleeve gastrectomy, *RYGB* roux-en-Y gastric bypass, *BPD-DS* biliopancreatic diversion with or without duodenal switch

anti-inflammatory properties, such as adiponectin. The resultant proin-flammatory environment contributes to a state of insulin resistance and altered glucose homeostasis which is characteristic of viscerally obese patients. Weight loss has been shown to be accompanied by a reduction in inflammatory cytokines, and an increase in anti-inflammatory mediators, such as adiponectin, alongside partial or complete resolution of coexisting metabolic diseases. A second mechanism by which a reduction in central adiposity contributes to an improvement in metabolic state is through decreasing IAP. Sugerman et al. first reported an important association between chronically raised IAP in obese individuals and various obesity-associated comorbidities. Chronically elevated IAP in this setting was shown to result in increased pleural pressure, cardiac filling pressures, femoral venous pressure, renal venous pressure, systemic blood pressure, intracranial pressure, and vascular resistance. It remains to be definitively proven that increased IAP and presumed pressure-related comorbidities are causally linked, but these data are compelling. Sugerman et al. subsequently demonstrated that surgically induced weight loss significantly lowered IAP (as measured by urinary bladder pressure), which was associated with decreases in sagittal abdominal diameter and obesity-related comorbidity.

C. Weight Independent Metabolic Effects of Bariatric Surgery

While weight loss certainly plays a major role in inducing improved glucose homeostasis following bariatric surgery, it appears that there are other mechanisms at play. An abundance of evidence exists to support this assertion. This includes the fact that leaner patients with type 1 diabetes experience similar antidiabetic effects without significant weight loss, and most patients' glucose control improves or normalizes almost immediately after surgery, well before any significant weight loss takes place. Many patients with T2DM are able to decrease, or even discontinue, insulin and oral hypoglycemics just days after undergoing RYGB. Furthermore, it has been observed that malabsorptive procedures in which GI anatomy has been altered result in significantly greater remission of metabolic comorbidities, such as T2DM, compared to other interventions with equivalent weight loss.

Various weight-independent antidiabetes mechanisms of bariatric surgery have been proposed over the last few years. Rubino et al. aptly summarized these as follows:

- Exclusion of the proximal duodenum and small intestine from nutrient flow, possibly downregulating unidentified anti-incretin factor(s).
- Increased postprandial secretion of distal gut hormones, such as glucagon-like peptide 1 (GLP-1), from enhanced and expedited distal intestinal nutrient delivery.
- Changes in intestinal nutrient-sensing mechanisms which affect insulin sensitivity.
- Impaired ghrelin secretion.
- Bile acid alterations.

As mentioned previously, the rapid normalization of glycemic control following gastric bypass surgery may be attributed to altered gut anatomy and resultant changes in gut hormone production. It is thought that exclusion of the duodenum and proximal jejunum from nutrient flow may reduce insulin resistance, and/or that exaggerated responses of the distal small bowel to nutrients results in a beneficial change in the release of gut hormones produced in the distal ileum, such as GLP-1 and peptide tyrosine tyrosine (PYY) post-RYGB. GLP-1, and other hormones secreted from the foregut, such as glucose-dependent insulinotropic polypeptide (GIP), act as incretins which stimulate pancreatic beta cells to restore normal first phase insulin responses.

Two main theories have been proposed to explain the rapid postoperative shift in hormone secretion and the improvement in glucose tolerance following bypass surgery. The "**distal bowel/hindgut hypothesis**," proposed by Mason et al., attributes improved glucose metabolism after RYGB to enhanced delivery of nutrients to the distal bowel stimulating intestinal L cells to release increased amounts of peptides, such as GLP-1 and PYY. Both of these peptides increase satiety and reduce food intake. Additionally, GLP-1 stimulates insulin secretion, decreases intestinal motility and gastric emptying, and improves β-cell function. They are also primarily responsible for the "ileal brake"; an inhibitory feedback mechanism which controls transit of a meal through the gastrointestinal tract in order to optimize nutrient digestion and absorption. Other gut hormones implicated in the hindgut hypothesis include enteroglucagon and neurotensin, both of which are thought to modulate intestinal motility and delay gastric emptying, thereby contributing to the tight neurohormonal control of the ileal brake. Rubino et al. have extensively evaluated the "**proximal bowel/foregut hypothesis**," which is based on the premise that exclusion of the proximal small bowel from nutrient exposure is primarily responsible for the beneficial effect of gastrointestinal bypass surgery on T2DM. In a nonobese rat model of type 2 diabetes (Goto–Kakizaki rat), Rubino and Marescaux performed duodenal jejunal bypass surgery and observed significant improvements in glucose tolerance compared with sham-operated rats, despite equal body weights in both groups. The mediators and precise mechanisms responsible for this effect are not fully understood. It is thought that bypassing the proximal bowel (duodenum and jejunum) may decrease the expression or secretion of a "diabetogenic signal." Rubino and colleagues propose that when the foregut of susceptible individuals is overstimulated with carbohydrates and fat it releases an unknown factor which contributes to the development of type 2 diabetes. Hormones which may contribute to this phenomenon include the gut peptide GIP, insulin-like growth factor 1, leptin and insulin itself. In addition to evidence of a defective enteroinsular axis in type 2 diabetes, the findings that RYGB in humans seems to selectively alter hormonal levels of diabetic patients, but not of nondiabetics, adds further credence to the foregut hypothesis.

Aside from significant alterations in hormone levels themselves, bariatric surgery results in **increased sensitivity to insulin** and **improved cellular uptake of glucose**. Following RYGB, the following results have been observed; the insulin sensitivity index increases four to fivefold, there is an associated elevation in levels of the insulin-sensitizing hormone adiponectin, the concentration of insulin receptors and markers of insulin signaling in muscle increase, as does the expression of the mitochondrial transcription cofactor PPARγ-coactivator-1 (PGC-1) and its target, mitofusin 2. Additionally, it has been shown that fatty acid metabolism in muscle is stimulated in response to increased insulin signaling and PGC-1 activity, resulting in decreased intramyocellular lipid levels. Since lipid accumulation in muscle is known to cause insulin resistance, this decrease in intramyocellular lipid levels after RYGB should increase insulin sensitivity. Pontiroli et al. present further data supporting a weight-independent effect on insulin sensitivity after GI surgery. The authors performed oral glucose tolerance testing on two cohorts of bariatric surgery patients within one week postoperatively; one group had undergone laparoscopic gastric banding while the other underwent BPD. Beneficial effects on fasting glucose levels, oral glucose insulin sensitivity, and insulin resistance scores were observed only in the BPD patients. Gumbs et al. attribute the improvement in insulin sensitivity and cellular uptake of glucose after bariatric surgery to other mechanisms, specifically the combined effects of caloric restriction and weight loss. They postulate that a decrease in fat mass significantly alters circulating levels of adipocytokines and inflammatory markers, which favorably modifies the degree of peripheral insulin resistance.

Evidence for an important role of **ghrelin** in mediating the antidiabetic effects of bariatric surgery is conflicting. Secreted from A cells in the oxyntic glands of the gastric fundus and duodenum, ghrelin stimulates appetite, increases food intake and gut motility, and decreases insulin sensitivity. However, it has been repeatedly observed that ghrelin levels are decreased in obese individuals. This downregulation may be a consequence of simultaneously elevated insulin or leptin levels, as fasting plasma ghrelin concentration has been shown to negatively correlate with fasting insulin and leptin, and may represent a physiological adaptation to the positive energy balance associated with obesity. It is generally accepted that fasting ghrelin levels increase after weight loss induced by calorie restriction (including after gastric banding); however, changes in this hormone after gastric bypass and other "rerouting" bariatric surgeries are less consistent. Cummings' group provided the first evidence to suggest that decreased secretion of this prodiabetic hormone may contribute to the anorexic and antidiabetic effects of RYGB. Given that more than 90% of ghrelin is produced by the stomach and duodenum, which are both altered or excluded by RYGB, this group hypothesized that ghrelin regulation would be disturbed after gastric bypass. Indeed, they observed that ghrelin levels in post-RYGB patients were extremely low throughout an entire 24-h period, compared to the normal ghrelin profile of preprandial surges followed by postprandial suppression. In a review of all related prospective studies of ghrelin expression after RYGB, Cummings found that eight other groups observed similar decreases in ghrelin levels after RYGB, and four cross-sectional studies confirmed abnormally low levels in post-RYGB patients compared with appropriate controls. For example, Morinigo et al. demonstrated a decrease in ghrelin as early as 2–6 weeks post-RYGB, and suggested that this particular effect was related to altered anatomy and nutrient flow rather than weight loss. Conversely, three other studies found no significant change in human ghrelin levels after RYGB although the respective authors interpreted this as an impairment in the expected increase of ghrelin with weight loss. Adding further controversy to this issue, four groups reported normal increases in ghrelin with RYGB-induced weight loss. It is possible that such highly variable findings may reflect differences in surgical techniques, particularly with regard to the treatment of the vagus nerve during the procedure, as this could affect ghrelin secretion from the gastric fundus. While it appears that ghrelin alone is clearly not responsible for immediate changes in insulin sensitivity following bariatric surgery, it may play a role as a cofactor in this phenomenon. The proposed mechanisms underlying the metabolic effects of the commonest bariatric procedures are summarized in Table 5.1.

In addition to playing an essential role in absorption of dietary lipids, **bile acids** have been recognized as important modulators of metabolism. In rodent studies where animals were administered high concentrations of bile acids, it was observed that energy expenditure in brown adipose tissue increased, preventing obesity and resistance to insulin. These beneficial effects of bile acids on metabolism were found to be mediated by binding of bile acids to the G-coupled receptor TGR5, leading to cAMP generation and activation of the intracellular type 2 thyroid hormone deiodinase. Altered gastrointestinal anatomy following gastric bypass has been shown to affect enterohepatic recirculation of bile acids. Patti et al. demonstrated that total serum bile acid concentrations and bile acid subfractions are higher in patients who have undergone RYGB compared to nonoperated overweight and severely obese individuals. Furthermore, it was found that total bile acids correlated inversely with 2-h post-meal glucose and fasting triglycerides, and correlated positively with adiponectin and peak GLP-1. Nakatani et al. reported similar results, which occurred within the first month postoperatively. These data support an important role for bile acids in the metabolic and antidiabetic effects of bariatric surgery.

D. Other Beneficial Effects of Bariatric Surgery

1. Cardiovascular Disease

Obesity is an important determinant of CVD and is associated with widespread alterations in cardiac and vascular structure and function. Two proposed mechanisms for this association, alluded to above, are as follows. First, the mass effect of central adiposity leads to a chronic increase in IAP with deleterious effects on the cardiovascular, renal, and pulmonary systems. Chronic intra-abdominal hypertension leads to secondary renal artery and vena cava compression, decreased venous return and renal hypoperfusion, which culminate in activation of the renin-angiotensin-aldosterone system. This may, at least in part, explain the pathogenesis of systemic hypertension in morbidly obese individuals. Second, the function of adipose tissue as an active endocrine and paracrine organ contributes to a state of low-grade inflammation, created by the host of proinflammatory cytokines and peptides secreted by adipose tissue which are thought to mediate the link between obesity and CVD. Bariatric surgery has been shown to have striking beneficial effects on a variety of risk factors for CVD, including hypertension, diabetes, and dyslipidemia. Three studies have measured Framingham risk score (FRS), before and after bariatric surgery; all authors observed a significant decrease in FRS postoperatively. Endothelial function and novel CVD risk factors, such as C-reactive protein, have also been shown to improve after surgically induced weight loss. These beneficial effects are thought to be mediated by the significant reduction in intra abdominal fat lowering IAP and decreasing the secretion of proinflammatory cytokines, as well as the aforementioned alterations in gut hormones and lipid metabolism seen after GI bypass surgeries.

2. Liver Disease

Nonalcoholic fatty liver disease (NAFLD) is one of the most prevalent liver diseases worldwide, mostly attributable to the obesity pandemic. Its major significance in this context is that it has the potential to progress to cirrhosis and hepatocellular carcinoma. NAFLD is also a major contributor to insulin resistance. Given these serious consequences, treating NAFLD is a high priority. To date, no pharmacologic treatment has been effective for NAFLD. Weight loss, achieved via bariatric surgery or subsequent to lifestyle modification/behavior therapy, remains the cornerstone in its treatment and has been shown to improve both metabolic parameters and liver histology, including inflammatory changes. A recent Cochrane review summarized the evidence to date regarding effects of bariatric surgery on NAFLD. Although there were no randomized controlled trials in this setting, 21 prospective or retrospective cohort studies all reported an improvement in steatosis or hepatic inflammation scores.

E. Adverse Metabolic Effects of Bariatric Surgery

While the benefits of bariatric surgery are indisputable, unfortunately it also has the potential to cause a variety of nutritional and metabolic complications. Malabsorptive procedures achieve greater weight loss and metabolic benefits than restrictive procedures; however, they are generally associated with more postoperative metabolic problems. These include micronutrient deficiencies, such as vitamin B12, iron, calcium, and vitamin D. At the most severe end of this spectrum, protein-calorie malnutrition and fat malabsorption can occur. These latter consequences usually occur only after malabsorptive procedures, such as the biliopancreatic diversion and jejuno-ileal bypass.

The main reason why the latter procedure has been abandoned in current practice is due to its long-term metabolic complications, including cirrhosis and oxalate nephropathy. Although the risk of severe nutritional deficiencies after bariatric surgery today is small, counseling, monitoring, and dietary supplementation are essential for the treatment and prevention of nutritional and metabolic complications after bariatric surgery.

Selected References

Adams TD, Gress RE, Smith SC, et al. Long-term mortality after gastric bypass surgery. N Engl J Med. 2007;357(8):753–61.

Buchwald H, Avidor Y, Braunwald E, et al. Bariatric surgery: a systematic review and meta-analysis. JAMA. 2004;292(14):1724–37.

Buchwald H, Estok R, Fahrbach K, et al. Weight and type 2 diabetes after bariatric surgery: systematic review and meta-analysis. Am J Med. 2009;122(3):248e245–56e245.

Cottam DR, Mattar SG, Barinas-Mitchell E, et al. The chronic inflammatory hypothesis for the morbidity associated with morbid obesity: implications and effects of weight loss. Obes Surg. 2004;14(5):589–600.

Cummings DE, Overduin J, Foster-Schubert KE. Gastric bypass for obesity: mechanisms of weight loss and diabetes resolution. J Clin Endocrinol Metab. 2004;89(6):2608–15.

Cummings DE, Overduin J, Shannon MH, Foster-Schubert KE. Hormonal mechanisms of weight loss and diabetes resolution after bariatric surgery. Surg Obes Relat Dis. 2005; 1(3):358–68.

Fried M, Ribaric G, Buchwald JN, Svacina S, Dolezalova K, Scopinaro N. Metabolic surgery for the treatment of type 2 diabetes in patients with BMI <35 kg/m2: an integrative review of early studies. Obes Surg. 2010;20(6):776–90.

Galic S, Oakhill JS, Steinberg GR. Adipose tissue as an endocrine organ. Mol Cell Endocrinol. 2010;316(2):129–39.

Gumbs AA, Modlin IM, Ballantyne GH. Changes in insulin resistance following bariatric surgery: role of caloric restriction and weight loss. Obes Surg. 2005;15(4):462–73.

Malinowski SS. Nutritional and metabolic complications of bariatric surgery. Am J Med Sci. 2006;331(4):219–25.

Mason EE. Ileal [correction of ilial] transposition and enteroglucagon/GLP-1 in obesity (and diabetic?) surgery. Obes Surg. 1999;9(3):223–8.

Nakatani H, Kasama K, Oshiro T, Watanabe M, Hirose H, Itoh H. Serum bile acid along with plasma incretins and serum high-molecular weight adiponectin levels are increased after bariatric surgery. Metabolism. 2009;58(10):1400–7.

Pillai AA, Rinella ME. Non-alcoholic fatty liver disease: is bariatric surgery the answer? Clin Liver Dis. 2009;13(4):689–710.

Pontiroli AE, Gniuli D, Mingrone G. Early effects of gastric banding (LGB) and of biliopancreatic diversion (BPD) on insulin sensitivity and on glucose and insulin response after OGTT. Obes Surg. 2010;20(4):474–9.

Pories WJ. Why does the gastric bypass control type 2 diabetes mellitus? Obes Surg. 1992;2(4):303–13.

Pournaras DJ, Osborne A, Hawkins SC, et al. Remission of type 2 diabetes after gastric bypass and banding: mechanisms and 2 year outcomes. Ann Surg. 2010;252(6):966–71.

Ronti T, Lupattelli G, Mannarino E. The endocrine function of adipose tissue: an update. Clin Endocrinol (Oxf). 2006;64(4):355–65.

Rubino F, Gagner M. Potential of surgery for curing type 2 diabetes mellitus. Ann Surg. 2002;236(5):554–9.

Rubino F, Gagner M, Gentileschi P, et al. The early effect of the Roux-en-Y gastric bypass on hormones involved in body weight regulation and glucose metabolism. Ann Surg. 2004;240(2):236–42.

Rubino F, Forgione A, Cummings DE, et al. The mechanism of diabetes control after gastrointestinal bypass surgery reveals a role of the proximal small intestine in the pathophysiology of type 2 diabetes. Ann Surg. 2006;244(5):741–9.

Rubino F, Schauer PR, Kaplan LM, Cummings DE. Metabolic surgery to treat type 2 diabetes: clinical outcomes and mechanisms of action. Annu Rev Med. 2010;61:393–411.

Schauer PR, Burguera B, Ikramuddin S, et al. Effect of laparoscopic Roux-en Y gastric bypass on type 2 diabetes mellitus. Ann Surg. 2003;238(4):467–84. discussion 484–465.

Shah M, Simha V, Garg A. Review: long-term impact of bariatric surgery on body weight, comorbidities, and nutritional status. J Clin Endocrinol Metab. 2006;91(11):4223–31.

Sjostrom L, Lindroos AK, Peltonen M, et al. Lifestyle, diabetes, and cardiovascular risk factors 10 years after bariatric surgery. N Engl J Med. 2004;351(26):2683–93.

Sjostrom L, Narbro K, Sjostrom CD, et al. Effects of bariatric surgery on mortality in Swedish obese subjects. N Engl J Med. 2007;357(8):741–52.

Sugerman HJ. Effects of increased intra-abdominal pressure in severe obesity. Surg Clin North Am. 2001;81(5):1063–75. vi.

Van Citters GW, Lin HC. The ileal brake: a fifteen-year progress report. Curr Gastroenterol Rep. 1999;1(5):404–9.

Vazquez LA, Pazos F, Berrazueta JR, et al. Effects of changes in body weight and insulin resistance on inflammation and endothelial function in morbid obesity after bariatric surgery. J Clin Endocrinol Metab. 2005;90(1):316–22.

6. Accreditation and Requirements for a Bariatric Program

Matthew M. Hutter, M.D., M.P.H., F.A.C.S.
Timothy D. Jackson, M.D., M.P.H., F.R.C.S.C.

A. Accreditation in Bariatric Surgery

Early reports of adverse outcomes following bariatric surgery prompted significant concerns over safety and quality of care in weight loss surgery.

In October 2005, Flum et al. (2005) reported a 2% 30-day mortality in Medicare patients undergoing gastric bypass. Following this report and others, the Centers for Medicare and Medicaid Services (CMS) issued a memorandum on November 25, 2005 proposing that it would no longer cover bariatric surgical procedures. After significant public appeal and data review, the CMS ultimately reversed the noncoverage decision on February 21, 2006 with specific conditions. Most importantly, CMS mandated that it would only reimburse bariatric procedures performed at facilities accredited as either a "Center of Excellence" by the American Society of Metabolic and Bariatric Surgery (ASMBS) or as a Level I accredited center by the American College of Surgeons Bariatric Surgery Center Network (ACS-BSCN). These two large National Surgical Associations had independently developed accreditation programs in an effort to improve the quality of bariatric surgical care. The programs have more similarities than differences: Both accreditation programs require bariatric surgery centers to meet certain standards of care, including a volume requirement of 125 cases per year. Both require accredited centers to have the necessary organization, facilities, and trained personnel. Both programs identify the collection of data and reporting of outcomes as an integral way to ensure delivery of high quality care.

N.T. Nguyen and C.E.H. Scott-Conner (eds.), *The SAGES Manual: Volume 2 Advanced Laparoscopy and Endoscopy*, DOI 10.1007/978-1-4614-2347-8_6, © Springer Science+Business Media, LLC 2012

1. ASMBS Bariatric Surgery Center of Excellence Program

Established in 2004 and run through the Surgical Review Corporation (SRC), the ASMBS Bariatric Surgery Center of Excellence Program (ASMBS BSCOE) offers accreditation to both inpatient and outpatient centers performing bariatric procedures. Requirements include an institutional commitment to excellence, having a designated medical director and meeting standards for surgeon experience, critical care support, and equipment, on call coverage, clinical pathways, bariatric nursing, physician extenders, program coordination, patient support groups, and long-term follow up. Bariatric surgical case volume must be 125 cases or greater per year. Outpatient facilities must also meet additional requirements for patient selection and facility licensing.

Facilities meeting these criteria may be accredited after a site visit.

Programs accredited within the ASMBS BSCOE program report outcomes data into the Bariatric Outcomes Longitudinal Database (BOLD). This was established in 2007 to help ensure ongoing compliance with BSCOE standards and for identification of quality improvement opportunities. Data are collected by participating surgeons or other caregivers during each patient encounter. National summary reports allow providers to compare their individual outcomes to other centers (Table 6.1).

Table 6.1. The ten requirements for ASMBS bariatric surgery center of excellence hospitals.

1.	Institutional commitment to excellence
2.	Surgical experience and volumes
3.	Designated medical director
4.	Responsive critical care support
5.	Appropriate equipment and instruments
6.	Surgeon dedication and qualified call coverage
7.	Clinical pathways and standardized operating procedures
8.	Bariatric nurses, physician extenders and program coordinator
9.	Patient support groups
10.	Long-term patient follow-up, including BOLD

2. *ACS-Bariatric Surgery Center Network*

Developed in 2005, the ACS-BSCN network was built on the success of prior accreditation programs provided by the American College of Surgeons for Trauma Care and Cancer Care. Similar to the ASMBS program, ACS-BSCN defines high standards of care for the delivery of bariatric surgical care. The program outlines necessary physical resources, personnel, clinical standards, and surgeon credentialing standards, with requirements based upon Betsy Lehman Center Weight Loss Surgery Recommendations.

For the ACS-BSCN program, hospitals are accredited as Level I, Level II, Level II New or Outpatient facilities, depending on hospital surgical volume and resources.

a.   **Level I** hospitals must perform over 125 cases per year, and demonstrate sufficient resources to care for the most challenging and complex patients. They are accredited to care for patients with/without stipulation as to age, comorbidities, or body mass index (BMI), and are accredited to perform elective revisional surgery.

b.   **Level II** hospitals have lower volume requirements—25 cases per year—and are accredited for the care of less complex obese patients. Level 2 centers may not perform elective revisional operations, or any elective primary procedure on high-risk patients. High-risk patients are defined as follows: non-ambulatory patients, patients over 60 years old, adolescents under the age of 18, high BMI patients (male patients may not have a BMI of 55 or greater and female patients may not have a BMI of 60 or greater), patients who have organ failure, an organ transplant, or are a candidate for a transplant, and patients with significant cardiac or pulmonary comorbid conditions.

c.   **Level II New** status was developed to facilitate the integration of newer programs, and features an expedited approval timeline.

d.   **Outpatient status** is for facilities that focus on outpatient surgery with adjustable gastric bands only.

The accreditation process includes an application and a subsequent site visit by a bariatric surgeon from the ACS-BSCN Accreditation Program to assess compliance with the accreditation requirements for structure, process, and outcomes. The program accredits hospitals, and the hospitals in turn privilege surgeon(s)—there is no specific surgeon accreditation by ACS-BSCN.

Table 6.2. ACS-BSCN Level I and level II centers.

Level I
- ≥125 cases per year.
- Full spectrum of hospital services required.
- Can operate on all patients including
  - Extremes of BMI.
  - Medically complex patients.
  - Elective revisional bariatric procedures.

Level II
- ≥25 cases per year.

Cannot operate on:
- Age >60 years old
- Males BMI>55, females BMI>60.
- Adolescents/pediatric patients.
- Significant cardiac or pulmonary issues.
- Transplant patients.
- Non-ambulatory patients.
- Elective revisional operation.

Participating centers are required to report outcomes data in the ACS-BSCN database. This collects prospective, longitudinal, bariatric-specific data on all patients undergoing bariatric surgery in a given program. The data collection program was designed to work either in conjunction with the ACS-NSQIP or as a stand-alone system for those not participating in the ACS-NSQIP. Data is entered by an independent trained data collector and validated to ensure quality of reporting. This high quality data is subjected to risk adjusted analysis for report generation. Results are reported back to participating centers to allow identification of opportunities to target quality improvement (Table 6.2).

B. Scope of the Problem

Obesity is a public health crisis. Current data indicates that 34.3% of the US population are obese (BMI>30) and 5.9% are morbidly obese (BMI>40). Obesity is associated with comorbidities that significantly decrease life expectancy. Estimates suggest that obesity accounts for upto 15% of all deaths annually in the USA and will soon emerge as the single leading cause of preventable death in the developed world. This escalating epidemic reflects failure of preventative and medical approaches. Bariatric surgery remains the only effective and durable treatment option for obesity resulting in long-term success and reversal of associated comorbidities.

With the increasing burden of obesity, the number of bariatric procedures performed annually has increased dramatically. 220,000 bariatric procedures were performed in the USA and Canada in 2008; a 113.6% increase from 5 years earlier. Significant improvements in safety and outcomes after bariatric surgery have occurred concurrently with increased clinical experience and the development centers of excellence for comprehensive bariatric surgical care and accreditation programs.

C. Essential Components of a Bariatric Surgery Program

Morbidly obese patients represent a high-risk surgical population. A comprehensive and organized approach to their care helps to maximize the opportunity for safe and effective outcomes.

D. Preoperative Assessment

1. Multidisciplinary Assessment

A multidisciplinary evaluation of obese patients is essential to assess appropriate indications for surgery and to identify and manage comorbidities. Patients should meet established National Institutes of Health (NIH) criteria and be of acceptable operative risk. Current NIH criteria include BMI > 35 kg/m^2 with the presence of serious associated comorbidities or BMI > 40 kg/m^2.

The decision to recommend surgery should include input from the surgeon, anesthesia, and internal medicine subspecialties as required do define medical and surgical risk and optimize comorbidities. In addition, an assessment by a psychologist or psychiatrist is often beneficial if associated psychiatric diagnoses are suspected that would affect outcome after a bariatric procedure.

High risks alone do not preclude a patient from having a bariatric surgical procedure. Potential operative risks have to be carefully weighed against the potential benefits. Though patients with super-obesity and/or significant weight related illnesses like diabetes, hypertension, hyperlipidemia, and obstructive sleep apnea can be high operative risks, they also have a lot to gain from bariatric surgery. A careful risk/benefit evaluation must be performed for each individual patient to optimize their care.

2. Patient Education and Counseling

Preoperative counseling and education are critical. Similar to the medical and surgical assessment, this is a multidisciplinary process requiring input from several groups of health professionals. This may include a dietician, social worker, nurse practitioner, physician assistant, or other dedicated bariatric team members. The goals are to provide patients with the best possible opportunity to understand surgical options and their risks and benefits, and to develop realistic expectations and tools for long-term success. Patients selected for a bariatric procedure should demonstrate a dedication to participate in long-term follow up.

E. Perioperative Care

1. Institutional Requirements

Bariatric surgical care may be provided in two distinct settings—outpatient (ambulatory) and inpatient (hospital) facilities. Procedures performed within outpatient facilities may be performed safely when patient and procedure selection is appropriate. This type of practice is limited to placement of laparoscopic adjustable gastric bands. Regardless of the type of setting, the institution in which the procedures are performed must have appropriate clinical resources, personnel, and equipment to ensure safety.

2. Selection of Bariatric Procedure

A comprehensive program should provide the bariatric patient with a range of standard surgical options to optimize outcome and accommodate patient preference. In general, these currently include the Roux-en-Y gastric bypass (RYB), and the laparoscopic adjustable gastric banding

(LAGB). The sleeve gastrectomy (SG) is a newer procedure and as long-term outcomes become better understood it may also become more prevalent. Other procedures like the biliopancreatic diversion with duodenal switch can be considered for centers with appropriate experience. Other procedures lacking suitable evidence should only be performed within the context of an Institutional Review Board (IRB) approved research protocol. A minimally invasive approach should be applied whenever possible. Elective revisional bariatric surgery should be performed only where expertise allows.

3. Surgeon Requirements

Adequate surgeon training and experience are required for any successful bariatric surgery program. This may be assessed by previous case volume, outcomes, or completion of an accredited bariatric fellowship program. A center must perform an adequate volume of procedures to ensure maintenance of expertise. Ideally, a center may benefit from having more than one trained bariatric surgeon to allow for additional surgical support and on call coverage. Active participation in continuing medical education and advanced laparoscopic skills are an additional requirement.

4. Personnel and Clinical Support

The complexity of the bariatric surgical patient necessitates a wide range of clinical expertise be accessible to provide safe care. Within the perioperative period, a multispecialty team comfortable with issues arising in higher BMI patients must be available. This includes anesthesiology, internal medicine and subspecialties, critical care, interventional radiology, and endoscopy. In addition to sufficient medical support, trained nurses, nutritionists, physiotherapists, and other allied health professionals should be actively involved in the program.

5. Facilities

Bariatric patients require specialized equipment to accommodate higher BMIs. Toward this end, operating room tables and equipment (long instruments, retractors, staplers, and others) must be available. Beyond the operating room, all other inpatient and outpatient areas used in the care of the bariatric patient should be suited for the morbidly obese. This includes recovery rooms, ICU, inpatient wards having appropriate beds, furniture, lifts, toilets, scales, and showers for patients. Outpatient clinic space must also be accessible to the bariatric patient.

F. Postoperative Care

All comprehensive bariatric surgical programs should have a mechanism in place for organization of discharge and follow up. This includes a commitment to postoperative rehabilitation and long-term adherence in a dedicated bariatric clinic. Follow up programs must incorporate monitoring for nutritional deficiencies, dietary counseling, promotion of healthy lifestyle and exercise. Ongoing psychological counseling, support, and education are also critical.

G. Processes of Care

1. Program Structure

A successful and efficient bariatric program will have leadership and organization to facilitate patient care and ensure optimization of resources. This often involves a bariatric surgery coordinator in addition to a medical and surgical director for a given program.

2. Outcomes Reporting

A comprehensive bariatric surgery program ideally should participate actively in outcomes reporting. Collection of relevant bariatric-specific endpoints may be accomplished by joining established accreditation programs. Subsequent risk adjusted analysis and feedback to providers allows for benchmarking and quality assurance.

3. Quality Improvement Programs

Participation in ongoing quality improvement is a necessary component of any high quality bariatric program. Identification and review of adverse events enables implementation of best practices and system changes to improve care and optimized patient safety.

4. Application of Best Practices and Clinical Pathways

A bariatric program should establish a set of procedure specific clinical pathways with order sets to guide care throughout the perioperative period. These need to reflect current evidence and incorporate best practices guidelines for care of the bariatric patient. Protocols must be reviewed and updated as appropriate.

H. Summary

Performing bariatric surgery within a comprehensive bariatric surgery program allows for the greatest opportunity for safety and the optimization of care. Within this setting, outcomes after bariatric surgery continue to improve. Accreditation programs offered by both the ASMBS and ACS have defined high standards of care allowing modern bariatric surgery to become a surgical quality improvement success story.

Selected References

ACS-BSCN. http://acsbscn.org. Accessed 18 Mar 2011.

ASMBS BSCOE. http://surgicalreview.org. Accessed 18 Mar 2011.

Blackburne G, Hutter MM, et al. Expert panel on weight loss surgery: executive report update. Lehman Center Wight Loss Surgery Expert Panel. Commonwealth of Massachusetts Betsy Lehman Center for Patient Safety and Medical Error Reduction. Obesity. 2009;17(5):842–62.

Buchwald H, Oien DM. Metabolic/bariatric surgery worldwide 2008. Obes Surg. 2009; 19(12):1605–11.

CMS Decision Memo for Bariatric Surgery for the Treatment of Morbid Obesity (CAG-00250R). http://www.cms.gov/medicare-coverage-database/details/nca-decision-memo.aspx?NCAId=160&ver=32&NcaName=Bariatric+Surgery+for+the+Treatment+of+Morbid+Obesity+(1st+Recon)&bc=BEAAAAAAEAgA. Accessed on 3 Apr 2011.

Encinosa WE, Bernard DM, Du D, Steiner CA. Recent improvements in bariatric surgery outcomes. Med Care. 2009;47(5):531–5.

Flum DR, Dellinger EP. Impact or gastric bypass operation on survival: a population based analysis. J Am Coll Surg. 2004;199:543–51.

Flum DR, Salem L, Elrod JA, Dellinger EP, Cheadle A, Chan L. Early mortality among medicare beneficiaries undergoing bariatric surgical procedures. JAMA. 2005; 294(15):1903–8.

Nguyen NT, DeMaria EJ, Ikramuddin S, Hutter MM, editors. The sages manual: a practical guide to bariatric surgery. New York: Springer; 2008.

NHANES Obesity Statistics. 2011. http://www.cdc.gov/nchs/data/hestat/overweight/overweight_adult.htm. Accessed 16 Mar, 2011.

Phurrough S, Salive ME, Brechner RJ, et al. Proposed coverage decision memorandum for bariatric surgery for morbid obesity. 23 November 2005. www.cms.hhs.gov/coverage/download/id160a.pdf. Accessed 3 Apr 2011.

Stewart ST, Cutler DM, Rosen AB. Forecasting the effects of obesity and smoking on U.S. life expectancy. N Engl J Med. 2009;361(23):2252–60.

7. The Role of Endoscopy in Bariatric Surgery

Bruce David Schirmer, M.D., F.A.C.S.

A. Indications

This chapter deals only with flexible upper endoscopy and its application to bariatric surgery. While the bariatric surgery patients may develop colonic pathology and need colonoscopy, that pathology is unrelated to the aspects of their bariatric operation or its sequelae, and thus is not be discussed.

Indications for performing flexible upper endoscopy can be grouped into three broad areas, relative to temporal relationship of the bariatric operation: **preoperative assessment** to determine preexisting pathology prior to performance of bariatric surgery, **operative endoscopy** to assist with or even perform part of a bariatric operation or confirm the security of anastomoses performed, and **postoperative endoscopy** to treat symptoms of pathologic conditions that arise after bariatric operations and are appropriately diagnosed and/or treated with flexible upper endoscopy.

1. Preoperative Indications

Preoperative indications to perform flexible upper endoscopy are based on the proposed bariatric operation as well as the patient's medical history.

a. Individuals who have a history of significant documented upper gastrointestinal tract pathology should almost always undergo screening upper endoscopy prior to any bariatric operation. Such conditions include previous history of malignancy, polyps, inflammatory conditions, especially peptic ulcer, and gastroesophageal reflux disease (GERD). The latter is probably

N.T. Nguyen and C.E.H. Scott-Conner (eds.), *The SAGES Manual: Volume 2 Advanced Laparoscopy and Endoscopy*, DOI 10.1007/978-1-4614-2347-8_7, © Springer Science+Business Media, LLC 2012

the most common preoperative pathology found in patients considering bariatric surgery.

b. Patients with GERD may develop Barrett's esophagus due to the chronic inflammation of their lower esophagus. Barrett's esophagus may progress to dysplasia and then to frank carcinoma. Although this is a gross oversimplification of the disease and there is still controversy about the progression and incidence of carcinoma developing from Barrett's esophagus, the relationship between Barrett's esophagus, dysplasia, and subsequent esophageal carcinoma is clear. Thus, a patient with known Barrett's esophagus and dysplasia would certainly not be a candidate for bariatric surgery unless the esophageal disease was adequately addressed.

c. Patients whose operation precludes subsequent visualization of portions of the gastrointestinal tract, such as laparoscopic Roux-en-Y gastric bypass (LRYGB), should undergo preoperative screening endoscopy.

There is ample evidence in the literature to support the practice of performing preoperative upper endoscopy on patients planning LRYGB. However, insurance companies in the USA have not uniformly approved such diagnostic evaluation unless documentation of symptoms suggestive of upper gastrointestinal tract disease exists or such disease itself has been previously established. This is in spite of considerable evidence in the literature regarding the efficacy of preoperative esophagogastroduodenoscopy (EGD) prior to bariatric surgery.

Sharaf et al. (2004) evaluated 195 patients by upper endoscopy prior to bariatric surgery, and found one or more lesions of the upper gastrointestinal tract in 89.7% of cases. Of these, 61.5% were felt to be clinically important. The most common findings were hiatal hernia (40%), gastritis (29%), esophagitis (9%), gastric ulcer (3.6%), Barrett's esophagus (3%), and esophageal ulcer (3%).

Verset et al. (1997) reported a 37% incidence of gastroduodenal lesions and a 31% incidence of esophagitis in a group of 159 patients undergoing routine flexible upper endoscopy prior to vertical banded gastroplasty (VBG). Most of these gastroduodenal lesions were asymptomatic, and the esophagitis was almost always associated with a hiatal hernia or incompetent lower esophageal sphincter.

Overall, the most common pathologies generally reported in series of patients screened by upper gastrointestinal endoscopy prior to bariatric surgery include hiatal hernia, gastritis, and esophagitis.

In addition, endoscopy may demonstrate pathology that causes the planned bariatric operation to be changed or modified. This percentage is much lower in most reported series, but may be more important than the group of patients discussed above. In our own experience at UVA, we endoscoped 767 patients prior to bariatric surgery between 1986 and 2001. In this series, 4.6% of patients had pathology that caused us to alter the operation. The most common pathologic findings which altered surgery were severe gastritis, duodenal ulcer, or duodenitis. For the majority of these patients, a distal gastrostomy was added to the planned gastric bypass. Less common causes for alteration of operation included gastric polyps, large hiatal hernia, and Barrett's esophagitis with dysplasia. Other articles in the surgical literature quote a varying rate of endoscopic pathology affecting the subsequent bariatric surgical procedure from under 5%, as our own experience, to as high as 15%.

Among the current common bariatric procedures, it is prior to LRYGB that most of the screening endoscopies are performed. A case could certainly be made to extending the need for preoperative screening to patients planning to undergo LAGB. The rationale for this suggestion is that if a patient has a hiatal hernia, it should be repaired at the time of LAGB to prevent slippage or prolapse of the band, a complication facilitated by the hernia. However, routine endoscopic screening prior to LAGB has not been routinely practiced in the past. In the USA, this is in part due to a lack of reimbursement.

d.   Other indications and value of preoperative endoscopy are as follows:

   i.   Another preoperative value to EGD prior to gastric bypass is the determination and treatment of *Helicobacter pylori* in the stomach of patients planning to undergo that operation. Our experience showed that the incidence of postoperative marginal ulcers after gastric bypass decreased from 6.8 to 2.4% when we initiated the practice of routine preop screening and treatment for patients who were found to have *H. pylori* on routine gastric biopsy during upper endoscopy.

ii.   Others have observed that foregut symptoms in patients after gastric bypass are decreased if *H. pylori* is tested for and treated prior to surgery.

iii.   Preoperative endoscopy is nearly essential, not just valuable, as part of the planning for **reoperative** bariatric surgery. Conversion of one type of bariatric operation to another is a technically much more demanding operation than initial surgery. Preoperative endoscopy helps to:

– Confirm the size of any previously created gastric pouch.

– Determine the integrity of any previous gastric staple lines.

– Discover the presence of any upper gastrointestinal pathology as a result of the previous operation.

– Improve outcomes for reoperative surgery by assessing these aspects of the anatomy preoperatively.

2. *Intraoperative Indications*

Use of upper endoscopy intraoperatively during bariatric surgery is a common practice among bariatric surgeons. Situations where endoscopy has been described include the following:

a.   Intraoperative esophagogastroscopy to test the patency and integrity of the gastrojejunostomy created during LRYGB.

b.   Determination of pouch size and staple line location in reoperative surgery.

c.   Use as a guide for creation of the gastric staple line during LSG.

d.   Test the integrity and patency of the duodenoileostomy during duodenal switch (DS) procedure.

Of the above indications, the most frequent is the first, since LRYGB is the most common bariatric operation performed in the USA, and intraoperative esophagogastrojejunoscopy (EGJ) to test the anastomosis is a technique used by many bariatric surgeons. However, of the above indications, probably the most essential use of endoscopy is for reoperative surgery. During reoperative surgery, the endoscope is used to identify previous staple lines and their location, and thus help avoid the creation of blind pouches, ischemic areas of stomach between adjacent staple lines, and other anatomic pitfalls of reoperative surgery.

3. Postoperative Indications

A large number of patients will develop symptoms after bariatric surgery that will require or use flexible endoscopy for their assessment. Endoscopy can provide the correct diagnosis and often allow immediate treatment of postoperative problems after bariatric operations. Such symptoms and their pathophysiology include the following:

a. Following LRYGB
   i. Progressive food intolerance 3 or more weeks after surgery (stenosis of the gastrojejunostomy).
   ii. Constant epigastric pain following surgery, even years later (marginal ulcer).
   iii. Mid-epigastric pain of moderate intensity worsened by food (gastric remnant gastritis or ulcers not amenable to endoscopic visualization and diagnosed by exclusion).
b. Following LAGB
   i. New onset of severe dysphagia, total food intolerance, or newly experienced heartburn (severe or moderate prolapse)—may also be treated with fluoroscopic studies and fluid removal.
   ii. Port site infection: Secondary to band erosion into lumen of stomach.
   iii. Persistent epigastric pain and low-grade inflammatory picture: Erosion of band into gastric lumen.
c. Following LSG.
   i. Progressive food intolerance (stenosis).
d. Following any operation, where weight regain has occurred.
   i. Investigation of the integrity of staple lines, the size of gastric pouch, and the size of all anastomoses needs to be determined to plan possible reoperative surgery.

Specifics of the diagnosis and treatment of these conditions that are suggested by the above symptoms are given in the sections below.

B. Patient Positioning and Room Setup

Standard endoscopic diagnostic techniques and setup are indicated for the bariatric patients as would be for most endoscopic patients. Where special considerations are needed, they are indicated. Greater details of general endoscopy principles, room setup, and patient monitoring are given in other chapters of this text. The following is a summary of generalized standard protocol measures:

1. Appropriate monitoring of patient for conscious sedation (EKG tracing, BP cuff, oxygen saturation probe).

2. Have the patient thoroughly gargle with viscous xylocaine solution for topical anesthesia of the posterior hypopharynx. Spray with direct contact agents may be preferred in less cooperative or alert patients.

3. Place the patient in the left-side-down lateral position, supported by posterior foam wedge.

4. Have a nurse focus on the patient, standing behind patient, to monitor vital signs and administer medications.

5. A technician stands at the head of bed, watching for any equipment issues, available to assist with biopsy, dilation, and other endoscopic procedures, and available to perform oral suctioning as needed.

6. Endoscopist stands at patient's side, facing patient, opposite side of nurse, and prepared to perform endoscopy.

7. Monitors ideally both at patient head (on endoscopy cart) as well as one screen on monitoring cart to the left of vital signs screen facing patient and above patient's leg.

8. Induce conscious sedation using fentanyl, midazolam, or other appropriate short-acting medications.

9. Place bite block in patient's mouth prior to introduction of scope.

C. Diagnostic Techniques

Performance of flexible upper endoscopy is operator dependent and experience dependent for achievement of competence. Adequate volume usually produces an efficient and competent endoscopist. There are no known numbers of procedures which ensure competence or expertise.

1. General Pointers for Successful Endoscopy

While greater detail is available in other chapters, the following serve as general guidelines and pointers to improve efficiency of the novice while learning the nuances of flexible endoscopy.

a. Use the right hand to torque, advance, and retract the scope. Hold the scope 6–8 in. from the bite block and use the right hand for gross manipulations of the scope into the generally optimal position for viewing.

b. Use the dials to perform slight adjustments of field focus or to make turns in areas, such as the transition between the first and second portions of the duodenum or for retroflexion.

c. Lock the dials only when performing a therapeutic procedure or multiple biopsies to prevent variance of field focus.

d. Learn to torque the scope to optimize the position of the working channel for biopsy, dilatation, or other therapeutic procedures.

e. Make smaller movements with the scope, dials, and right hand than you think you should, especially in the beginning. Oversteering and overcompensation are common errors of the novice endoscopist.

f. "Pink screens" occur when the scope is against the mucosal surface. Back up, insufflate slightly, and reorient. Nothing is accomplished with the pink screen.

2. Introduction of the Scope

For upper endoscopy, the most difficult portion of the standard diagnostic EGD is usually the safe and smooth introduction of the scope into the proximal esophagus. The following are overall guidelines and suggestions to achieve this maneuver.

a. **Direct Vision Introduction**: This is the most common technique used and, if the endoscopist masters only one, is the most important because it can be universally applied in all situations. Awake or anesthetized patients are amenable to this approach.

   i.   Advance the scope, with a slight flexion of the tip, over the tongue to visualize the vocal cords.

   ii. Advance the scope to the crease of mucosal tissue formed by the ridge of tissue beneath the vocal cords.

   iii. Apply direct gentle pressure to allow the scope to pass through the crycopharyngeal sphincter. If the patient is awake enough to cooperate, swallowing facilitates this passage.

b. **Blind Awake Passage**: Less commonly used, this technique is employed by experienced upper endoscopists only. It does require excellent sedation of the patient and patient cooperation.

i.   The tongue is depressed by the endoscopist's index finger of the left hand. The finger is placed just to the middle of the tongue, on the patient's right side.

ii. The scope is placed adjacent to the index finger, and then advanced as the finger pulls the tongue forward and the patient swallows. The coordinated motion of these actions allows easy passage of the scope into the upper esophagus. The bite block, present higher up on the scope, is then slid over the scope and positioned between the patient's teeth.

iii. The endoscopist does risk injury from the patient biting if the patient is uncooperative or inadequately sedated and frightened by the passage of the scope. Hence, this technique is generally not recommended, except for very experienced endoscopists.

3. Biopsy Technique

a.   The biopsy forcep emerges from the 7 o'clock position. Position this portion of the field of view over the lesion.

b.   Maneuver the scope so that the surface to be biopsied is as *en face* as possible to allow good penetration of the biopsy forceps.

4. Special Considerations in Performing EGD in the Bariatric Patient Population

There are some particularly important issues and measures which must be taken in performing EGD in the bariatric patient population.

a.   Conscious sedation in the patient with obstructive sleep apnea (OSA) or Pickwickian syndrome: such patients are at high risk for apnea with intravenous sedation. A 200-kg man with severe OSA may develop near-respiratory arrest with 4 mg of midazolam. Careful and slow titration of any sedation is indicated in patients with a history of such pulmonary problems. Availability of narcan (to reverse the fentanyl) and flumazenil (to reverse the midazolam) is necessary. It is highly recommended to avoid the use of any other sedating drugs, such as benadryl, since they do not have a readily available antidote.

b.   A mask for ventilation, intubation kit, and appropriate intuba-
     tion equipment should be part of any endoscopy unit and must
     be readily available for these high-risk patients.
c.   Consider using a very small bore endoscopic tube, which may
     be introduced with nearly no sedation, using topical anesthetic
     only, via the nasopharynx. Such small bore tubes have been
     shown to be highly successful in performing diagnostic upper
     endoscopy for patients at high risk for conscious sedation.
     Figure 7.1. illustrates such a small bore tube in place during a
     diagnostic upper endoscopy of a noted SAGES endoscopist.
d.   Intravenous access in bariatric patients is often difficult. It
     should not be tenuous, as a situation of apnea requiring narcan
     and flumazenil may arise.

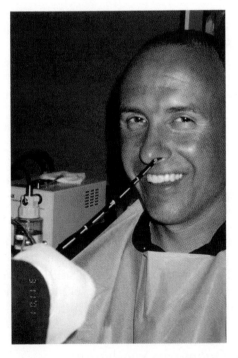

Fig. 7.1. Use of a small bore upper endoscope for performance of awake esophagogastroduodenoscopy. Exam being performed on noted SAGES author and
endoscopist Dr. Brian Dunkin (used with permission of Dr. Dunkin).

D. Pathologic Findings

A large variety of pathologic findings may be encountered on upper endoscopy in the non-bariatric patient, all of which are of course potentially possible in the bariatric patient. In addition, the bariatric patient is predisposed to other procedure-related pathology which the endoscopist must be experienced enough to interpret correctly.

1. Esophageal Pathology: Non-bariatric

a. Esophagitis: Graded from mild (erythema only) to severe (coalesced ulcers and severe erosions).
b. Thrush: Whitish exudative deposits on the surface of the mucosa.
c. Diverticulae: Located in the crycopharyngeal area, associated with food trapping and symptoms, less commonly in the distal esophagus (epiphrenic).
d. Barrett's esophagus: Salmon-pink fingers of tissue projecting upward from the Z-line.
e. Distal esophageal web: Usually a very thin membrane located several cm above the Z-line.
f. Esophageal stricture: Secondary to an inflammatory process.
g. Neoplasms: Malignant or benign.

2. Esophageal Pathology: Bariatric

a. Chronic or acute distal esophagitis: (Fig. 7.2). Seen often in obstructive processes after LRYGB, prolapsed after LAGB, and mini gastric bypass.
b. Esophageal dilatation after LAGB: Secondary to incorrect band placement on esophagus or GE junction and chronic obstruction of esophagus.

3. Gastric Pathology: Non-bariatric

a. Ulcers: May be benign or malignant, location determines type, always involve biopsy.

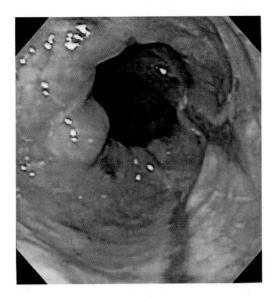

Fig. 7.2. Distal esophagitis and erosions after previous gastric bypass.

b. Gastritis: Graded mild (erythema) to severe (diffuse ulcers and inflammation).

c. Polyps: Benign fundic gland, hyperplastic, tubular, and villous types.

d. Tumors: Malignant or benign, including submucosal GIST tumors and lipomas.

e. Hiatal hernias, both sliding and paraesophageal and combined.

f. Dieulafoy's ulcer: Proximal bleeding source with minimal mucosal ulceration.

4. Gastric Pathology: Bariatric

a. Gastric outlet obstruction: Secondary to stenosis of gastrojejunostomy after LRYGB (Fig. 7.3) or LAGB with prolapse, or after VBG due to stenosis of band.

b. Atrophic gastritis: Found in gastric remnant after LRYGB (not normally accessible by endoscope).

c. Breakdown of gastric staple lines after LRYGB: Ability to navigate scope into distal stomach. Breakdown of gastric staple lines after VBG: Large opening into proximal stomach not through band area.

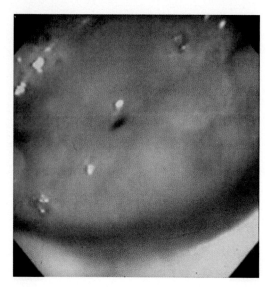

Fig. 7.3. Stenosis of gastrojejunal anastomosis after laparoscopic Roux-en-Y gastric bypass.

d. Marginal ulcer: Occurs at the edge of gastrojejunostomy following LRYGB; (Fig. 7.4) may result in gastric outlet obstruction secondary to edema; if chronic in nature, may result in gastrogastric fistula to distal stomach; if acute, may cause bleeding.

e. Gastric pouch dilatation: Following LRYGB, VBG, or LAGB, where there has been chronic obstruction present; may be associated with retained food, gastroparesis, and gastritis.

f. Band erosion into stomach: After LAGB, may be evident on endoscopy.

g. Proximal gastric blind pouch: After LAGB with associated chronic prolapse.

h. Bleeding from gastrojejunostomy after LRYGB.

5. Duodenal Pathology: Non-bariatric

a. Duodenitis, varying in grade from mild (erythema) to severe (coalesced ulcers).

b. Duodenal ulcer.

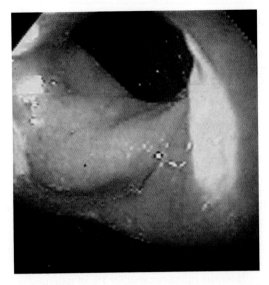

Fig. 7.4. Marginal ulcer at gastrojejunostomy after laparoscopic Roux-en-Y gastric bypass.

   c.   Duodenal obstruction due to peptic stricture.

   d.   Duodenal neoplasms, of both duodenum and ampulla of Vater.

   e.   Crohn's disease.

   f.   Diverticulae, often adjacent to ampulla of Vater.

6. Duodenal or Jejunal Pathology: Bariatric

   a.   Marginal ulcer after LRYGB, may be actively bleeding.

   b.   Redundant jejunal blind limb after LRYGB: Retained food in this dilated blind limb may cause intermittent pain and obstructive symptoms relieved by position change.

   c.   Jejunal obstruction after LRYGB: May occur at the site of the transverse colon mesentery in retrocolic Roux limb placement.

   d.   Ischemia of Roux limb after LRYGB secondary to internal hernia, torsion.

E. Treatment Procedures

There are five major areas, where flexible endoscopy may prove useful for therapeutic intervention after bariatric surgery. They are listed below, with descriptions of varieties of procedures and settings, where they are commonly performed under each broad category.

1. Hemorrhage

Bleeding may occur after any bariatric operation. It is least common after LAGB, where there is no division of the alimentary tract. It is more common after other bariatric procedures.

a. Acute hemorrhage at the gastrojejunal anastomosis after LRYGB.
   i. It occurs in approximately 1% of patients.
   ii. It may be self-limited, but usually is manifested by vomiting bright red blood soon after surgery.
   iii. This symptom produces such alarm in the patient that intervention is usually indicated.
   iv. Return to the operating room for endoscopic injection with epinephrine, clip placement, as preferred options. Energy sources, such as heater probe, are less favored at the site of a freshly constructed anastomosis.
b. Hemorrhage from marginal ulcer days to months after LRYGB.
   i. Endoscopy indicated for active bleeding as therapeutic intervention.
   ii. Range of endoscopic measures to correct bleeding may be employed.
   iii. May require retreatment for recurrence, stenosis.
   iv. Biopsy for *H. pylori* indicated.
c. Hemorrhage from LSG acutely after surgery.
   i. Percentages in series to date 1–3% of cases.
   ii. May be self-limited, but if endoscopic intervention needed small bore scope often necessary due to size of channel.
   iii. Injection and clipping preferred to avoid energy injury to staple line.

2. Stenosis/Obstruction

a. Stenosis after LAGB is usually secondary to prolapse, and normally endoscopic treatment is not needed or effective.

b. Stenosis soon (3–12 weeks) after LRYGB is usually at the gastrojejunostomy.

    i. Endoscopy is diagnostic and therapeutic.

    ii. Endoscopic balloon dilatation with an 18-mm balloon is performed (Fig. 7.5).

    iii. Care is taken only to insert the balloon 2 cm or less into the stenosis to prevent potential injury to the back wall of the jejunum.

    iv. Dilation of the anastomosis to allow a smaller bore scope with a working channel through the stenosis is optimal: the scope is then withdrawn to just distal to the anastomosis, the balloon extended deflated, the scope pulled back so the midaspect of the balloon is directly situated at the stenosis, and then the balloon fully inflated and held in place for 60 seconds.

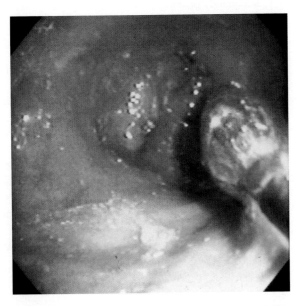

Fig. 7.5. Dilating a stricture of the gastrojejunostomy after gastric bypass using an endoscopic balloon.

    v.   Two or three such balloon dilatations during the endoscopy are often more effective than a single one.

    vi.   Repeat balloon dilatation 2 weeks later may be needed. If further dilatation is needed, consider fluoroscopic dilatation with a guide wire and a larger balloon.

    vii.   Success rates for serial endoscopic dilatations have been reported in the 90% range. Most failures are secondary to the presence of marginal ulcers with their associated scarring.

c.   Late stenosis after LRYGB and associated with marginal ulcer is a more difficult treatment.

    i.   Endoscopy is important to confirm the diagnosis, sample for *H. pylori*, and dilate the anastomosis.

    ii.   A fistula to the lower stomach should be evaluated and, if a suspicious opening is seen, a follow-up contrast study is performed to determine its presence.

    iii.   Any other etiology of the marginal ulcer, such as suture material, should be treated endoscopically with removal if possible.

    iv.   Medical therapy is front line as long as the anastomosis is adequately patent.

    v.   Surgery is reserved for stenosis not amenable to dilation, and ulcers associated with a gastrogastric fistula or chronicity of ulceration.

    vi.   Stenting has had limited value in this setting, but may offer value in select cases.

d.   Stenosis after LSG is usually acute, within the first week of surgery.

    i.   It is amenable to endoscopic dilatation with varied success.

    ii.   Few reports in the literature give anything but case reports or small numbers of patients involved in such dilations.

    iii.   Success is mixed, depending on the nature of the stenosis. Edema is treatable; ischemic scarring from too narrow a lumen is less likely to be correctable.

    iv.   Stenting has been performed in a very few cases with case reports of success.

3. Leakage or Fistula

a. Leak from a staple line after LRYGB:
   i. Most common sites are gastrojejunostomy followed by proximal gastric pouch staple line and then distal gastric pouch staple line.
   ii. Endoscopic measures to treat leakage or fistula include clipping, stenting acutely and injection of fibrin glue for chronic fistula tract, or stenting for chronic fistula.
   iii. Best success for stenting is at gastrojejunostomy due to approximation of surface of stent with leak site and ability of flange proximal to stenosis to prevent migration in most cases.
   iv. Expandable covered stents are the most common variety used; noncovered stents are not indicated in benign condition.
   v. Stent migration may occur and require early stent removal or stent may pass.
   vi. Usual duration of stent is 4–8 weeks.
   vii. Clipping acutely and fibrin glue chronically are less successful.
b. Erosion of band into stomach after LAGB:
   i. Essentially the same as a fistula.
   ii. May have surprisingly few systemic inflammatory symptoms.
   iii. If band erosion full thickness enough, may have formed enough fibrous capsule to allow endoscopic division of band and removal intraluminally.
   iv. If systemic symptoms arise or occur, operative treatment indicated.
c. Leakage of staple line after LSG:
   i. Similar in treatment to that after LRYGB.
   ii. Incidence in the 2–3% range in most series.
   iii. Proximal staple line leaks tend to be the most chronic and most difficult to treat, and may be best candidates for stenting.

4. Placement of Enteral Access

a. Need for enteral access distally after LRYGB:
   i. Proximal staple line leak or chronic stenosis may be indication.
   ii. Most such access issues should be and are performed at surgery.
   iii. Can on occasion have antecolic Roux limb that allows simultaneous percutaneous and endoscopic-guided placement of feeding jejunostomy tube.

5. Access to the Biliary Tree after LRYGB

a. Limited in nature to LRYGB, but may also be needed after DS or biliopancreatic diversion (BPD), less commonly performed malabsorptive operations that also have no direct endoscopic access to the duodenum due to diversion or Roux limb (LRYGB).
   i. Most common indications for endoscopic need to access duodenum after LRYGB, DS, or BPD include choledocholithiasis or pancreatitis.
   ii. Some reported endoscopic success reaching duodenum after LRYGB using double-balloon enteroscopy. However, front-viewing scope is not optimal for performing therapeutic biliopancreatic endoscopy, which is best done via a side-viewing scope.
   iii. Operative intervention to place distal gastric gastrostomy after LRYGB is now being advocated either as a single procedure accompanied by intraoperative endoscopy or less preferably as a staged procedure with endoscopy later once the gastrostomy has matured.

6. Interventions to Produce Weight Loss

An entire chapter could be devoted to the performance of new and innovative endoscopic treatments for production of weight loss in the morbidly obese patient population or the patient populations that have had bariatric surgery and have regained weight after the index operation.

These interventions shall be, thus, grouped into two categories, though some have been used in both situations.

a. Primary Weight Loss Operations

There have been several endoscopic procedures to produce weight loss in morbidly obese patients as *de novo* and initial procedures. Unfortunately, none has proven durable or effective over the longer term. The procedures tried to date and their results include the following.

    i. Garren–Edwards Bubble: An intragastric balloon that proved transiently popular for 2 years until sham-control trials proved no efficacy above that of the diet and exercise. Had a high incidence of balloon migration, intolerance, and complications.

    ii. Intragastric balloon: Despite the Garren-Edwards' failure, there are still companies today and in the recent past that have championed an intragastric balloon for weight loss.

      – Most of the studies have been done outside the USA.

      – Recent randomized controlled trial comparing two balloons showed 20% removed in one group due to intolerance, almost one-third in other group needed endoscopic or surgical removal, and weight loss was 12–14 kg with concurrent 1,000 kcal/day diet at 6 months.

    iii. ROSE procedure: Prototype for primary weight loss via an endoscopic approach for bariatric surgery. Company who championed this has recently gone out of business.

      – Limited short-term weight loss of under 9 kg at 3 months

      – Success in 17 of 20 patients attempted

      – No long-term efficacy proven

7. Revisional Endoscopic Procedures

There is another more prevalent recent belief that an endoscopic approach may be effective in producing durable weight loss in patients who have undergone a restrictive bariatric operation and who have failed because of dilation of the anastomosis. Specifically, since RYGB has been performed for so long, there are a large number of patients who have regained some weight over the years after the index procedure.

There is no evidence in the bariatric surgical literature over the past several decades that a reoperation for these patients that featured decreasing the size of the gastrojejunostomy produced new and durable weight loss as a reoperative procedure. In fact, the failures of such attempts are known but generally unpublished. Now, there is a new movement to attempt to decrease the anastomosis of the gastrojejunostomy to produce weight loss in patients that have regained weight after LRYGB or RYGB. Published studies with the best results for this concept to date are the following.

a. Endoscopic suturing of anastomosis of previous RYGB patients, eight patients (Thompson et al. 2006). These patients had 11 kg weight loss over 3–6 months (23% excess weight loss). No larger follow-up studies published to date.

b. Plication of gastric pouch volume using an endoscopic device (StomaphyX) (Fig. 7.6). Largest US series reported 1-year weight loss of 10 kg (19.5% excess weight loss) for 39 patients.

While these endoscopic measures do generally have good safety records, their long-term efficacy has yet to be proven and the lack of long-term reports following some of the initial procedures suggests that such efficacy is likely lacking.

However, this text does not mean to discourage or diminish the continued new efforts at potentially developing endoscopic bariatric treatment options for patients with morbid obesity. Such procedures would undoubtedly prove highly popular and would likely produce an exponential increase in demand for bariatric procedures as was seen when laparoscopic options became available. However, to date, none have proven long-term efficacy.

F. Complications

1. Diagnostic Endoscopy

a. Complications are relatively rare, on the order of 0.4%.
   i.   Most common involve conscious sedation and its complications.
   ii. Perforation is rare if simple diagnostic test is being performed.

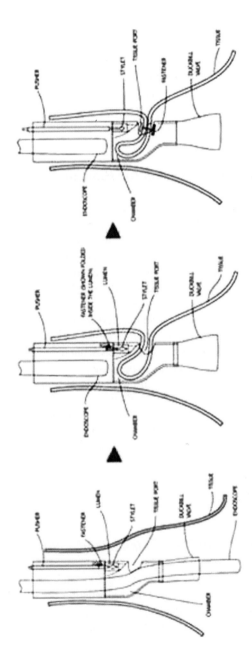

Fig. 7.6. The StomaphX device used to endoscopically place plastic fixation devices to reduce gastric pouch size after previous gastric bypass.

    iii.   Bleeding, infection, and reaction to medication all reported, but all well under 1% each.

    iv.   Aspiration is a risk if stomach is not empty—need to intubate the patient in any situation where this is in question, such as acute bleeding.

    v.   Loose teeth are a risk and patient should be made aware.

    vi.   Elderly, frail, pulmonary compromised, and sleep apnea patients at the highest risk for conscious sedation.

2. Therapeutic Intervention for Bleeding

a.   Airway management to avoid aspiration and pulmonary complications.

b.   Adequate volume resuscitation before embarking on procedure.

c.   Hemodynamic stability—if not, needs operative treatment.

d.   Blood available for transfusion as well as blood products.

e.   Coagulopathy ruled out or treated.

f.   Perforation due to heat source <1%.

g.   Rebleeding up to 50% if visible vessel.

h.   Failure to stop bleeding depends on source: Most common for large arterial bleeding sources, such as duodenal ulcer, bleeding gastric varices with portal hypertension.

i.   Direct injection of epinephrine in blood vessel may produce hemodynamic reaction.

j.   Perforation of anastomosis from procedure is possible, but uncommon.

k.   Worst complications arise from poor attention to patient systemic symptoms, volume repletion, hemodynamic instability, vascular access, inadequate monitoring, or inadequate resuscitation.

3. Therapeutic Stenting of Stenosis or Leak

a.   Inadequate attention to airway and oversedation may occur.

b.   Attention needed to be certain that patient is not in septic shock and hemodynamically unstable.

c.   Stent should be placed, where migration is a minimal risk.

d.   Migration itself may be benign but could cause obstruction or injury.

e. Be certain that guide wire location is in appropriate lumen and not extraluminal to cause worse injury/leak.

f. Intolerance of stent by patient is the most common complication after migration; may be due to migration; even if no migration, may complain of pain and food intolerance; incidence of 20% in some series.

4. Therapeutic Balloon Dilatation for Stenosis

a. Only major complication is blind insertion of stiff balloon dilator into small stenotic lumen and through back wall of jejunum causing perforation in end-to-side anastomosis; 1–3% incidence in literature.

b. Rare minor site bleeding and minor discomfort by patient.

c. Lack of efficacy for single treatment 50%, overall 10–20% based on etiology.

5. Access to the Biliary Tree

a. Complications typical for those involving intervention gastrointestinal procedure.

b. For the surgery: Bleeding, site infection, tube dislodgement, and leakage all reported at low rates.

c. For endoscopy: Pancreatitis, sepsis, stent dislodgement and obstruction, and bleeding and perforation from sphincterotomy all seen in standard ERCP and therapeutic biliopancreatic endoscopy reported in similar percentages to those seen otherwise for these procedures.

Selected References

Alami RS, Schuster R, Friedland S, et al. Transnasal small-caliber esophagogastroduodenoscopy for preoperative evaluation of the high-risk morbidly obese patient. Surg Endosc. 2007;21:758–60.

Champion JK, Hunt T, DeLisle N. Role of routine intraoperative endoscopy in laparoscopic bariatric surgery. Surg Endosc. 2002;16:1663–5.

DeCastro ML, Morales MJ, Del Campo V, et al. Efficacy, safety, and tolerance of two types of intragastric balloons placed in obese subjects: a double-blind comparative study. Obes Surg. 2010;20:1642–6.

Go MR, Muscarella P, Needleman BJ, et al. Endoscopic management of stomal stenosis after Roux-en-Y gastric bypass. Surg Endosc. 2004;18:56–9.

Mikami D, Needleman B, Narula V, et al. Natural orifice surgery: initial U.S. experience using the StomaphyX device to reduce gastric pouches after Roux-en-Y gastric bypass. Surg Endosc. 2010;24:223–8.

Mullady DK, Lautz DB, Thompson CC. Treatment of weight regain after gastric bypass when using a new endoscopic platform: initial experience and early outcomes (with video). Gastrointest Endosc. 2009;70:440–4.

Schirmer B, Erenoglu C, Miller A. Flexible endoscopy in the management of patients undergoing Roux-en-Y gastric bypass. Obes Surg. 2002;12:634–8.

Schwartz ML, Drew RL, Roiger RW, Ketover SR, Chazin-Caldie M. Stenosis of the gastroenterostomy after laparoscopic gastric bypass. Obes Surg. 2004;14(4):484–91.

Sharaf RN, Weinshel EH, Bini EJ, Rosenberg J, Sherman A, Ren CJ. Endoscopy plays an important preoperative role in bariatric surgery. Obes Surg. 2004;14:1367–72.

Thompson CC, Slattery J, Bundga ME, Lautz DB. Peroral endoscopic reduction of dilated gastrojejunal anastomosis after Roux-en-Y gastric bypass: a possible new option for patients with weight regain. Surg Endosc. 2006;20:1744–8.

Vance PL, de Lange EE, Shaffer Jr HA, Schirmer B. Gastric outlet obstruction following surgery for morbid obesity: efficacy of fluoroscopically guided balloon dilatation. Radiology. 2002;222:70–2.

Verset D, Houben J-J, Gay F, Elcheroth J, Bourgeois V, Van Gossum A. The place of upper gastrointestinal tract endoscopy before and after vertical banded gastroplasty for morbid obesity. Dig Dis Sci. 1997;42:2333–7.

8. Novel Endoscopic Approaches to Obesity

Rabindra R. Watson, M.D.
Christopher C. Thompson, M.D., M.Sc., F.A.C.G., F.A.S.G.E.

Principles of Patient Selection, Choice of Procedure, and Perioperative Care

A. Indications

Obesity is a complex metabolic disease that is associated with significant comorbid illnesses. It is a growing global pandemic that is now more prevalent than malnutrition from hunger. A series of consensus conferences of the National Institutes of Health have defined and categorized obesity based on the concept of increasing morbidity with increases in body mass index (BMI). Based on these categories, surgical eligibility has traditionally required obesity class III (BMI ≥ 40) or class II (BMI ≥ 35) with significant associated comorbid illnesses.

While the number of bariatric surgeries performed has increased to treat this burgeoning population, only a small percentage of eligible patients ultimately undergo surgery due to a variety of factors, including prohibitive comorbidities and patients' aversion to surgery. Additionally, despite the presence of obesity-associated health risks, a large group of obese and overweight patients do not meet surgical eligibility requirements. These patients are left to medical and pharmacologic therapies that in large part are ineffective. This growing population of overweight and obese patients has resulted in increased demand for effective, safe, and minimally invasive approaches to obesity therapy.

Rapid advances in flexible endoscopic technology have led to the pursuit of novel applications to address conditions traditionally within

N.T. Nguyen and C.E.H. Scott-Conner (eds.), *The SAGES Manual: Volume 2 Advanced Laparoscopy and Endoscopy*, DOI 10.1007/978-1-4614-2347-8_8, © Springer Science+Business Media, LLC 2012

Table 8.1. Potential advantages and disadvantages of the endoscopic approach.

Advantages	Disadvantages
Lack of incisional complications (hernias, wound infections, etc.)	Uncertain efficacy
Lower cost	Durability
Faster postoperative recovery	Reimbursement issues
Cosmesis	
Reversibility and modification	

the purview of laparoscopy, such as the treatment of gastrointestinal (GI) epithelial neoplasia, pancreatic debridement, and palliation of malignant intestinal or biliary obstruction. The possibility of lower complication rates, faster recovery time, and lower costs makes endoscopic methods an attractive approach (Table 8.1). Moreover, as only a small percentage of obese patients undergo surgery due to concerns of procedural invasiveness and surgical risk, a minimally invasive option is sorely needed. As our understanding of the neurohormonal and physiologic effects of bariatric surgery has grown, there has been a recent proliferation of devices and procedures that act to modify preexisting postsurgical anatomy or as de novo therapies to treat a variety of obese patient populations. While still within its infancy, endoscopic treatment of obesity will likely continue to play a significant role in combating the obesity epidemic.

B. Patient Selection and Therapeutic Targets

The low-risk profile of endoscopic bariatric procedures opens the possibility of a variety of roles in the treatment of obesity. Currently, devices are being developed that may impact obesity through several different mechanisms allowing for a broad range of applications. As such, the identification of target patient populations and therapeutic goals is paramount. While there are no standardized guidelines addressing this topic, the categorization of endoscopic interventions a priori aids in the definition of such criteria (Table 8.2).

Procedures from these categories may be used in combination or in sequence to treat obesity and associated metabolic conditions through multiple mechanisms. The application of this rubric may aid the clinician

Table 8.2. Procedure categories.

Early intervention	IGB, DJBS
Bridge to surgery	IGB, DJBS
Metabolic	DJBS
Primary	EVG, TERIS, TOGA
Revision	Sclerotherapy, IOP, OverStitch, Endocinch, Stomaphyx

IGB intragastric balloon, *DJBS* duodenal-jejunal bypass sleeve, *EVG* endoscopic vertical gastroplasty, *TERIS* transoral endoscopic restrictive implant system, *TOGA* transoral gastroplasty device, *IOP* incisionless operating platform

in aligning the patient with the appropriate intervention based on the given clinical scenario. The below categories have been suggested, and an individual device may apply to one or more specific categories based on its particular attributes.

1. Early interventions: Provide weight loss or stabilization to those patients who do not as yet qualify for bariatric surgery (overweight, obesity class I, obesity class II without comorbidities).

2. Bridge to surgery: Reduces obesity-related risk factors prior to various surgical interventions.

3. Metabolic: Primarily addresses the metabolic derangements associated with obesity, such as diabetes, irrespective of impact on weight loss.

4. Primary: Acts as a first-line treatment for obesity as an alternative to traditional surgery.

5. Revision: Repairs failed surgeries and treats insufficient weight loss.

C. Preoperative and Postoperative Care

1. *Preoperative Care*

A multidisciplinary team is critical to the management of the obese patient and the standard bariatric work-up will likely apply to most emerging endoscopic therapies. An assessment of diet and diet education should be provided by a nutritionist, and a period of time in a specific nutrition/diet program may be recommended prior to certain procedures. Psychological evaluation is also important to provide proper care for patients with eating disorders and prevent inappropriate procedures.

As is the case with bariatric surgery, all patients should be subjected to a thorough history and physical examination. Due to the prevalence of cardiopulmonary comorbidities in obese patients such as coronary artery disease, hypertension, congestive heart failure, obstructive sleep apnea, and pulmonary hypertension, appropriate preprocedural tests should be obtained, such as an echocardiogram and pulmonary function testing. Device- and procedure-specific concerns should also be addressed. For some devices, evaluation of the upper gastrointestinal tract may be important to exclude hiatal hernia or assure that the tissue is healthy for device implantation. Care should be taken to clearly explain the nature of the procedure and the procedure-specific treatment goals with the patient, as well as relevant risks and alternatives.

2. Postoperative Care

In the immediate postoperative period, the patient may experience pain requiring narcotics as well as nausea. It is important to avoid repeated bouts of emesis as this may result in dislodgement of endo-scopically placed devices or stitches. This may be combated with peripro-cedural use of a combination of decadron, scopolamine patches, and intravenous antiemetics, such as ondansetron, prochlorperazine, and metoclopramide. Patients infrequently require narcotics postprocedure; liquid preparations of opiates and acetaminophen may be given.

The patient may be discharged home the same day of endoscopy for many procedures, though overnight observation may be required for the assessment and treatment of postprocedural symptoms.

Postprocedure dietary recommendations vary based upon the proce-dure performed and written instructions should be provided and explained. Early postprocedure follow-up may comprise a telephone call or brief office visit within the first week after the endoscopic procedure to assess patient symptoms. Additionally, weight loss goals and dietary modifications may be reinforced during subsequent visits.

D. Instrumentation, Room Setup, Patient Preparation, and Adjuncts

These aspects vary considerably depending on the procedure and specific devices being used. The following measures are commonly taken when endoscopic suturing is performed for revision of dilated gastrojejunal anastomosis and have also been used in primary endoscopic obesity procedures. However, as these procedures continue to evolve, so too will these aspects of patient management.

1. A bowel preparation is administered the night prior to endoscopy.

2. The patient is positioned in the left lateral or supine position, depending upon the endoscopist's preference and anatomical or device considerations.

3. Carbon dioxide insufflation is preferable to air due to more rapid reabsorption with less postprocedure distention, nausea, and vomiting. Simethicone may also be instilled at the start of the procedure to help alleviate discomfort from gaseous distention.

4. Appropriate equipment for endoscopic hemostasis should be available, including dilute epinephrine, injection needles, and hemostatic clips. Additional adjuncts, including argon plasma coagulation for mucosal ablation, prior to endoscopic sewing and fibrin glue to aid in sealing may also be utilized.

5. Procedures may be performed in a standard endoscopy room or operating room. Arrangements for an appropriate bed may need to be made for those procedures performed in endoscopy units unaccustomed to managing bariatric patients.

6. Periprocedural antibiotics are not specifically indicated, though should be given based upon published perioperative guidelines.

Endoscopic Bariatric Procedures

A. Intragastric Balloon

1. Introduction

The deployment of an intragastric balloon to restrict oral intake was one of the earliest developed endoscopic treatments of obesity. The theorized mechanism of action is to enhance the sensation of satiety and inhibit gastric accommodation, essentially functioning as an artificial bezoar. It is also reasonable to believe that such devices impact the regulation and release of ghrelin, an appetite-regulating hormone released from gastric tissue, though early studies have yielded conflicting results.

Early versions of intragastric balloons first appeared in the 1980s. These devices were hampered by course external surfaces that resulted in mucosal irritation, smaller balloon volumes than recent iterations, and significant loss of follow-up. Consequently, early studies of these devices were unfavorable due to insignificant weight loss and high complication rates. Current balloons are generally spherical with smooth surfaces and manufactured with silicone components. There are several devices available (though none FDA approved), with the Bioenterics Intragastric Balloon (BIB) (Allergan, Irvine, CA), the most extensively studied.

Advantages of intragastric balloons include short procedure length, reversibility with device removal, and low complication rates. Published studies of this technology are limited to 6-month device implantation lengths per study protocols.

2. Technique

Placement of the device may be performed under deep intravenous sedation with endoscopic guidance using a standard gastroscope. A dual-channel endoscope can also facilitate device manipulation within the stomach using through-the-scope forceps, graspers, snares, and nets. The device is placed in the fundus, body, or antrum, depending on the specific model. The BIB is inflated by instilling 500–700 mL of saline or methylene blue. Deflation may be performed using available endoscopic needles, and the device is removed using a custom grasper or snare.

3. Outcomes

A large retrospective analysis of 2,515 patients with a mean BMI of 44.8 ± 7.8 kg/m^2 undergoing BIB placement demonstrated successful placement in 99.92% and a mean %EWL of 33.9 ± 18.7 at 6-month follow-up. Notably, improvement or resolution of hypertension and diabetes was observed in 93.7% and 86.9% of patients, respectively. The mean time of positioning was recorded as 15 ± 2 min in a second study.

A recent meta-analysis estimated a mean weight loss of 12.2% with a %EWL of 32.1% with the BIB. However, only one of the three published randomized controlled trials have demonstrated a significant improvement in weight loss and comorbid conditions compared with a sham procedure.

The role of the BIB in super obese patients was explored in a series of 26 patients with a mean BMI of 65.3 ± 9.8 who were deemed too high risk to undergo primary bariatric surgery. Mean %EWL was 22.4 ± 14.5 at 6-month follow-up, with improvement or resolution of hypertension and diabetes in 83 and 81% of patients, respectively. Significant improvements in serum glucose, insulin, low-density lipoprotein cholesterol, triglycerides, metabolic syndrome, diastolic blood pressure, c-reactive protein levels, and obstructive sleep apnea have also been demonstrated. Additional improvements in quality of life measures have been seen in uncontrolled studies.

4. Complications

Early device removal has been required in 2.8% of patients with the BIB mainly due to patient intolerance. Common symptoms include gastroesophageal reflux in over half of patients, nausea and vomiting (8.6%), and abdominal cramps (5%). Symptoms are most commonly encountered in the first several days after placement, and may be managed with antiemetics, acid suppression, and analgesics. Other minor complications include mucosal injury (2.1%) and migration (2.5%), both of which may be managed by medical and endoscopic means. Severe complications are rare but have been reported, including gastric perforation in 5 (0.19%) patients resulting in 2 deaths in 1 study of over 2,500 patients. The majority of these patients had prior gastric surgery, and this should be considered a contraindication to balloon placement. Aspiration pneumonia leading to death was also reported in another study.

5. Conclusions

Current evidence does not support the use of the intragastric balloon as an alternative to bariatric surgery. Furthermore, its durability is limited as it is typically removed after 6 months. Intragastric balloons are likely best utilized as a bridge to surgery, providing initial weight loss in the super obese. Additionally, their ease of insertion, removal, and low-risk profile may be well suited for an early intervention strategy in some overweight patients.

B. Duodenal-Jejunal Bypass Sleeve

1. Introduction

The first endoscopically delivered device designed to bypass the duodenum and proximal jejunum is the Endobarrier (GI Dynamics Inc., Watertown, Massachusetts). The mechanism of action is analogous to roux-en-y gastric bypass (RYGB) surgery, whereby biliopancreatic secretions are prevented from mixing with ingested nutrients in the proximal small bowel. Delivery of bile salts and undigested nutrients to the distal small bowel may also alter incretin pathways.

The device utilizes an impermeable 60-cm polyethylene sleeve that is extended from the duodenum into the proximal jejunum. The proximal sleeve consists of a nickel–titanium alloy self-expandable anchor designed to engage the tissue of the proximal duodenum to prevent sleeve migration (Fig. 8.1).

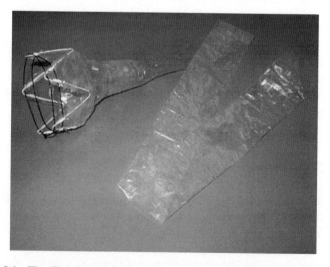

Fig. 8.1. The EndoBarrier DJBS comprises an impermeable fluoropolymer sleeve of 60 cm and a nitinol anchor with barbs. The polypropylene drawstring is necessary for removal of the device (reprinted with permission from Mullady DK, Jonnalagadda S. Primary endoscopic obesity procedures. Techniques in Gastrointestinal Endoscopy. 2010;12 (3):167–76).

2. *Technique*

The device is delivered with a wire-guided catheter system under fluoroscopic guidance. The inner sheath is pushed into the proximal jejunum releasing the sleeve. The duodenal anchor is then released into the duodenal bulb. Drawstrings at the proximal anchor are used for device removal.

3. *Outcomes*

The first human trial included 12 patients (mean BMI 43 kg/m^2), in whom the Endobarrier was placed successfully in all patients with a mean procedure time of 26.6 min. The device remained in place for 12 weeks, though two patients required early removal due to refractory abdominal pain attributed to poor device placement. All devices were successfully removed in mean time of 43.3 min. At 12 weeks, the mean %EWL was 23.6%.

A recent open-label randomized controlled trial compared sleeve placement in 25 patients versus low-calorie diet in 14 controls. Sleeve placement was tolerated in 20 patients over 12 weeks, and all were successfully removed. At 12 weeks, the device resulted in a mean %EWL of 22% versus 5% among controls. An FDA-approved clinical trial is currently underway.

4. *Complications*

Complications associated with sleeve placement and removal are not uncommon with the current device, although they are generally considered minor. Mucosal tears involving the oropharynx and esophagus have been reported in two patients during device removal. Injuries resulting from sleeve-induced mucosal inflammation have resulted in gastrointestinal bleeding in three patients as well as functional pain syndromes. Sleeve migration and occlusion have also been reported.

5. *Conclusions*

Proximal enteral bypass has a well-documented history of success with respect to weight loss in the bariatric literature. Perhaps, most intriguing is the emerging data reporting rapid improvement in glucose metabolism following diversion of the duodenal and proximal jejunal mucosa from gastric secretions and ingested nutrients. Such metabolic effects represent an exciting therapeutic target for endoscopic interventions, and further physiologic studies are eagerly anticipated. The role of the duodenal-jejunal bypass sleeve (DJBS) is currently being defined in ongoing studies, and questions remain as to its safety, tolerability, and durability. Possible roles include primary metabolic therapy, bridge to surgery, or perhaps as an early intervention in some patients.

C. Transoral Endoluminal Vertical Gastroplasty

1. Introduction

Initial experience with the creation of endoscopic gastric tissue plications was first explored as a treatment for GERD with the Endocinch device (C. R. Bard, Murray Hill, NJ). It has failed to gain widespread use for this application due in part to its lack of durability and incomplete control of GERD symptoms. The Endocinch was subsequently applied for bariatric revision procedures, and this is discussed in detail in the revision section. More recently, the Endocinch has been studied as a primary treatment for obesity through gastric volume restriction.

The suturing device consists of a hollow needle contained within a cap mounted on the tip of a gastroscope. Tissue is aspirated into the cap using suction, and a T-tag suture is deployed through the aspirated tissue via the needle. The device must then be removed from the patient and the needle reloaded to take subsequent bites. After a second or multiple sutures are deployed, a suture anchor is then passed to lock the sutures in place.

2. Technique

The technique of endoluminal vertical gastroplasty (EVG) was first described by Fogel et al. (2008). The procedure is performed under general anesthesia. After a diagnostic upper endoscopy has been performed to define anatomy and plan suture placement, an esophageal overtube is placed to facilitate endoscope removal and reinsertion. The Endocinch device is then mounted on the endoscope and a 3–0 polypropylene T-tag suture is loaded into the cap.

The first bite of tissue is taken on the anterior surface of the proximal fundus followed by a second bite taken on the anterior surface of the distal aspect of the rugal folds of the body. The third bite is placed 1–2 cm

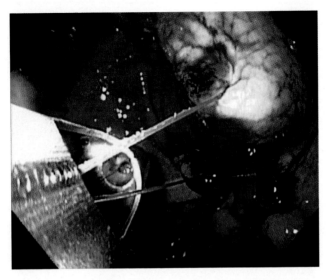

Fig. 8.2. Endoluminal vertical gastroplasty: Gastric plications are created to approximate the anterior and posterior gastric walls to achieve restriction of the upper stomach [reprinted with permission from Brethauer et al. (2010)].

proximal to the second stitch on the posterior wall (Fig. 8.2). Two to four additional bites are taken working proximally on alternating surfaces of the stomach. A second endoscope is then used to tighten and cinch the cross-linked plications, resulting in apposition of the anterior and posterior surfaces (Fig. 8.3). Excess suture is cut and removed.

3. Outcomes

The initial study by Fogel et al. (2008) was performed in 64 patients with a mean BMI of 39.9 ± 5.1 k/m^2. Procedure time was roughly 45 min, and patients were discharged within 3 h of endoscopy. Mean %EWL was an impressive $58.1 \pm 19.9\%$ at 12-month follow-up. Additionally, the superobese subgroup experienced a significantly greater %EWL than less obese subjects. Long-term follow-up was recently published in abstract form by the original investigators. Of 233 patients, 24-month follow-up was available for 45 patients, in whom %EWL remained significant at $49 \pm 28\%$ comparable to that observed with bariatric surgical procedures.

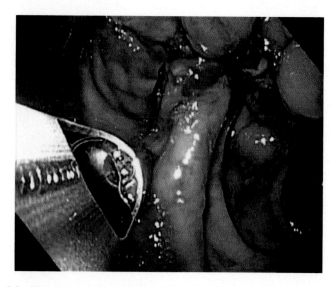

Fig. 8.3. Plications continued from distal to proximal toward angle of His and fastened (reprinted with permission from Brethauer et al. (2010).

A new version of the Endocinch that allows for deeper tissue bites and eliminates the need for device exchange was subsequently used for functional gastric outlet reduction in a multicenter trial. The procedure was also substantially different and involved the placement of multiple complex stitches in the gastric body and fundus, instead of creating a gastric "sleeve" with one running stitch. Short-term results showed good early weight loss, however, not as substantial as in earlier publication.

4. Complications

No serious adverse events have been reported. Two patients reported transient reflux symptoms, and one case of self-limited postprocedure nausea and vomiting occurred. While not reported in this study, bleeding remains a risk with this procedure. Additionally, suture disruption may be caused by postprocedure vomiting; therefore, aggressive use of anti-emetics is encouraged.

5. Conclusions

The experience with the Endocinch device in the treatment of GERD has led to questions regarding the durability of bariatric procedures that use this device. Concerns remain regarding inadequate suture depth and subsequent dehiscence over time, particularly since the plications are used to restrict gastric distention. Nonetheless, initial data regarding its bariatric applications are encouraging. These techniques may be envisioned as a primary obesity therapy or as an early intervention in overweight patients. Further randomized, sham-controlled studies with long-term follow-up are needed to corroborate the encouraging initial results.

D. Transoral Gastroplasty

1. Introduction

Increasing attention has been directed toward devices that create full-thickness gastric plications for primary obesity therapy. Transoral gastroplasty (TOGA) (TOGA System; Satiety Inc, Palo Alto, CA) is the first endoscopic platform to accomplish this. A transoral stapler is used to create a vertical gastric sleeve in the proximal stomach. Encouraging results have been published in two prospective uncontrolled pilot studies while a multicenter randomized, sham-controlled trial is ongoing in the USA.

2. Technique

The procedure is performed under general anesthesia in the supine position. The device is introduced into the stomach over a guide wire, in some cases after prior esophageal dilatation. A gastroscope is then passed within the device and retroflexed within the stomach for visualization. An expandable wire/sail is used to separate the anterior and posterior surfaces of the stomach, which are then brought within the stapling device using suction pods. Once fired, serosal apposition is achieved with titanium staples in parallel to the lesser curve. The stapler is removed and reloaded, and a second firing distally extends the sleeve to 8 cm from the angle of His. Using the TOGA Restrictor, a single suction pod stapler, the sleeve lumen of 20 mm is further reduced to roughly 12 mm, approximating that achieved with surgical techniques.

3. Outcomes

Results have been published in two studies involving a total of 33 patients. The mean BMI was above 40 kg/m^2 in both studies and all patients underwent TOGA successfully in a procedure length of approximately 131 min. Procedures were generally well tolerated.

Using an early generation device, an intact staple line was seen in only 5 of 21 patients at 6 months. The second-generation device achieved intact staple lines in 7 of 11 subjects at 6 months. Nonetheless, the %EWL at 6-month follow-up was 24.4% for the first-generation device and 46.0% for the second-generation device. Significant improvements in quality of life measures (p <0.05) were also seen, and hospital stays were limited to one night on average. A multicenter randomized, sham-controlled trial was recently completed and results are pending.

4. Complications

No serious adverse events have been reported. The most common adverse events include nausea, vomiting, and abdominal pain limited to the first week post procedure.

5. Conclusions

The TOGA device creates full-thickness tissue apposition, which may result in greater durability of gastric restriction than that achieved with the Endocinch device; however, it is likely working by a different mechanism than that of the functional gastric volume reduction procedure that involves stitching of the fundus. The stapling procedure can be achieved in a reasonable time, and there are no major complications reported. Despite the somewhat frequent occurrence of staple dehiscence, significant weight loss has been achieved, albeit in short-term follow-up. Additionally, as with the Endocinch device, one must question the durability of gastric partitioning procedures, given the poor long-term results with vertical banded gastroplasty and the well-documented limitations of the sleeve gastrectomy. The results of a multicenter randomized, sham-controlled US study should further elucidate the efficacy of this primary obesity therapy.

E. Transoral Endoscopic Restrictive Implant System

1. Introduction

The transoral endoscopic restrictive implant system (TERIS) is designed to mimic laparoscopic gastric banding through the implantation of a silicone restrictor diaphragm, although the exact mechanism may be quite different. Gastric plications are created in the gastric cardia along with anchor placement followed by implantation of the restrictor diaphragm, resulting in a restrictive pouch with a 10-mm orifice. A Phase I trial has recently been completed.

2. Technique

The procedure is performed under general anesthesia with the patient in the supine position with the head tilted slightly backward. A 22-mm overtube is placed. With the endoscope in the retroflexed position, the stapler is used to create five circumferential transmural plications in the cardia approximately 3 cm below the gastroesophageal junction. Five tissue anchors are then pulled through the plications using a steerable grasping forceps. A multiple-lumen guide is used to place five custom anchor graspers which facilitate locking of the restrictor diaphgram in place. The anchors are then pulled through the restrictor diaphragm one at a time.

Per trial protocol, all patients were admitted for overnight observation, and an upper GI study was performed in all patients to confirm the absence of a gastric leak.

3. Outcomes

The Phase I trial involved 13 patients with a mean BMI of 42.1 kg/m^2 at enrollment. Device implantation was completed in 12 patients in a mean time of 142 min. Ten patients were hospitalized for one night; the longest stay was three nights. The median %EWL was 28% at 3 months. Improvements in the physical component summary of the Short Form-36 were significant ($p < 0.01$), though the mental component summary remained unchanged.

4. Complications

Three serious adverse events occurred, resulting in an alteration in the study protocol. One patient suffered a gastric perforation caused by the stapler itself, which required laparoscopic conversion and repair. Two patients developed pneumoperitoneum, with one patient developing respiratory compromise requiring needle decompression. Following these complications, the stapler was modified and tested in animal studies prior to continuation of the study. Carbon dioxide insufflation was also adopted.

Other common adverse events included abdominal pain, fever, nausea, vomiting, and throat pain.

5. Conclusions

The TERIS provides another mechanism through which endoscopic interventions may mimic bariatric surgery, in this instance through gastric restriction by creation of a type of gastric banding. Three serious adverse events did occur in the Phase I trial, though two could have likely been averted through the initial use of pressure-controlled CO_2 insufflation. The secondary outcome of weight loss was acceptable, and theoretically this device is removable. The procedure requires further refinement before larger studies are justified.

F. Notes

Peritoneal access through natural orifices may provide the benefits of reductions in anesthesia, analgesia, hospital stay, complications, and improved cosmesis. The application of NOTES techniques to the treatment of obesity is a logical step in the reduction of periprocedural complications in this high-risk patient cohort.

A hybrid sleeve gastrectomy was first reported in a porcine model using transgastric and transrectal access aided by minilaparoscopy and gastric retraction using the Endostitch device (Auto-Suture, Norwalk, CT). The procedure length was 2.5 h and suture lines remained intact at autopsy, though closure of the rectal defect was not performed.

This was followed by the first human experience in four patients in Brazil. Transvaginal endoscopy was performed, with two abdominal trocars and one umbilical trocar required for stapling. Procedures were completed without complication in 90–100 min. Sutures were used for staple line reinforcement and vaginal closure. Drains were placed for 5 days while hospital stay was 2 days. No detailed follow-up was reported.

Additional cadaveric studies have been published exploring NOTES gastrojejunal anastomoses. Difficulties were encountered in placing the stapler shaft and anvil in the small bowel and docking of the stapler with endoscopic instruments while several perforations occurred. These studies, along with previous reports of other NOTES applications, emphasize the need for development of NOTES-specific tools and training.

Endoscopic Revision Procedures

A. Introduction

Weight regain or insufficient weight loss following RYGB may occur in up to 20% of patients. Dilation of the gastrojejunal anastomosis has been shown in multivariate analysis to be a significant predictor of weight regain. Various techniques for endoscopic anastomotic reduction have been examined due to the significant morbidity and mortality associated with surgical RYGB revision.

B. Sclerotherapy

1. Introduction

Sclerotherapy involves the submucosal injection of sodium morrhuate circumferentially around the gastric aspect of the gastrojejunal anastomosis. The proposed mechanism of action is reduction of the stomal diameter due to expansion of the submucosal layer of the gastric mucosa and scar formation (Fig. 8.4).

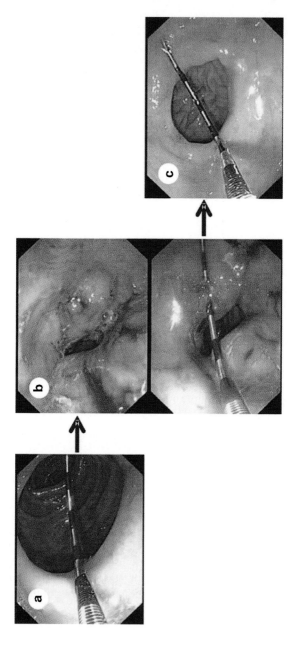

Fig. 8.4. Gastrojejunostomy anastomosis (**a**) before, (**b**) immediately after sclerotherapy injections, and (**c**) 3 months post procedure (reprinted with permission from Woods KE, Abu Dayyeh BK, Thompson CC. Endoscopic post-bypass revisions. Tech Eastroint Endo. 2010;12 (3):160–6).

2. Technique

The procedure may be performed under conscious sedation, with the patient in the left lateral position. A diagnostic endoscopy is performed to exclude the presence of fistulae or ulcers. Fistulae may be responsible for weight gain, and should be managed appropriately prior to sclerotherapy. Ulcers are a contraindication to sclerotherapy, and should be medically managed and healing confirmed prior to treatment.

Due to the rare occurrence of systemic reactions, benadryl is often administered prior to injection. In addition, sclerotherapy has been associated with bacteremia; therefore, an intravenous antibiotic should also be given, such as ciprofloxacin.

Using an injection needle, a 1–2-mL test dose should be administered and the patient's hemodynamics monitored for several minutes. Subsequently, 1–2-mL aliquots are injected circumferentially around the anastomosis. Care should be taken to avoid superficial injection; this may be appreciated by blanching of the overlying mucosa. Superficial injection results in early mucosal necrosis, which may result in hemorrhage. Similarly, the injection needle should be withdrawn as the injection bleb increases in size to avoid burying the needle within the bleb which may also result in bleeding through the mucosal defect. Six to thirty cc of sodium morrhuate may be injected in a single session. Patients should be discharged with 5 days of an oral liquid antibiotic.

Repeat sessions may be performed as needed, typically every 12 weeks. Subsequent injections are often more difficult due to mural scarring. Ideally, subsequent injections should be placed proximal to the prior injection sites to create an appropriate bleb. One must avoid injection in proximity to the gastroesophageal junction due to the risk of mediastinitis.

3. Outcomes

A retrospective study of 71 patients with weight regain in an average of 2.9 years following RYGB demonstrated weight stability or weight loss in 72% of subjects at 12 months. The mean anastomotic diameter was 2.3 cm, and an average of 13 mL of sodium morrhuate was injected. Repeat injection was performed in 49% of patients, and no complications or hospitalizations occurred. High BMI at endoscopy was found to be the only factor predictive of response.

A second study of 32 patients demonstrated weight loss in 56%, stabilization in 32%, and continued weight gain in 9% of patients at 12 months. A third study demonstrated a reduction in stomal diameter of 5.7 mm with an average of 2.3 injections. Sclerotherapy was successful in 18 of 28 patients, with a modest reduction of stomal diameter of 1.9 mm in treatment failures. Those in the success group lost an average of 26 kg while "failures" lost an average of 8.8 kg.

4. Complications

Complications are relatively minor, with most patients reporting postinjection abdominal pain responsive to non-narcotic medication. Bleeding requiring endoscopic injection of epinephrine is not uncommon, and shallow ulceration at follow-up endoscopy is also commonly seen. One patient developed an anastomotic stricture which required endoscopic dilation. Systemic effects of injection may also rarely be seen, manifested by hypertensive urgency. Early recognition is key, and intravenous administration of toradol quickly blunts this effect.

5. Conclusions

The endoscopic injection of sodium morrhuate for gastrojejunal anastomotic reduction is a relatively simple and safe intervention with favorable outcomes. The main limitation of this method is the limited number of injections that can be performed due to progressive mural scarring. The response is also variable, which may be due to unpredictable tissue effects. Additionally, it is unclear whether subsequent surgical or endoscopic interventions may be performed safely. The durability of this intervention is unknown, and further study is warranted.

C. Endoscopic Suturing

Endoscopic suturing has been available for several years, with significant recent improvements in device technology driving its dissemination among endoscopists. Stomal and pouch reduction using sutures theoretically may provide improved user control.

1. Endocinch

a. Introduction

The Endocinch (C. R. Bard, Murray Hill, NJ) device has been studied as both a primary obesity therapy as well as in the treatment of weight regain following RYGB. Results of a recently completed large, multi-center, randomized, sham-controlled study are encouraging.

b. Technique

The procedure is performed under general anesthesia. A diagnostic endoscopy is performed, and an esophageal overtube placed. The tissue around the anastomosis is thermally ablated using argon plasma coagulation (APC) to promote tissue apposition at the suture sites (Fig. 8.5). The number of stitches placed varies, though typically at least two stitches are placed with a goal stomal diameter of 5–8 mm (Fig. 8.6 a, b).

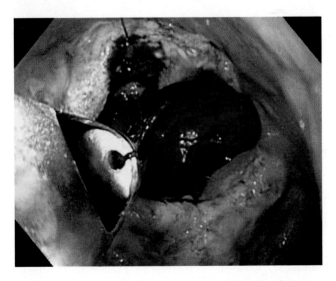

Fig. 8.5. Argon plasma coagulation is used around the rim of the stoma and suturing begins top to bottom, left to right (images provided by Dr. Christopher C. Thompson).

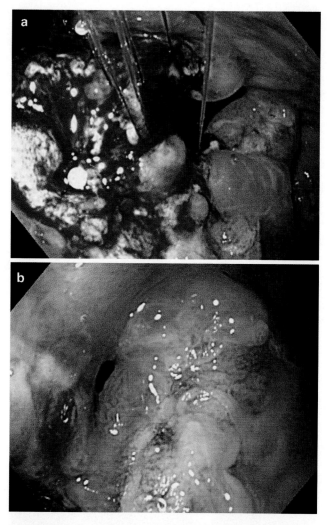

Fig. 8.6. (a) Each pair of sutures is fastened in order of placement. (b) Final diameter of 5–8 mm, reinforced with fibrin glue (images provided by Dr. Christopher C. Thompson).

c. Outcomes

The Randomized Evaluation of Endoscopic Suturing Transorally for anastomotic Outlet Reduction (RESTORe) study, a prospective multicenter, randomized, blinded, sham-controlled trial, tested the

Endocinch device in the treatment of weight regain after RYGB due to dilation of the gastrojejunal anastomosis to >20 mm. Technical success, defined as stomal reduction to <10 mm in diameter, was achieved in 89% of the 48 intervention patients in a mean procedure length of 107 min. Weight loss or stabilization was achieved in 96% of suture patients versus 78% in the sham group ($p = 0.019$). In per protocol analysis, mean weight loss at 6 months in the intervention group was $4.2 \pm 5.4\%$ versus $1.9 \pm 5.2\%$ in the sham group ($p = 0.041$). A significant reduction in blood pressure and trend toward improved metabolic indices were also observed in the intervention group.

d. Complications

No serious adverse events occurred in the RESTORe trial. One gastric mucosal tear was reported, and common patient complaints included pharyngeal pain, nausea, and vomiting in the early postoperative period.

e. Conclusions

The application of the Endocinch device to stomal reduction following RYGB has yielded positive results in a randomized, sham-controlled study. The improvement of obesity-associated hypertension and metabolic indices is an intriguing benefit of this technique, suggesting a robust physiologic effect. Long-term results are needed to confirm durability.

2. OverStitch

a. Introduction

The OverStitch device (Apollo Endosurgery, Austin, TX) is an FDA-approved endoscopic suturing system designed to create full-thickness plications in the GI tract. The device utilizes a curved needle and anchor exchange mounted on the end of the endoscope (Fig. 8.7). Multiple stitches may be placed without peroral device removal. It is currently being studied in a variety of applications directed toward repair of post-RYGB complications, including fistula closure, ulcer oversew, and stomal reduction.

b. Technique

The cap-based system is mounted on a dual-channel gastroscope. As with the Endocinch device, the procedure is performed under general anesthesia and the stomal mucosa is ablated with APC. A tissue anchor

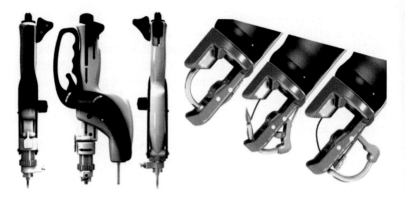

Fig. 8.7. OverStitch (Apollo Endosurgery, Austin, TX. Used with permission).

and suture are loaded into the system handle mounted on the working channel of the gastroscope and passed to the needle by squeezing the handle grip and plunging the handle.

Tissue is positioned between the curved needle and anchor exchange; a tissue grasper may be used to facilitate this step. The needle is then passed to the anchor exchange through the interposed tissue by squeezing the handle grip and plunging the system handle. After two bites of tissue are taken, the tissue anchor is released. A suture cinch is then passed down the handle and used to approximate the tissue and complete the stitch. Tension should be maintained on the free end of the suture to avoid looping and entrapment in the needle gears. Typically, at least two stitches are placed at the stoma, and additional stitches may be placed in the distal pouch for pouch reduction.

c. Outcomes

Pilot data has recently become available regarding feasibility and safety. Nine patients with a mean stomal diameter of 26 mm underwent outlet reduction in a mean procedure length of 36 min. An average of three stitches were placed, resulting in a reduction of stomal diameter of 71.8%. At 1 month, mean total body weight loss was 6.9%.

d. Complications

One case of self-limited bleeding was reported. Three patients suffered self-limited intolerance of liquids, one patient required balloon dilation, and one patient suffered persistent emesis and bleeding with endoscopy revealing torn stitches.

e. Conclusions

The OverStitch device represents an important advance in endoscopic suturing. A second-generation device is forthcoming, which boasts a more streamlined design, suture loading, and cinching. The use of the OverStitch for primary obesity therapy is currently being evaluated in animal models.

D. Endoscopic Plication

The endoscopic creation of tissue plications in the gastric pouch and along the stoma presents another mechanism through which pouch and stomal reduction may be achieved. Such procedures have utilized a variety of endoscopic devices and fasteners in the pursuit of durable plications and a low-procedural-risk profile.

1. Stomaphyx

a. Introduction

The use of endoscopically placed H-fasteners hold the promise of creating tissue plications for reduction of the gastric pouch and anastomotic diameter in a relatively simple procedure. The Stomaphyx device (EndoGastric Solutions, Redmond, WA) uses polypropylene T-fasteners, is FDA approved, and is currently being evaluated in the USA.

b. Technique

The device is passed transorally, with a gastroscope passed within the device. Tissue is aspirated into a tissue port on the side of the device, and a T-fastener is deployed, securing the tissue. The device may be reloaded and fired multiple times with a single transoral passage. Multiple fasteners are required for adequate pouch reduction.

c. Outcomes

The largest study to date evaluating the Stomaphyx device in the treatment of weight regain included 39 patients (BMI 39.8 kg/m^2) at a single center. The study suffered from poor follow-up, with a %EWL of 17% in 14 patients and 19.5% in 6 patients. A second smaller study reported an average procedure time of 50 min. A multicenter randomized, sham-controlled US study is underway.

d. Complications

No major complications occurred, with sore throat and abdominal pain the most common patient complaints.

e. Conclusions

The endoscopic placement of T-fasteners presents a minimally invasive option for the treatment of weight regain, with a short procedure length and low-risk profile. It is unclear whether such fasteners will provide comparable durability compared with transmural sutures, and given the advances in endoscopic suturing technology the placement of T-fasteners risks the possibility of obsolescence.

2. Incisionless Operating Platform

a. Introduction

The use of endoscopically delivered basket-type tissue anchors for transmural tissue plication may provide increased durability and avoid tissue pull-through due to the distribution of force over a greater surface area. USGI Medical (San Clemente, CA) has created such an endoscopic platform, the Incisionless Operating Platform (IOP), that includes the g-Prox tissue approximation device, g-Lix tissue grasper, and g-Cath tissue anchor delivery catheter (Fig. 8.8). The anchors are made of nitinol mesh connected by a braided polyester suture.

b. Technique

The platform is mounted on the working channel of the endoscope. The g-Prox device is advanced into the stomach and a bite of tissue is grasped between the jaws. The needle deployment tube is then advanced through the tissue, and the first tissue anchor is deployed. The needle is then withdrawn from the tissue, a second anchor delivered, and the suture is cinched and cut to complete the plication. Multiple plications can be placed around the stoma or in the pouch for volume reduction (Fig. 8.9).

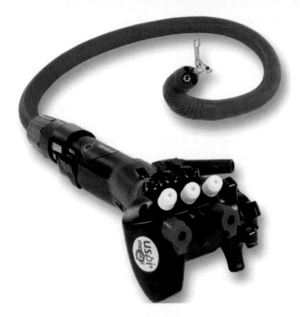

Fig. 8.8. Incisionless Operating Platform (IOP) (USGI Medical, San Clemente, CA. Used with permission).

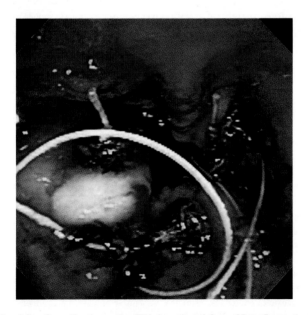

Fig. 8.9. After five plications, the GJA is reduced from 28 to 5 mm (reprinted with permission from Mullady DK, Lautz DB, Thompson CC. Treatment of weight regain after gastric bypass surgery when using a new endoscopic platform: initial experience and early outcomes. Gastrointest Endosc. 2009;70(3):440–4).

c. Outcomes

The Restorative Obesity Surgery Endoscopic (ROSE) trial is a multi-center US feasibility study with 6 months data on 116 patients recently published. Inclusion criteria included documented weight loss followed by weight regain after RYGB and a stomal diameter of at least 20 mm measured endoscopically. Anchors were successfully placed in 97% of patients in an average of 87 min. In 88 patients, weight gain ceased, and 96% of these patients experienced an average of 18% %EWL. Those who were most successful in postoperative weight loss benefited most from endoscopic revision, with a mean %EWL of 29%. Endoscopy at 12 months demonstrated intact anchor placement.

d. Complications

No major complications were reported in the trial. Adverse events were minimal, including abdominal pain and nausea.

e. Conclusions

The USGI device has demonstrated durable tissue anchor placement and short-term weight loss following weight regain after RYGB. The application of this device to primary obesity therapy is an intriguing concept that merits further study.

Selected References

Abu Dayyeh BK, Lautz DB, Thompson CC. Gastrojejunal stoma diameter predicts weight regain after Roux-en-Y gastric bypass. Clin Gastroenterol Hepatol. 2011;9:228–33.

Brethauer SA, Chand B, Schauer PR, Thompson CC. Transoral gastric volume reduction for weight management: technique and feasibility in 18 patients. Surg Obes Relat Dis. 2010;6:689–94.

Catalano MF, Rudic G, Anderson AJ, et al. Weight gain after bariatric surgery as a result of a large gastric stoma: Endotherapy with sodium morrhuate may prevent the need for surgical revision. Gastrointest Endosc. 2007;66:240–5.

Cote GA, Edmundowicz SA. Emerging technology: endoluminal treatment of obesity. Gastrointest Endosc. 2009;70:991–9.

De Jong K, Mathus-Vliegen EM, Veldhuyzen EA, et al. Short-term safety and efficacy of the trans-oral endoscopic restrictive implant system for the treatment of obesity. Gastrointest Endosc. 2010;72:497–504.

Deviere J, Ojeda Valdes G, Cuevas Herrera L, et al. Safety, feasibility and weight loss after transoral gastroplasty: First human multicenter study. Surg Endosc. 2008;22: 589–98.

Fogel R, De Fogel J, Bonilla Y, et al. Clinical experience of transoral suturing for an endoluminal vertical gastroplasty: 1-year follow-up in 64 patients. Gastrointest Endosc. 2008;68:51–8.

Gersin KS, Rothstein RI, Rosenthal RJ, et al. Open-label, sham-controlled trial of an endoscopic duodenojejunal bypass liner for preoperative weight loss in bariatric surgery candidates. Gastrointest Endosc. 2010;71:976–82.

Herron DM, Birkett DH, Thompson CC, et al. Gastric bypass pouch and stoma reduction using a transoral endoscopic anchor placement system: a feasibility study. Surg Endosc. 2008;22:1093–9.

Imaz I, Martinez-Cervell C, Garcia-Alvarez EE, et al. Safety and effectiveness of the intragastric balloonfor obesity. a meta-analysis. Obes Surg. 2008;18:841–6.

Loewen M, Barba C. Endoscopic sclerotherapy for dilated gastrojejunostomy of failed gastric bypass. Surg Obes Relat Dis. 2008;4:539–42.

Mikami D, Needleman B, Narula V, et al. Natural orifice surgery: initial US experience utilizing the stomaphyx device to reduce gastric pouches after Roux-en-Y gastric bypass. Surg Endosc. 2010;24:223–8.

Moreno C, Closset J, Dugardeyn S, et al. Transoral gastroplasty is safe, feasible, and induces significant weight loss in morbidly obese patients: results of the Second Human Pilot Study. Endoscopy. 2008;40:406–13.

Ramos AC, Zundel N, Neto MG, et al. Human hybrid notes transvaginal sleeve gastrectomy: initial experience. Surg Obes Relat Dis. 2008;5:660–3.

Ryou M, Mullady DK, Lautz DB, et al. Pilot study evaluating technical feasibility and early outcomes of second-generation endosurgical platform for treatment of weight regain after gastric bypass surgery. Surg Obes Relat Dis. 2009;5:450–4.

Schouten R, Rijs CS, Bouvy ND, Hameeteman W, et al. A multicenter, randomized efficacy study of the endobarrier gastrointestinal liner for presurgical weight loss prior to bariatric surgery. Ann Surg. 2010;251:236–43.

Spaulding L, Osler T, Patlak J. Longterm results of sclerotherapy for dilated gastrojejunostomy after gastric bypass. Surg Obes Relat Dis. 2007;3:623–6.

Thompson CC. Endoscopic therapy of obesity: a new paradigm in bariatric care. Gastrointest Endosc. 2010;77:505–7.

Thompson CC, Roslin MS, Chand B, et al. RESTORE: Randomized evaluation of endoscopic suturing transorally for anastomotic outlet reduction: a double-blind, sham-controlled multicenter study for treatment of inadequate weight loss or weight regain following Roux-en-Y gastric bypass. Gastroenterology. 2010;138:S-388.

Thompson CC, Slattery J, Bundga ME, et al. Peroral endoscopic reduction of dilated gastrojejunal anastomosis after Roux-en-Y gastric bypass: a possible new option for patients with weight regain. Surg Endosc. 2006;20:1744–8.

9. Single-Site Access Bariatric Surgery: Principles and Techniques

Julio A. Teixeira, M.D., F.A.C.S.
John N. Afthinos, M.D.

A. Single-Incision Laparoscopic Surgery Principles

Laparoendoscopic single-site (LESS) surgery is not a new concept. Navarra and others first described the technique in the late 1990s, but the concept never gained popularity. More recently, natural orifice transluminal endoscopic surgery (NOTES) arose out of the continued goal of less invasive approaches to surgery. Initial enthusiasm was tempered with caution as questions were raised with regards to the safety and durability of visceral access and closure methods. This led many investigators to revisit the concept of LESS and a resurgence of interest resulted. The instrumentation and technology used in LESS are more readily available and the approach has now gained considerable popularity. The potential benefits include less pain, faster recovery, better cosmesis, and fewer wound complications, but they have remained largely unconfirmed. Please see Vol. I, Chap. 7, for further discussion of LESS.

Operations that best lend themselves to the single incision approach are procedures that require a slightly larger incision for extraction of a bulky specimen or the implantation of a device. Certain bariatric procedures, such as the vertical sleeve gastrectomy (VSG) and laparoscopic adjustable gastric banding (LAGB), fit this profile. The LESS approach maximizes the use of these larger incisions. Concealing the singular incision within the umbilicus is particularly appealing to the bariatric patient population due to the increased awareness of body image and scarring. An additional potential benefit of LESS is the ability to maintain bariatric surgery as a personal matter, as there is significant associated social

N.T. Nguyen and C.E.H. Scott-Conner (eds.), *The SAGES Manual: Volume 2 Advanced Laparoscopy and Endoscopy*, DOI 10.1007/978-1-4614-2347-8_9, © Springer Science+Business Media, LLC 2012

stigma. The LESS approach can create significant challenges. In this chapter, we describe patient selection, instrumentation, and techniques to overcome these challenges.

1. Access Choices.
   a. Incision choices.
      i. Periumbilical technique.
         1. A semicircular incision is made along the rim of the umbilicus and dissection proceeds down to the level of the fascia.
         2. This allows maximal dissection and exposure of the fascia, accommodating virtually any approach or device; however, the cosmetic result may not be the most advantageous.
      ii. Transumbilical technique.
         1. An incision is made through the base of the umbilicus. The skin edges are grasped with heavy-toothed forceps, elevated anteriorly, and the skin is detached from its posterior attachments using a scalpel.
         2. This may have a better cosmetic result, but may not be the most ideal incision for LESS gastric banding.
   b. Single-access device, single fascial incision.
         1. The larger fascial incision needed to accommodate a prefabricated device is well suited for bariatric procedures as a larger fascial incision is needed to accommodate the placement of an adjustable gastric band or the extraction of a sleeve gastrectomy specimen.
         2. After the incision is made, blunt dissection proceeds down to the level of the umbilical stalk. It is grasped by a Kocher clamp, elevated anteroinferiorly, and the fascia is cleared of subcutaneous tissue in a cephalad direction. The midline fascia 1.5 cm cephalad is also grasped and the resulting tissue ridge is incised vertically. Alternatively, the native umbilical defect can be found, and the fascia incised centered on this.

3. The peritoneum is grasped between two clamps and incised sharply, verifying peritoneal access.

c. Multiple access devices, multiple fascial incisions.

1. This approach requires a larger fascial area to be cleared of subcutaneous tissue to accommodate the placement of multiple trocars through the same skin incision.

2. An area of fascia, cephalad to the umbilicus, large enough to accommodate up to four trocars is cleared of subcutaneous tissue and a Veress needle is used to insufflate the peritoneal cavity.

3. A clear-tipped dilating trocar is advanced into the peritoneal cavity using a laparoscope for direct vision.

4. A total of three or four low-profile ports are then introduced through separate fascial punctures.

2. Port Devices.

a. The SILS™ port (Covidien, Norwalk, CT) is a soft pliable port which can accommodate three 5-mm low-profile trocars, one of which can be exchanged for a 12- or 15-mm trocar. It also has built-in insufflation tubing. The port can be inserted in a fascial opening of no more than 2 cm.

b. The Olympus TriPort™ or QuadPort™ (Olympus, Center Valley, PA) can accommodate three or four instruments through its ports. Each prefabricated elastic port has a gel valve to create a seal with instruments and can accommodate different size instruments. The port itself can fit 1.5- to 2.5-cm incision lengths and abdominal wall thicknesses of up to 10 cm.

c. The GelPoint™ access platform (Applied Medical, Rancho Santa Margarita, CA) consists of a wound protector, a GelSeal™ cap, and access trocars designed to prevent slippage through the cap. This creates a pseudo-abdomen above the level of the fascia which allows for more room between instruments externally. This accommodates slightly larger incisions and is placed in the manner of a hand-assist device.

d. Alternatively, a group of three to four low-profile ports can be placed in a fascial area that has been cleared of subcutaneous tissue.

> e. Other improvised devices have been described using sterile gloves and standard laparoscopic trocars.

3. Visualization—Several Alternatives Exist, and Each Has Advantages and Disadvantages.

> a. A 50 cm long, 5 mm telescope with right-angle light cable prism (Karl Storz, El Segundo, CA): This instrument experiences a degree of light loss due to the angled light cable prism and, as a result, the image is small and can be somewhat dim. The length is helpful for maintaining the camera head and assistant's hand out of the working area.
>
> b. A flexible tip 5 mm laparoscopic camera (LTF-VP, Olympus): This is perhaps the most ideal instrument as it permits the camera holder to have his/her hand on the drapes and away from the external working cylinder. The image quality is excellent and the mobile tip permits the surgeon to look from virtually any angle.
>
> c. A standard 5-mm laparoscope can be used and the image quality is very good; however, this is least desirable because the camera head and assistant's hand will occupy the same space in the external working cylinder as the other instruments, making the ergonomics more challenging.

4. Instrumentation.

> a. The goal is to choose instruments with low profiles to minimize external collisions within the external working cylinder.
>
> > i. Regular and/or bariatric length laparoscopic instruments are the easiest and probably the cheapest to obtain.
> >
> > > 1. They can be disposable or nondisposable.
> > > 2. If nondisposable, they should have small rotating wheels and, in most instances, a non-ratcheted handle so as to have the lowest possible profile.
> >
> > ii. Flexible-tip graspers.
> >
> > > 1. One type is a roticulating grasper whose instrument tip flexes and locks into that position (Covidien). Although the instrument flexes, it cannot do so in a dynamic fashion.
> > > 2. Another type is a grasper which is truly flexible in a dynamic fashion (Cambridge Endoscopic Devices, Framingham, MA). As the surgeon

   moves his/her wrist, the tip responds to that movement.

   3. The ability to angle the grasper tip enables the recreation of working angles that are achieved in multiport laparoscopy.

  iii. Laparoscopic instruments which are made with a preformed curvature instead of a straight shaft (Olympus): These instruments would function along the same lines as flexible-tip graspers; however, the preformed curve may limit the working angles that can be achieved.

5. Accessory Instruments and Tools.

  a. LESS is often challenged by the lack of a second assistant to provide appropriate exposure. Accessory tools and instruments can be used to minimize abdominal wall trauma while maximizing exposure.

  b. Microlaparoscopic instruments can be introduced transabdominally and used as retraction adjuncts without having to use additional trocars. The nick in the skin can be closed with liquid skin adhesive.

  c. A Carter-Thomason fascial closure needle can be used as a grasping device to provide retraction from a small accessory incision.

  d. Percutaneous sutures can be placed to provide intracorporeal retraction without occupying a trocar.

  e. Intracorporeally placed sutures can provide the surgeon with static retraction, again without occupying a trocar.

  f. Extracorporeal sutures can be used to provide dynamic retraction, but must pass through a trocar.

  g. Penrose drain can be employed as retraction adjuncts, as can red rubber catheters and other drain tubing.

6. General Ergonomic Considerations.

  a. Due to the position of the port and angle needed to reach the stomach or gastroesophageal junction, the operating room table may need to be in a slightly different reverse Trendelenburg angle than usual.

  b. The use of a flexible-tip laparoscope in combination with other instruments is perhaps the most advantageous approach. It enables the camera head and assistant's hand to be resting on the drapes, allowing the surgeon to make full use of the working cylinder.

    c.   Staggering instrument lengths reduce crowding in the external working cylinder by keeping the bulkiest parts of the instruments at different distances from the trocar.

        i.   For example, one could use the extra-long bariatric 5-mm laparoscope, a bariatric-length instrument, and a regular-length instrument to maintain the handles at different distances and maintain maximal working space around the surgeon's and assistant's hands.

7.   Liver Retraction.

    a.   Liver retractors can be placed either through a multiport device, adjacent to such a device, but within the same skin incision or away from the central access incision altogether.

        i.   Through a port device:

            1.   A self-retaining liver retractor can be placed through a trocar in a multiport device, but this can limit the versatility of the access platform.

        ii.   Adjacent to a port device:

            1.   Alternatively, the retractor can be placed through a separate trocar adjacent to the multiport access device. Although there is a separate fascial puncture, it spares a trocar.

        iii.   Through an accessory incision:

            1.   A 5-mm subxiphoid skin incision can be made and a Nathanson liver retractor can be inserted.

            2.   Sutures can be passed through the access device and then retrieved transabdominally.

    b.   A self-retaining liver retractor does not need to be used in every procedure and should be determined on a case-by-case basis. Furthermore, it may not even be required for the entire procedure.

        i.   There are instances when the use of the liver retractor may help for a certain part of the procedure and actually hinder in another. Its effectiveness needs to be continually reassessed with every step and if it is not helping, removing it may actually permit improved exposure.

        ii.   If a self-retaining liver retractor is used, the attachment holding the instrument to the bed rail should be placed on the patient's left side and the arm should extend relatively parallel to the ground across to meet the retractor itself. Placement on the patient's right side will interfere with the working space and will also not properly retract the liver.

c. Other methods of liver retraction have been described using combinations of sutures, Penrose drains, red rubber catheters, and other improvised devices. These can be used without occupying a port or placed through a separate nick in the skin. Any of these are probably acceptable, depending on the familiarity of the surgeon.

d. When a self-retaining liver retractor is not used, flexible instruments can be used as to retract the liver while simultaneously grasping. An example of this is the use of a flexible grasper to retract the greater curvature of the stomach during a sleeve gastrectomy. While this is being done, the bent shaft of the instrument or the stomach itself can be used to retract the liver and provide adequate exposure while the short gastric vessels are ligated.

8. Operative Strategies and Techniques.

a. The basic surgical principles of traction-countertraction and retraction are accomplished with in-line movements, in a coaxial direction with respect to the instruments.

   i. Lateral traction and countertraction require instruments to cross over each other in order to re-establish the triangulation of a multiport laparoscopic procedure.

b. In the very beginning of the procedure, it is imperative to establish the working relationships among the instruments contained within the imaginary surgical cylinder in order to maximize ergonomics (see Fig. 9.1). If the initial relationship does not afford maximal range of motion, then the relationship should be reevaluated. This will often require instruments to be moved to different ports.

   i. This reevaluation should be done at every step of the procedure.

c. Each movement must be minimal, calculated, and efficient.

d. Resistance and external collisions of the instruments and the camera should be resolved by pulling the camera back until the resistance is released. The camera can then be advanced forward through a new path to allow better

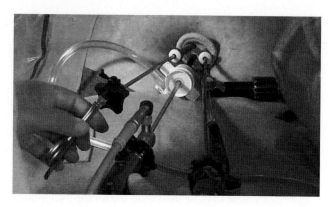

Fig. 9.1. External view of instrument configuration during LESS surgery.

mobility of the instruments. If resistance cannot be resolved, then this should prompt a reevaluation of the instrument relationships.

e. Intracorporeal suturing is most efficiently performed by grasping and positioning the needle with a one-handed technique. To avoid this problem, the Endostitch™ (Covidien) could be used, but this necessitates the placement of a 12-mm trocar.

f. Knot tying is most easily and efficiently accomplished extracorporeally; however, intracorporeal tying can certainly be performed.

9. Special Cautions.

a. Electrocautery.

i. Extreme care should be exercised when this energy source is used in LESS. The active tip is in very close proximity to metal instruments and the possibility of arcing current and causing injury is increased.

b. Air leaks.

i. Continuous leakage of pneumoperitoneum can occur through the instruments themselves, trocars, or a poor seal with the access device against the fascia. The danger here is that a sudden drop or loss of pneumoperitoneum will degrade exposure and lead to an injury.

        ii.   The surgeon must remain aware of changes in pneumoperitoneum and make adjustments accordingly.

            1. If leakage cannot be mitigated, the pressure can be increased.

    c.   Exposure.

        i.   If exposure degrades at any point during a LESS procedure, it must be remedied to avoid morbidity. If it cannot be remedied, then conversion to a multiport laparoscopic procedure should be considered.

        ii.   Pneumoperitoneum can be increased to increase the working space.

        iii.   Accessory tools can be employed as retraction adjuncts to enhance exposure.

10.   Patient Preparation.

        i.   As in all bariatric surgery candidates, patients must undergo a detailed multidisciplinary evaluation in the preoperative period. They must fit the criteria set in the NIH guidelines (see Chap. 1).

        ii.   A detailed history and physical are mandatory, with particular attention paid to symptoms or signs of gastroesophageal reflux or dysphagia.

        iii.   Nutritional and psychological evaluations also assist in evaluating patients for potentially detrimental binging or purging behaviors, eating disorders, or potentially serious psychiatric disorders, such as severe depression, psychoses, and bipolar disorders.

        iv.   Routine chest X-ray and liver ultrasound are performed as part of the workup to evaluate liver size. If the liver is beyond 20 cm, patients are required to begin a high-protein diet to reduce the liver size preoperatively.

        v.   The patients are instructed to be on clear liquids diet for at least 48 h and to take a bottle of magnesium citrate or other bowel preparation the night before.

        vi.   Routine upper endoscopy should be considered for patients considering sleeve gastrectomy, particularly if they have symptoms of reflux, history of peptic ulcer disease, or gastric tumors.

11. Contraindications to single-incision laparoscopic bariatric surgery: These are relative and they may prove to be more or less important based on the level of experience.
    a. Males.
    b. Central obesity.
    c. Presence of hiatal hernia.
    d. Prior abdominal surgery.
        i. Diaphragmatic hernia repair.
        ii. Umbilical hernia repair with mesh.
        iii. History of open abdomen closed with biologic mesh.
    e. Umbilical hernia.
    f. Enlarged liver (greater than 20 cm in greatest dimension).
    g. Prior splenectomy.
12. Patient Position and Room Setup.
    a. Place the patient supine on the operating room table with the arms out.
        i. The modified lithotomy position can also be used for LESS bariatric surgery.
    b. The surgeon can stand at either side of the patient with the assistant on the opposite side.
    c. Place the monitors at the head of the bed and close to the operating room table, as in a laparoscopic cholecystectomy.
    d. Patients receive 5,000 U of subcutaneous heparin, sequential compression devices, and a dose of prophylactic antibiotics before the procedure begins.

B. Single-Incision Laparoscopic-Adjustable Gastric Banding

1. Criteria for qualification are the same as the NIH criteria. Recently, the FDA has approved the use of the band in patients whose body mass index (BMI) is greater than 35 kg/m^2 or greater than 30 kg/m^2 with one comorbidity.
2. The ideal characteristics of a patient who would tend to benefit the most from the single incision approach include younger female patients, perhaps even teenagers, who have no prior abdominal surgical history and have low BMI.
3. Single-incision laparoscopic-adjustable gastric banding technique.

    i.   Create an umbilical as described above. We prefer the vertical approach when feasible, but this can be difficult in a very deep umbilicus.

    ii.   Once the fascia is opened and access to the peritoneal cavity is secured, use an army-navy retractor to elevate the abdominal wall at the 1 o'clock position. Pass the gastric band, which has been prepared in the usual manner, entirely into the left upper quadrant with a laparoscopic grasper.

        1.   This maneuver avoids having to upsize one of the 5-mm trocar sleeves to a 15-mm trocar sleeve. This decreases operative time and cost.

    iii.   At this time, introduce the SILS™ port into the opening using a large Kelly clamp.

        1.   Once secure, pass the accompanying trocars into their preformed slots and insufflate the abdomen to 15 mmHg.

        2.   Rotate the port such that the insufflation tubing exits at the 4 o'clock position.

    iv.   Use a 5-mm laparoscope to inspect the abdomen before beginning any portion of the procedure.

    v.   Place a fourth 5-mm trocar within the left lower quadrant of the incision, outside of the SILS™ port.

1.   Pass a self-retaining liver retractor through this trocar, and expose the gastroesophageal junction. Ensure that the attachment affixing this retractor to the operating room table rail is on the left side to avoid crossing in front of the working cylinder.

    a.   Inspect the diaphragmatic hiatus for the presence of a hiatal hernia. At this time, if there is one present, the surgeon may opt to convert to a multiport procedure, depending on his/her level of comfort with the LESS approach.

        i.   In our experience, we have been able to reproducibly repair small-to-moderate Type I sliding hernias with a formal posterior approximation of the crura using permanent suture. Larger hernias typically prompt us to convert to a multiport procedure.

    b.   Bluntly dissect the gastroesophageal junction and angle of His using rigid fenestrated laparoscopic graspers.

    c.   Direct attention to the pars flaccida approach of the gastrohepatic ligament, and incise it with hook electrocautery. Take care to avoid injuring a replaced or accessory left

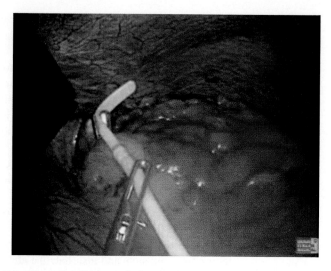

Fig. 9.2. The adjustable gastric band tubing is being passed to the flexible grasper, which is traversing posterior to the stomach.

hepatic artery and arcing to any nearby instruments or liver retractor.

d. Identify the right arm of the right crus and open the perito-neum anterior to the inferiormost portion of the crus.

   i.   Pass the left grasper bluntly through this plane, stay-ing anterior and exiting through the site of the prior dissection on the left side. Accomplish this maneuver with the absolute minimum of dissection to maintain a low rate of posterior slippage.

   ii. This grasper can be a rigid fenestrated or flexible-tip laparoscopic grasper.

e. Pass the tip of the gastric band to this grasper and pass the band around the stomach (see Fig. 9.2).

   i.   Do not completely fasten the band unless it is very loose. Extract the tip from the right-upper trocar site in the SILS™ port. Replace the trocar, pinning the tubing against the channel of the SILS™ port. This is used to retract the band inferiorly while sutures are placed.

   ii. Place gastro-gastric sutures of full-length 2–0 polyes-ter to create an adequate pouch. Knots are most effi-ciently tied using the extracorporeal technique.

    f.   After the last suture is placed, fasten the band and rotate it as usual.

    g.   Remove the self-retaining liver retractor and the insufflation, trocars, and SILS™ port.

    h.   Use a short right-angle clamp to puncture the fascia 1 cm cephalad from the superior apex of the original fascial incision. Bring the band tubing out through this to avoid kinking and entrapment in the fascial closure.

    i.   Close the fascia with a running #0 absorbable suture.

    j.   Create a subcutaneous pocket adjacent to the fascial incision to accommodate the port. Dissection proceeds in the usual manner until the anterior fascia is clearly visible. Connect the port to the tubing and anchor the port to fascia with four 2–0 polypropylene sutures.

    k.   Close the incision in layers with absorbable suture and apply a sterile dressing.

    l.   The band may be adjusted at the time of operation, depending on surgeon preference.

4.   Technical considerations.

    a.   Liver retraction.

        i.   We usually employ a self-retaining liver retractor to enable visualization of the gastroesophageal junction. It is important to ensure that a preoperative ultrasound is obtained to measure the liver. Any dimension greater than 20 cm should prompt the bariatric nutritionist to place the patient on a high-protein diet to decrease the size, 1 month prior to surgery.

5.   Complications.

    a.   Slippage.

        i.   The band can slip out of position. If there is no gastric wall compromise, it can be repositioned; however, the likelihood of recurrence is higher once repositioning has been attempted.

        ii.   Anterior slippage (1.5–2.2%) with consequent gastric wall herniation can occur early if there is severe vomiting or inadequate fixation. If this occurs, immediate deflation of the band and laparoscopic exploration should be performed.

        iii.   Posterior slippage with consequent gastric wall herniation was once high (~20%) with the perigastric technique. With the pars flaccida technique now being the most common, the slippage rate is very low (2.5%). The same course of action is needed as in anterior slippage.

b. Band erosion.

    i. The band can, in rare cases, erode through the stomach (1.5%). This is frequently present with dysphagia and PO intolerance or with a port-site infection as infection tracks along the tubing from the site of the leak.

    ii. This complication is diagnosed best by endoscopy, though contrast esophagography may also demonstrate it.

    iii. If the erosion is chronic depending on the patient's hemodynamics, clinical status, and ability to eat, it may be managed expectantly. If the patient is not absolutely asymptomatic, afebrile with a normal white blood cell count, and then exploration is warranted, with removal of the eroded band, repair of the perforation, wide drainage, antibiotics, and enteral feeding access.

c. Port dysfunction (0.5–7%).

    i. This includes flipping and angulation of the port. This can occur from improperly placed sutures at the first operation or a subclinical infection which allowed the sutures to pull through the fascia. The port becomes increasingly difficult to access percutaneously, even under fluoroscopic guidance and can eventually require revision.

d. Tubing breakage (0.5–2%).

    i. The tube can break or fracture. Symptoms can include focal abdominal pain due to irritation of the peritoneum. Radiography may demonstrate the free tubing lying within the pelvis on the side of the pain reported by the patient. This requires laparoscopic exploration, inspection of the tubing, and reattachment to the port in a different subcutaneous site. The tubing position, once it exits the port, should have a gentle curve to prevent fracture.

e. Port-site infection and erosion (0.4–4%).

    i. Rarely, the site of port placement can become infected, requiring removal of the port and replacement at another operation once the wound is healed and the infection has resolved.

1. If an infection is seen at the port site late, band erosion must be ruled out by endoscopy.
2. The port can erode through the skin, particularly if the patients' belt line sits right on the port. It is important to note where the patients place their belt preoperatively and site the port above this area to avoid this postoperative issue.

f. Electrocautery injury.

   i. The surgeon should use increased caution when electrocautery is being used during a LESS procedure. The electrocautery tip is now in greater proximity to metal instruments and arcing is more of a concern.

g. Visceral and vascular injuries.

   i. Vascular injuries are rare occurrences and most require conversion to multiport laparoscopic or open procedure to control or repair.

   ii. Perforation of the gastroesophageal junction is a rare and potentially life-threatening injury and one with a protracted recovery time due to the watershed blood supply in the area and the difficulty in diverting the food/saliva stream.

      1. This requires conversion to a multiport laparoscopic, if not open, procedure to address the injury.

h. Incisional hernia

   i. The incidence of incisional hernia is at this point unknown. Most studies show a very low incidence. This is not isolated to LESS procedures only, as it has been reported in multiport laparoscopic-adjustable gastric banding.

C. Single-Incision Vertical Sleeve Gastrectomy

1. Criteria for performing a sleeve gastrectomy are the same as for any other bariatric procedure. This procedure is particularly well suited to patients who have certain comorbidities who otherwise would not be candidates for Roux-en-Y gastric bypass. Some examples are patients with HIV on HAART therapy,

significant abdominal surgical history, or chronic hepatitis B or C infection.

2. Single-Site Vertical Sleeve Gastrectomy Technique.

    i. Gain access as described above with an incision at the umbilicus. Once access is assured, place the SILS™ port in position and insufflate the abdomen.

    ii. Ideally, a flexible-tip laparoscope is used to evaluate the peritoneal cavity before the procedure is begun. Place the camera in the trocar at the 2 o'clock position.

        1. This allows the instruments to have a better vertical working room, as these are the movements required to perform the first portion of the procedure.

    iii. Evaluate the liver and decide whether or not a self-retaining liver retractor will be needed. If the greater curvature of the stomach is visible and the lobe is relatively thin, then a retractor may not be necessary.

        1. If one is to be placed, it is placed as in the LESS lap band approach with the bed-rail attachment on the patient's left side.

    iv. Identify the pylorus by the vein of Mayo and measure a distance of 4 cm proximal to that along the greater curvature. It is at this distance, where we begin our division of the greater omentum.

        1. Here, a flexible-tip laparoscopic grasper is ideal, but not necessary. Use the grasper to retract the greater curvature of the stomach anteriorly to begin the dissection of the greater omentum.

        2. We prefer the use of the LigaSure™ Advance (Covidien) in this situation. It provides a surer grip on the tissue being ligated, though the Harmonic Scalpel™ (Ethicon) performs well, also.

    v. The dissection proceeds along the greater curvature until the short gastric vessels are reached (see Fig. 9.3). Divide these until the left crus is seen. Take care to avoid injuring the spleen.

    vi. Use the bent shaft of the grasper as a liver retractor. The use of a liver retractor can be avoided if the greater curvature can be seen under the unretracted liver and the liver is relatively thin.

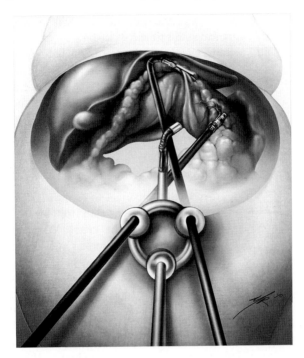

Fig. 9.3. Position of instruments and camera during division of short gastric vessels (reused with permission from Marie Rossettie, Continuum Health Partners).

1. As our experience has grown, we have found that most cases can be performed without a liver retractor.

2. When approaching the area containing the short gastric vessels, the shaft must be retracting the stomach anteromedially to hold the liver edge anteriorly and the greater curvature anteromedially. This allows for triangulation between the energy source and the grasper to be recreated. This is an important relationship to reestablish using the LESS technique in this portion of the procedure as uncompromised visibility and proper traction-countertraction allow for safe dissection and ligation of the short gastric vessels.

vii. Once the left crus is reached, the greater curvature of the stomach is then rotated medially to expose the posterior gastric wall. Any posterior attachments are divided at this time.

viii. At this juncture of the procedure, have the anesthesiologist remove the orogastric tube and advance a 32 Fr. Bougie under direct vision. Place an instrument flat on the stomach near the lesser curvature to guide the bougie and visualize its passage toward the beginning of the greater omentum dissection.

1. Lifting the greater curvature of the stomach anteriorly again reveals the position of the bougie tip.

2. It is vitally important to follow the path of the bougie as it is inserted to prevent it from positioning along the greater curvature of the stomach. This is dangerous as it could lead to transection of the bougie.

3. Alternatively, a gastroscope can be used as a bougie, with the added advantage of visualization of the staple line for integrity and hemostasis.

ix. The next step is to remove the camera from the 2 o'clock trocar and place it at the 5 o'clock position. Dilate the trocar at the 10 o'clock position up to a 15-mm trocar. To do this, place a lubricated 12-mm trocar in the 5-mm trocar slot and then exchange it for a 15-mm trocar with a reducer cap. This allows for the use of the linear cutting stapler.

1. The switch in instrument positions now allows for horizontal freedom of movement, which is essential to perform the stapling portion of the procedure.

x. We prefer a 60-mm linear cutting stapler with absorbable buttress material (EndoGIA Duet™, Covidien).

xi. Use green loads for the first two applications in order to accommodate the thicker antral tissue. Use blue cartridges for the subsequent applications to accommodate thinner tissue.

1. Reevaluate the position of the bougie before stapling begins.

2. Use the instrument through the lower trocar of the LESS port to provide traction on the stomach as the staple is fired.

xii. When the incisura angularis is reached, make a deliberate adjustment in the stapling line to avoid creating an obstruction. The staple line should be parallel to the lesser curvature at all points.

    1. It is imperative that a flat, planar staple line is created.

xiii. Once stapling is complete, check the integrity of the staple line and hemostasis. Any bleeding points along the staple line can be sutured, but large clips are usually sufficient. We do not routinely oversew the staple line.

xiv. Exchange the bougie for an orogastric tube and perform an air leak test.

    1. If there is any concern for the staple line or pouch shape, perform an intraoperative endoscopy to evaluate the internal anatomy. This can also visualize the level of hemostasis and reduce the risk of staple line dehiscence by the passage of the stiff orogastric tube.

xv. Place the specimen in a specimen bag. Remove the instruments, port, insufflation, and specimen bag. Close the fascia with #0 absorbable suture, typically in interrupted fashion. Close the subcutaneous tissue in layers and apply a sterile dressing.

3. Variations in technique.

   a. Energy sources.

      i. Different energy sources can be used to ligate the short gastric vessels, depending on preference:

        1. Harmonic scalpel™ (Ethicon).

        2. LigaSure™ (Covidien).

   b. Two techniques have been described.

      i. Division of the short gastric vessels is performed first and then the pouch is formed. This technique lends itself to the LESS approach due to the inherent limited exposure.

     ii. Alternatively, the pouch can be formed first with subsequent division of the short gastric vessels.

   c. Staple cartridge choices.

      i. Stapler cartridges can come with a buttressing material or without. Buttress materials decrease the bleeding rate, but do not affect the leak rate.

d. Oversewing of staple lines.
   i. This is also a major area of variation among surgeons. Some prefer to oversew their staple lines completely, some oversew where staple lines intersect, and others not at all. Oversewing may decrease bleeding if no buttress material is used in the stapler cartridges.

e. Bougie size.
   i. Considerable differences exist over which bougie size is used. There is no study that has yet demonstrated, in the long term, superiority of results of one size over another. One study showed that by 18 months post sleeve gastrectomy the weight loss was equivalent, though in the initial months of follow-up there was a greater degree of weight loss with a smaller bougie size.

f. Distance to pylorus.
   i. Reports in the literature vary widely on the distance used. Some authors staple right up to the pylorus, removing a significant portion of antrum. There is no convincing data on what distance should be used.

4. Complications.
   a. There have been no studies demonstrating that complications are higher with the LESS approach. In fact, most have reported a very low rate of complications.
   b. Bleeding (~1%) can arise from an ineffectively ligated short gastric vessel, staple line, or spleen.
   c. Leaks (~2%).
      i. Leaks are commonly found at the gastroesophageal junction. The mechanism is unclear, but some authors suggest that it may be related to ischemia.
         1. Leaks are usually managed with reoperation, repair of the leak, wide drainage, and placement of a distal feeding tube. The recovery time for a high leak can be very protracted and enteral access is a must.
         2. In very select stable patients, stenting is a possibility. The stents employed for this task are designed for palliating esophageal cancer. They tend not to seat well and can migrate distally.

        ii.   Lower leaks behave more like typical staple line leaks. They are still overall problematic given the pouch size constraints and inability to enterally feed the patient during healing.

  d.   Splenic injury (0.1%).

        i.   This rate increases if there is a history of prior surgery in the area. Meticulous care should be taken in the region of the spleen. If prior surgery or an intimate anatomic relationship with the stomach exists, one should strongly consider conversion to a multiport procedure.

        ii.   If the spleen is injured apart from a superficial capsular tear, a splenectomy should be performed, as the bariatric patient population does not physiologically tolerate surgical stress very well.

  e.   Incisional hernia—It is unknown what the true rate of incisional hernia is. It is a known entity in multiport sleeve gastrectomy and multiport laparoscopic-adjustable gastric banding.

  f.   Gastroesophageal reflux (GER) appears to worsen in observational studies, but the degree to which this occurs is unknown.

Selected References

Gagner M, et al. The second international consensus summit for sleeve gastrectomy, March 19–21, 2009. Surg Obes Relat Dis. 2009;5(4):476–85.

Navarra G, et al. One-wound laparoscopic cholecystectomy. Br J Surg. 1997;84(5):695.

Saber AA, El-Ghazaly ET, Dewoolkar AV, Slayton SA. Single-incision laparoscopic sleeve gastrectomy versus conventional multiport laparoscopic sleeve gastrectomy: technical considerations and strategic modifications. Surg Obes Relat Dis. 2010;6(6): 658–64.

Shi X, et al. A review of laparoscopic sleeve gastrectomy for morbid obesity. Obes Surg. 2010;20:1171–7.

Stroh C, et al. Fourteen-year long-term results after gastric banding. J Obes. 2011 (in press). doi:10.1155/2011/128451.

Teixeira J, McGill K, Koshy N, McGinty J, Todd G. Laparoscopic single-site surgery for placement of adjustable gastric band-a series of 22 cases. Surg Obes Relat Dis. 2010; 6:41–5.

Part II
Benign and Malignant Esophageal Disease

10. Laparoscopic Treatment of Gastroesophageal Reflux Disease and Associated Sliding Hiatal Hernia

Jeffrey H. Peters, M.D., F.A.C.S.

A. Indications and Preoperative Evaluation

1. Laparoscopic Fundoplication

Laparoscopic fundoplication is indicated for the treatment of objectively documented, relatively severe gastroesophageal reflux disease (GERD). Prior to consideration of antireflux surgery, most patients will have been treated with proton pump inhibitors (PPIs) for years, and most will have persistent symptoms despite PPI therapy. Neither, however, is absolutely necessary prior to consideration of surgery. Guidelines published by the American Gastroenterology Association recommend "antireflux surgery for patients with an esophageal GERD syndrome with persistent troublesome symptoms, especially regurgitation, despite PPI therapy." Careful patient selection and preoperative evaluation are essential for good results. Patients with gastroesophageal reflux and any of the following may be considered candidates for the procedure:

 a. Esophageal complications, such as erosive esophagitis, stricture, and/or Barrett's esophagus

 b. Respiratory complications, such as recurrent pneumonia or bronchiectasis

 c. Dependence upon PPIs for relief of symptoms, particularly if dose escalation is required, and in the young

 d. Cough, hoarseness, and respiratory symptoms with a good response to PPI therapy

N.T. Nguyen and C.E.H. Scott-Conner (eds.), *The SAGES Manual: Volume 2*   151
Advanced Laparoscopy and Endoscopy, DOI 10.1007/978-1-4614-2347-8_10,
© Springer Science+Business Media, LLC 2012

2. The Common Therapeutic Approach

The common therapeutic approach to patients presenting for the first time with symptoms suggestive of gastroesophageal reflux includes an initial trial of PPI therapy. Many patients will already have sought relief with readily available over-the-counter agents, modified their diets and altered behavior (such as not eating immediately before bedtime).

a. **Failure of PPIs** to control heartburn, suggests either that the diagnosis is incorrect or that the patient has severe disease. Regurgitating and respiratory symptoms often respond poorly to PPI therapy even when caused by GERD.

b. **Endoscopic examination** at this stage of evaluation provides the opportunity for assessing the severity of mucosal damage and the presence of Barrett's esophagus (see Part II, Chapters on indications for upper gastrointestinal endoscopy).

3. Appropriate Preoperative Evaluation

Appropriate preoperative evaluation should then be undertaken. **The diagnostic approach** to patients suspected of having GERD and being considered for antireflux surgery has three important goals (Table 10.1).

Symptoms thought to be indicative of gastroesophageal reflux disease, including heartburn or acid regurgitation, are very common in the general population and should not be used alone to guide therapeutic decisions, particularly when one is considering antireflux surgery. These symptoms, even when excessive, are not specific for gastroesophageal reflux and can be caused by other diseases (such as achalasia, diffuse spasm, esophageal carcinoma, pyloric stenosis, cholelithiasis, gastritis, gastric or duodenal ulcer, and coronary artery disease).

Table 10.1. Goals of diagnostic evaluation for possible antireflux surgery.

- To determine that gastroesophageal reflux is the underlying cause of the patient's symptoms
- To evaluate the status of esophageal body, and occasionally gastric function
- To determine the presence or absence of esophageal shortening
- To exclude alternate diagnoses especially named esophageal motility disorders

The most precise approach to define GERD is to measure the basic pathophysiologic abnormality of the disease, that is, increased exposure of the esophagus to gastric juice. Preoperative evaluation consists of the following:

a. **24-h pH monitoring**, to confirm the presence of significant GERD and assess the degree and pattern of esophageal exposure to gastric juice. A positive 24-h pH study is the single most important predictor of a successful surgical outcome.

b. **Manometric examination** of the lower esophageal sphincter and esophageal body. This excludes named esophageal motility disorders, such as achalasia, as the cause of the patient's symptoms and provides insight into the reasons for reflux (i.e., sphincter incompetence) as well as the function of the esophageal body.

c. **Assessment of the type and size of hiatal hernia and complications including strictures.** Repetitive injury causes scarring and fibrosis (stricture) which results in anatomic shortening of the esophagus. This compromises the ability to do an adequate repair without tension and may lead to an increased incidence of breakdown or thoracic displacement of the repair.

   i. Esophageal length is best assessed using video roentgenographic contrast studies and endoscopic findings.

   ii. Endoscopically, hernia size is measured as the difference between the diaphragmatic crura, identified by having the patient sniff, and the gastroesophageal junction, identified as the upper extent of the gastric rugal folds. Concern for esophageal shortening should be raised if there is a large (>5 cm) hiatal hernia, particularly in the presence of an esophageal stricture.

   iii. **Selection of a partial versus complete fundoplication**, is based upon on an assessment of esophageal contractility and length. Laparoscopic fundoplication is used in the majority of patients unless a very large (>5–6 cm) hiatal hernia or intrathoracic stomach is present, in which case an open approach may be reasonable. Recent data would suggest that in the absence of a named motility disorder, such as achalasia or scleroderma, most patients with reflux disease will tolerate a properly constructed 360-degree Nissen fundoplication without an increased incidence of dysphagia.

B. Patient Positioning and Room Setup

1. Position the patient supine, in a split leg or modified lithotomy position. In the lithotomy position, it is important that the knees be only slightly flexed, to avoid limiting mobility of the surgeon and the instruments (Fig. 10.1).
2. The surgeon stands between the legs and works with both hands. This allows the right- and left-handed instruments to approach the hiatus from the respective upper abdominal quadrants.
3. Use 30–45% reverse Trendelenburg to displace the transverse colon and small bowel inferiorly, keeping them from obstructing the view of the video camera.

C. Trocar Position and Principles of Exposure

1. Five 10-mm ports are utilized (Fig. 10.2); 5-mm ports may be substituted in the subxiphoid and right subcostal access sites.
2. **Place the camera** above the umbilicus, one third of the distance to the xiphoid process. In most patients, if the camera is placed in the umbilicus, it will be too low to allow adequate visualization of the hiatal structures once dissected. A transrectus location is preferable to midline to minimize the prevalence of port site hernia formation. An open Hasson technique works well. Access starts with a 1 in. vertical incision carried down to the anterior rectus fascia which is incised with electrocautery. The rectus muscle split with s-retractors and the posterior rectus fascia incised carefully with electrocautery. The abdomen can then be opened under direct vision.
3. **Place two lateral retracting ports** in the right and left anterior axillary lines, respectively. Position the trocar for the liver retractor in the right midclavicular line, at or slightly below the camera port. This allows the proper angle toward the left lateral segment of the liver and thus the ability to push the instrument toward the operating table, lifting the liver. Place the second retraction port at the level of the umbilicus, in the left anterior axillary line. Placement of these ports too far lateral or too low on the abdomen will compromise the excursion of the instruments and thus the ability to retract.

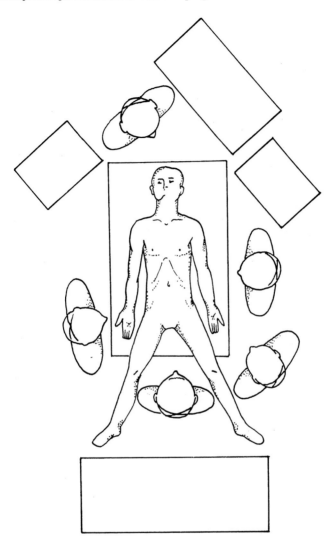

Fig. 10.1. Patient positioning and room setup for laparoscopic fundoplication. The patient is placed with the head elevated 45° in the modified lithotomy or split leg position. The surgeon stands between the patient's legs. One assistant, on the surgeon's right, retracts the stomach; the second assistant, on the surgeon's left, manipulates the camera.

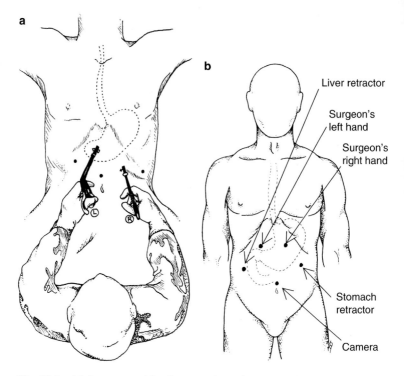

Fig. 10.2. (**a**) Surgeon position between the patients legs with left hand accessing the subxiphoid port and right hand the left subcostal port. (**b**) Trocar placement for laparoscopic antireflux surgery. Five 10-mm trocars are generally used The camera is place paramedian and trans rectus approximately one third the distance above the umbilicus, a left mid abdominal retraction port approximately even with the camera and in the midclavicular line, and a right mid abdominal liver retraction port approximately even with the camera and in the midclavicular line. The surgeons right handed port is placed left subcostal area so it lies between the camera and left sided retraction port and the surgeon right had subxiphoid. The author prefers 10mm ports although nearly all can be 5mm depending upon surgeon preference and instrument selection.

4. **Place the left-sided operating port (surgeon's right hand)** 1–2 in. below the costal margin approximately at the lateral rectus border. This allows triangulation between the camera and the two instruments, and avoids the difficulty associated with the instruments being in direct line with the camera. The right-sided operating port (surgeon's left hand) is placed last, after the right lateral segment of the liver has been retracted. This prevents "sword fighting" between the liver retractor and the left-handed instrument. The falciform ligament hangs low in

many patients and provides a barrier around which the left-handed instrument must be manipulated.

5. **Initial retraction** is accomplished with exposure of the esophageal hiatus. A fan retractor is placed into the right anterior axillary port and positioned to hold the left lateral segment of the liver toward the anterior abdominal wall. We prefer to utilize a table retractor to hold this instrument once properly positioned. Trauma to the liver should be meticulously avoided because subsequent bleeding will obscure the field. Mobilization of the left lateral segment by division of the triangular ligament is not necessary. Place a Babcock clamp into the left anterior axillary port and retract the stomach toward the patient's left foot. This maneuver exposes the esophageal hiatus (Fig. 10.3). Commonly, a hiatal hernia will need to be reduced. Use an atraumatic clamp, and take care not to grasp the stomach too vigorously, as gastric perforations can occur.

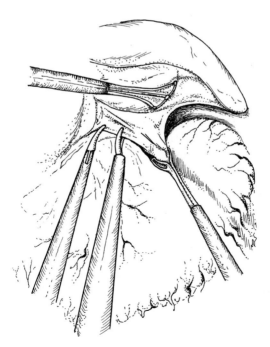

Fig. 10.3. Laparoscopic exposure of the esophageal hiatus. A fan-type retractor (placed through the right subcostal port) elevates the left lateral hepatic segment anterolaterally. A Babcock clamp (placed through the left lateral port) retracts the stomach caudad. This places the phrenoesophageal membrane on traction.

D. Technique of Nissen Fundoplication

The critical elements of laparoscopic Nissen fundoplication are enumerated in Table 10.2.

1. The Dissection

The dissection begins with identification of the right crus. Metzenbaum-type scissors and fine grasping forceps are preferred for dissection. In all except the most obese patients, there is a very thin portion of the gastrohepatic omentum overlying the caudate lobe of the liver (Fig. 10.4).

   a. Begin the dissection by incising this portion of the gastrohepatic omentum above and below the hepatic branch of the anterior vagal nerve (which the author routinely spares although this is not necessary).

   b. A large left aberrant hepatic artery arising from the left gastric artery will be present in up to 25% of patients. It should be identified and avoided. A right crural branch will occasionally be seen and can be divided.

   c. After the gastrohepatic omentum has been incised, the outside of the right crus will become evident. Incise the peritoneum overlying the anterior aspect of the right crus with scissors and electrocautery, and dissect the right crus from anterior to posterior as far as possible.

   d. The medial portion of the right crus leads into the mediastinum and is entered by blunt dissection with both instruments.

   e. At this juncture, the esophagus usually becomes evident. Retract the right crus laterally and perform a modest dissection of the

---

Table 10.2. Elements of laparoscopic Nissen fundoplication.

1. Crural dissection, identification, and preservation of both vagi, including the hepatic branch of the anterior vagus
2. Circumferential dissection and mobilization of the esophagus
3. Crural closure
4. Fundic mobilization by division of short gastric vessels
5. Creation of a short, loose fundoplication by enveloping the anterior and posterior wall of the fundus around the lower esophagus

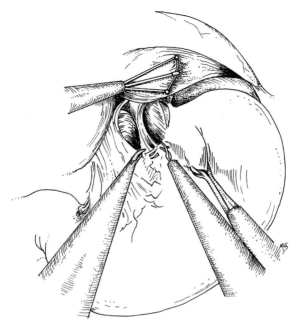

Fig. 10.4. Initial dissection of the esophageal hiatus. The right crus is identified and dissected toward its posterior confluence with the left crus.

tissues posterior to the esophagus. Do not attempt to dissect behind the gastroesophageal junction at this time.

f.   Meticulous hemostasis is critical. Blood and fluids tend to pool in the hiatus and are difficult to remove. Irrigation should be avoided. Take care not to injure the phrenic artery and vein as they course above the hiatus. A large hiatal hernia often makes this portion of the procedure easier because it accentuates the diaphragmatic crura. On the other hand, dissection of a large mediastinal hernia sac can be difficult.

g.   Following dissection of the right crus, attention is turned toward the anterior crural confluence. Use the left-handed grasper to hold up the tissues anterior to the esophagus, and sweep the esophagus downward and to the right, separating it from the left crus.

h.   Divide the anterior crural tissues and identify the left crus. The anterior vagus nerve often "hugs" the left crus and can be injured in this portion of the dissection if not carefully searched for and protected (Fig. 10.5).

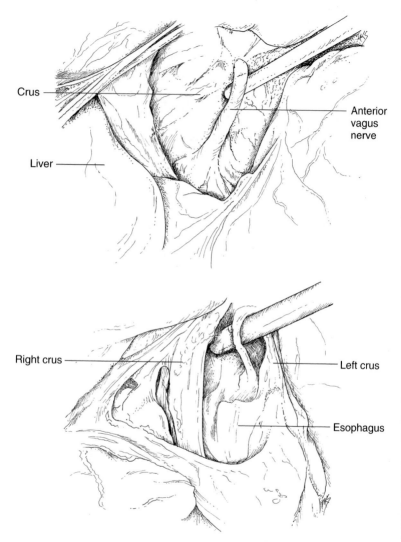

Fig. 10.5. Anterior dissection of the esophageal hiatus. The anterior (*left*) vagus nerve often "hugs" the inside of the left crus and can be injured if not dissected off before crural dissection.

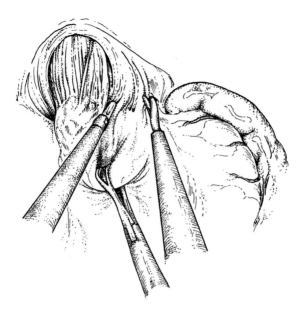

Fig. 10.6. Dissection of the left crus. The left crus is dissected as completely as possible, and the attachments of the fundus of the stomach to the diaphragm are taken down.

i.   Dissect the left crus as completely as possible, including taking down the angle of His and the attachments of the fundus to the left diaphragm (Fig. 10.6). A complete dissection of the lateral and inferior aspect of the left crus and fundus of the stomach is the key maneuver allowing circumferential mobilization of the esophagus. Failure to make a complete dissection will result in difficulty in encircling the esophagus, particularly if approached from the right. Repositioning of the Babcock retractor toward the fundic side of the stomach facilitates retraction for this portion of the procedure. The posterior vagus nerve may be encountered in the low left crural dissection. It should be looked for and protected.

2. Circumferential Dissection of the Esophagus

Circumferential dissection of the esophagus is achieved by careful dissection of the anterior and posterior soft tissues within the hiatus.

If the crura have been completely dissected, then dissection posterior to the esophagus to create a window will not be difficult.

a. From the patient's right side, use the left-handed instrument to retract the esophagus anteriorly. This allows the right hand to perform the dissection behind the esophagus. Reverse this maneuver for the left-sided dissection.

b. The posterior vagus should be identified, left on the esophagus and kept out of harm's way.

c. Identify the left crus and keep the dissection caudad to it. There is a tendency to dissect into the mediastinum and left pleura.

d. In the presence of severe esophagitis, transmural inflammation, esophageal shortening, and/or obese patients with a large posterior fat pad, this dissection may be particularly difficult. If unduly difficult, abandon this route of dissection and approach the hiatus from the left side by dividing the short gastric vessels at this point in the procedure rather than later.

e. After completing the posterior dissection, pass a grasper (via the surgeon's left-handed port) behind the esophagus and over the left crus. Pass a Penrose drain around the esophagus, secure it with an Endoloop and use this as an esophageal retractor for the remainder of the procedure.

3. Fundic Mobilization

Complete fundic mobilization allows construction of a tension-free fundoplication.

a. Suspend the gastrosplenic omentum anteroposteriorly, in a clothesline fashion via two Babcock forceps, and enter the lesser sac approximately one third the distance down the greater curvature of the stomach (Fig. 10.7). Sequentially dissect and divide the short gastric vessels with the aid of ultrasonic shears (Ethicon Endo-Surgery, Cincinnati, OH). An anterior–posterior rather than medial-to-lateral orientation of the vessels is preferred, with the exception of those close to the spleen. The dissection includes pancreaticogastric branches posterior to the upper stomach and continues until the right crus and caudate lobe can be seen from the left side (Fig. 10.8). With caution and meticulous dissection, the fundus can be completely mobilized in virtually all patients although this can be one of the most

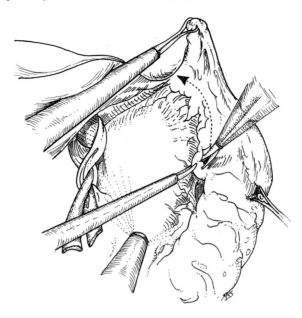

Fig. 10.7. Proper retraction of the gastrosplenic omentum facilitates the initial steps of short gastric division.

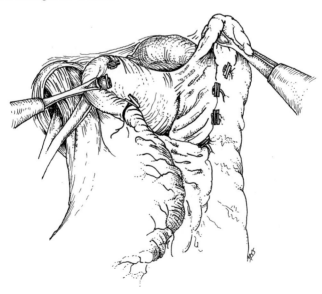

Fig. 10.8. Retract the stomach rightward and the spleen and omentum left and downward to complete mobilization of the fundus. These maneuvers open the lesser sac and facilitate division of the high short gastric vessels.

difficult portions of the procedure. Dissection and division of the high short gastric vessels toward the superior pole of the spleen is facilitated by retraction of the stomach rightward and toward the appendix. This is best done by pushing it with a Babcock forceps inserted into the left lower trocar. Grasping the posterior fundus and retraction can result in posterior serosal tears or perforation. Although generally possible via the right- and left-handed surgeon's access ports, occasionally this dissection will require removal of the liver retractor and placement of a second Babcock forceps through the right anterior axillary port to facilitate retraction during division of the short gastric vessels.

4. Esophageal Mobilization

The esophagus is mobilized into the posterior mediastinum for several centimeters to provide maximal intra-abdominal esophageal length. Posterior and right lateral mobilization is readily accomplished. Take care during the anterior and left lateral mobilization not to injure the anterior vagus nerve. Gentle traction on the Penrose drain around the gastroesophageal junction facilitates exposure. The right and left pleural reflections often come into view and should be avoided. If the pleura are opened, it is generally well tolerated. Communicate this fact to the anesthesia team and observe the airway pressures for excess elevation.

5. Crural Closure

Continue the crural dissection to enlarge the space behind the gastroesophageal junction as much as possible.

a.   Holding the esophagus anterior and to the left, approximate the crura with two to four interrupted figure-of-eight 0-gauge Ethibond sutures, starting just above the aortic decussation and working anterior (Fig. 10.9).

b.   The author prefers a large needle (CT1) passed down the left upper 10-mm port to facilitate a durable crural closure.

c.   Because space is limited, it is often necessary to use the surgeon's left-handed (nondominant) instrument as a retractor, facilitating placement of single bites through each crus with the

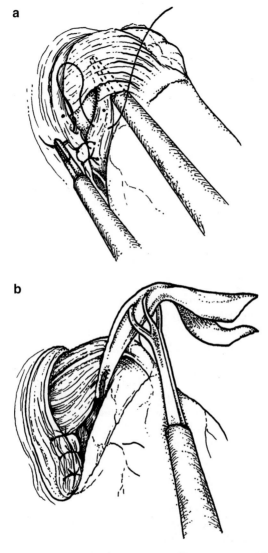

Fig. 10.9. (**a**) Three to six interrupted 0-gauge silk sutures are used to close the crura. (**b**) Exposure of the crura and posterior aspect of the esophagus is facilitated by traction on a Penrose drain encircling the gastroesophageal junction.

surgeon's right hand. The aorta might be punctured while suturing the left crus. Identification of its anterior surface and often retracting the left crus away from the aorta via the left handed grasper will help avoid inadvertent aortic puncture.

d. The author prefers extracorporeal knot tying using a standard knot pusher or a "tie knot" device, although tying within the abdomen is perfectly appropriate.

e. The crura should be approximated until the esophagus lies comfortably in the opening when "off tension," i.e., not retracted. Bougie sizing for crural closure is not necessary and may make it more difficult.

6. Create a Short, Loose Fundoplication

Create a short, loose fundoplication with particular attention to the geometry of the wrap.

a. Grasp the posterior fundus and pass it left to right rather than pulling right to left. This assures that the posterior fundus is used for the posterior aspect of the fundoplication. This is accomplished by placing a Babcock clamp through the left lower port, and grasping the midportion of the posterior fundus (Fig. 10.10). Gently bring the posterior fundus behind the esophagus to the right side with an upward, rightward, and clockwise twisting motion. This maneuver can be difficult particularly for the novice. If so, placing a 0 silk suture in the midposterior fundus and grasping it from the right side makes it easy to bring the posterior fundus around to create the fundoplication.

b. Bring the anterior wall of the fundus anterior to the esophagus above the supporting Penrose drain.

c. Manipulate both the posterior and anterior fundic lips to allow the fundus to envelope the esophagus without twisting (Fig. 10.11). Laparoscopic visualization has a tendency to exaggerate the size of the posterior opening that has been dissected. Consequently, the space for the passage of the fundus behind the esophagus may be tighter than thought and the fundus relatively ischemic when brought around. If the right lip of the fun-

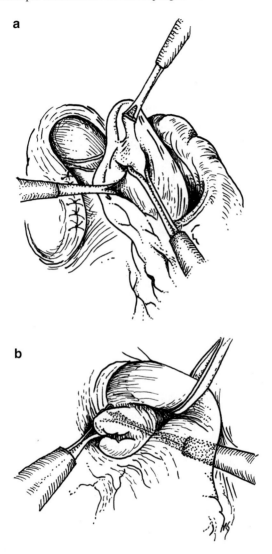

Fig. 10.10. (**a**) Placement of Babcock clamp on the posterior fundus in preparation for passing it behind the esophagus to create the posterior or right lip of the fundoplication. To achieve the proper angle for passage, place the Babcock through the left lower trocar. (**b**) Pass the posterior fundus from left to right and grasp it from the right with a Babcock clamp (passed through the right upper trocar).

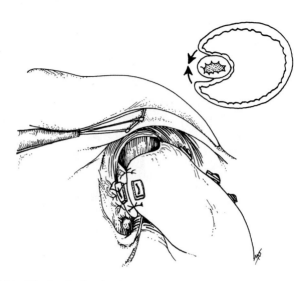

Fig. 10.11. The fundoplication is sutured in place with a single U-stitch of 2–0 Prolene pledgeted on the outside. A 60-French mercury-weighted bougie is passed through the gastroesophageal junction prior to fixation of the wrap to assure a floppy fundoplication. Inset illustrates the proper orientation of the fundic wrap.

doplication has a bluish discoloration, the stomach should be returned to its original position and the posterior dissection enlarged.

d. Pass a 60-French bougie to properly size the fundoplication, and suture it utilizing a single U-stitch of 2–0 Prolene buttressed with felt pledgets. The most common error is an attempt to grasp the anterior portion of the stomach to construct the right lip of the fundoplication rather than the posterior fundus. The esophagus should comfortably lie in the untwisted fundus prior to suturing.

e. Place two anchoring sutures of 2–0 silk above and below the U-stitch to complete the fundoplication. When finished, the suture line of the fundoplication should be facing in a right anterior direction.

f. Irrigate the abdomen, assure hemostasis, and remove the bougie and Penrose drain.

E. Laparoscopic Partial Fundoplication

Although the orientation of partial fundoplication may be either anterior, posterior, or lateral, the most commonly performed laparoscopic partial fundoplication is the modified Toupet procedure, a 270° posterior hemifundoplication.

1. **Patient positioning**, trocar placement, hiatal dissection, crural closure, and fundic mobilization are performed exactly as for laparoscopic Nissen fundoplication.

2. **Fixation of the fundoplication** is the only portion of the procedure that differs from that of Nissen fundoplication. The posterior lip of the fundoplication is created as described for Nissen fundoplication.

3. With adequate fundic mobilization the posterior fundus should lie comfortably on the right side of the esophagus prior to suturing it in place.

4. Place a Babcock clamp on the superior aspect of the right lip and suture the posterior fundus to the crural closure with three interrupted sutures of 2–0 silk.

5. Rather than bringing the lips together (as in a Nissen fundoplication), suture the right limb of the fundoplication to the esophageal musculature at the 11 o'clock position and the left at the 1 o'clock position on the esophagus (Fig. 10.12). Three interrupted sutures of 2–0 silk are placed along the lower esophagus just above the gastroesophageal fat pad to fix each limb (see also Chapter 23, in which Toupet and Dor fundoplications are discussed in the context of laparoscopic cardiomyotomy).

F. Postoperative Considerations

Recovery is more rapid than usual after the corresponding open procedure, and several aspects of postoperative management are correspondingly different.

1. **A nasogastric tube** is not necessary.

2. **Pain** is managed with parenteral narcotics or ketorolac for the first 24 h and oral hydrocodone thereafter as necessary.

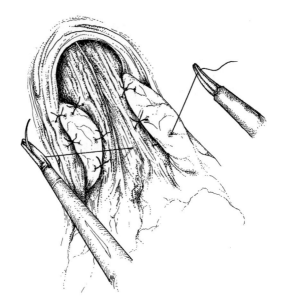

Fig. 10.12. Completed 270-degree posterior hemifundoplication (Toupet fundoplication).

3. **A Foley** catheter is placed following induction of anesthesia and left in place until the morning after surgery. The incidence of urinary retention is approximately 10–25% if bladder decompression is not used.
4. **A diet** of clear liquids ad libitum is allowed the morning following surgery. Soft solids are begun on the second postoperative day and continued for 2 weeks. The patient should be instructed to eat slowly, chew carefully, and avoid bread and meats for a minimum of 2 weeks.

G. Complications

The safety of laparoscopic fundoplication has now been established. **Mortality** is rare following an elective antireflux procedure, whether open or closed, estimated at 1–2 per 1,000. The complication rate of laparoscopic is similar to that of open fundoplication, averaging 10–15%, but the spectrum of the morbidity has changed. Complications associated with surgical access and postoperative recovery has improved. With the exception of a reduction in the number of splenic injuries and splenectomies performed during laparoscopic fundoplication, intraoperative complications, such as gastric or esophageal perforation, are slightly higher. Initial concern of the possibility of an increased incidence of pulmonary embolism has not proven true. Cumulative results suggest an incidence of pulmonary embolism of 0.49%, similar to that of open fundoplication.

Several excellent reports of the outcome of laparoscopic fundoplication have been published. These reports document the ability of laparoscopic fundoplication to relieve typical symptoms of gastroesophageal reflux, that is, heartburn, regurgitation, and dysphagia, in over 90% of patients. Atypical respiratory and laryngeal symptoms are relieved less reliably improving on average in 65–80% of patients.

Long-term outcome studies (10 years and beyond) and a single randomized trial comparing laparoscopic Nissen to esomeprazole have also been published. Comparison to PPI therapy favors antireflux surgery, although symptom control is similar in both groups. Most surgical studies show a small but definite incidence of recurrent reflux, with 80–85% of patients free of reflux symptoms at 5 years. Patients with long-segment Barrett's esophagus and those with hiatal hernias larger than 5 cm may be at higher risk of recurrence, although even in this population most will enjoy long-lasting reflux control.

A few complications are particularly noteworthy and are described briefly here.

1. **Pneumothorax and surgical emphysema** have occurred in 1–2% of patients. This is most likely related to excessive hiatal dissection and should decrease with increasing experience of the surgical team.

2. **Unrecognized perforations of esophagus or stomach** are the most life-threatening problems. Perforations of the esophagus and stomach occur during hiatal dissection should be rare and are likely related to operative experience. Intraoperative recognition and repair is the key to preventing life-threatening problems.

3. Although uncommon, **acute paraesophageal herniation** has been noted by a number of authors and usually results in early reoperation.

Selected References

American Gastroenterologic Association medical position statement on the management of gastroesophageal reflux disease. Gastroenterology 2008; 135:1383–91.

Attwood SEA, Lundell L, Ell C, Galmiche JP, Hatlebakk J, Fiocca R, Lind T, Eklund S, Junghard O. Standardization of surgical technique in antireflux surgery: the LOTUS trial experience. World J Surg. 2008;32:995–8.

Campos GMR, Peters JH, DeMeester TR, et al. Multivariate analysis of the factors predicting outcome after laparoscopic Nissen fundoplication. J Gastrointest Surg. 1999;3: 292–300.

Carlson MA, Frantzides CT. Complications and results of primary minimally invasive antireflux procedures: a review of 10,735 reported cases. J Am Coll Surg. 2001;193: 428–39.

DeMeester TR, Bonavina L, Albertucci M. Nissen fundoplication for gastroesophageal reflux disease—evaluation of primary repair in 100 consecutive patients. Ann Surg. 1986;204:9.

Horgan S, Pohl D, Bogetti D, Eubanks T, Pellegrini C. Failed antireflux surgery; what have we learned from reoperations? Arch Surg. 1999;134:809–17.

Horvath KD, Swanstrom LL, Jobe BA. The short esophagus; pathophysiology, pre- sentation and treatment in the era of laparoscopic antireflux surgery. Ann Surg. 2000;282: 630–40.

Hunter JG, Trus TL, Branum GD, Waring JP, Wood WC. A physiologic approach to laparoscopic fundoplication for gastroesophageal reflux disease. Ann Surg. 1996;223: 673–87.

Kelly JJ, Watson DI, Chin KF, Devitt PG, Game PA, Jamieson GG. Laparoscopic Nissen fundoplication: clinical outcmes at 10 years. J Am Coll Surg. 2007;205:570–5.

Lundell L, Attwood S, Ell C, Fiocca R, Galmiche JP, Hatlebakk J, Lind T, Junghard O. Comparing laparoscopic antireflux surgery with esomeprazole in the management of patients with gastroesophageal reflux disease; a 3-year interim analysis of the LOTUS trial. Gut. 2008;57:1207–13.

Jamieson GG, Watson DI, Britten-Jones R, Mitchell PC, Anvari M. Laparoscopic Nissen fundoplication. Ann Surg. 1994;220:137–45.

Peters JH, Heimbucher J, Kauer WKH, Incarbone R, Bremner CG, DeMeester TR. Clinical and physiologic comparison of laparoscopic and open Nissen. J Am Coll Surg. 1995; 180:385–93.

Peters MJ, Mukhtar A, Uunis RM, Kahn S, Pappalardo J, Memon B, Memon MA. Meta-analysis of randomized clinical trial comparing open and laparoscopic anti-reflux surgery. Am J Gastroenterol. 2009;104:1548–61.

Reardon PR, Matthews BD, Scarborough TK, Preciado A, Marti JL, Kamelgard JI. Geometry and reproducibility in 360° fundoplication. Surg Endosc. 2000;14:750–4.

Purdy M, Nykoop TK, Kainulainen S, Paakkonen M. Division of the hepatic branch of the anterior vagus nerve in fundoplication: effects on gallbladder function. Surg Endosc. 2009;23:2142–6.

Waring JP, Hunter JG, Oddsdottir M, Wo J, Katz E. The preoperative evaluation of patients considered for laparoscopic antireflux surgery. Am J Gastroenterol. 1995;90:35–8.

Watson D, Balgrie RJ, Jamieson GG. A learning curve for laparoscopic fundoplication: definable, avoidable or a waste of time? Ann Surg. 1996;224:198–203.

Watson DI, de Beaux AC. Complications of laparoscopic antireflux surgery. Surg Endosc. 2001;15:344–52.Figure 10.2. (**a**) Surgeon position between the patients legs with left hand accessing the subxiphoid port and right hand the left subcostal port. (**b**) Trocar placement for laparoscopic antireflux surgery. Five 10-mm trocars are generally used The camera is place paramedian and trans rectus approximately one third the distance above the umbilicus, a left mid abdominal retraction port approximately even with the camera and in the midclavicular line, and a right mid abdominal liver retraction port approximately even with the camera and in the midclavicular line. The surgeons right handed port is placed left subcostal area so it lies between the camera and left sided retraction port and the surgeon right had subxiphoid. The author prefers 10mm ports although nearly all can be 5mm depending upon surgeon preference and instrument selection.

11. Laparoscopic Heller Myotomy and Partial Fundoplication for Esophageal Achalasia[*]

Brian Bello, M.D.
Roberto Gullo, M.D.
Marco G. Patti, M.D.

Achalasia is a primary esophageal motility disorder of unknown origin, characterized by lack of esophageal peristalsis and failure of the lower esophageal sphincter (LES) to relax appropriately in response to swallowing. The LES is hypertensive in about 50% of patients.

The treatments of esophageal achalasia are palliative and they are based on the elimination of the outflow resistance at the level of the gastroesophageal junction caused by the nonrelaxing LES. There is no definitive evidence that even early and successful treatment is followed by return of normal esophageal peristalsis. Emptying of the esophagus is therefore based on gravity.

The use of laparoscopy over the past two decades has caused a major shift in the treatment of esophageal achalasia. During the 1970s and 1980s, pneumatic dilation was widely accepted as the primary treatment modality, reserving a myotomy for patients who had persistent or recurrent dysphagia after dilatation. Today, a laparoscopic Heller myotomy with a partial fundoplication is considered the best modality of treatment by most gastroenterologists and surgeons. This procedure is associated to a short hospital stay, minimal postoperative pain, and a relatively fast recovery time. Clinical results of the larger series of laparoscopic Heller myotomy with partial fundoplication (Toupet or Dor fundoplication) are shown in Table 11.1. Relief of dysphagia is consistently obtained in

---

[*]This chapter was contributed by Margret Oddsdottir MD in the previous edition.

N.T. Nguyen and C.E.H. Scott-Conner (eds.), *The SAGES Manual: Volume 2 Advanced Laparoscopy and Endoscopy*, DOI 10.1007/978-1-4614-2347-8_11, © Springer Science+Business Media, LLC 2012

Table 11.1. Laparoscopic Heller Myotomy and partial fundoplication.

Author/year	No. of patients	Type of surgery	Excellent/good results (%)
Perrone 2004	92	LHM+T	97
Yashodhan 2005	121	LHM+T	91
Patti 2005	151	LHM+D	91
Rosen 2007	101	LHM+T	95
Rebecchi 2008	71	LHM+D	97
Zaninotto 2008	400	LHM+D	97
Chen 2010	125	LHM+D	90
Total	**1,061**		**94**

Abbreviations: *LHM+T* laparoscopic Heller myotomy and Toupet fundoplication, *LHM+D* laparoscopic Heller myotomy and Dor fundoplication

about 90% of patients and no mortality has been reported. These excellent results are equally obtained in young and elderly patients.

The following review describes our approach for the treatment of esophageal achalasia by a laparoscopic Heller myotomy and Dor fundoplication.

A. Preoperative Evaluation

All patients who are candidates for laparoscopic Heller myotomy and partial fundoplication should have a thorough evaluation:

1. *Symptomatic evaluation.* Dysphagia is present in more than 90% of patients and it is usually the main complaint. Regurgitation is present in about 80% of patients, heartburn in 50%, and chest pain in 40%. Approximately one third will have experienced weight loss. Respiratory symptoms secondary to aspiration are present in about 50% of patients. Symptoms alone do not distinguish achalasia from gastroesophageal reflux disease (GERD). In one study, Fisichella et al. reported that 65 (45%) of 145 patients with achalasia had been initially treated with acid reducing medications on the assumption that GERD was the cause of the symptoms.

2. *Barium esophagogram.* This test usually demonstrates narrowing of the gastroesophageal junction (bird beak). It also defines the esophageal axis (straight or sigmoid), the diameter of the esophagus, and associated pathology, such as an epiphrenic

diverticulum. These findings are important for adequate preoperative planning.

3. *Upper endoscopy.* Although endoscopy suggests achalasia in only 50% of patients, the test is important in patients with dysphagia to rule out mechanical causes, such as a peptic stricture or cancer.

4. *Esophageal manometry.* This test is the gold standard for the diagnosis of achalasia. The typical findings are lack of peristalsis and incomplete relaxation of the LES in response to swallowing. Contrary to what was previously thought, the LES is hypertensive only in about 50% of patients. It is important to remember that the manometric picture of achalasia can also be given by cancer, most often located at the level of the gastroesophageal junction. This is defined as "pseudoachalasia" or "secondary achalasia." It should be suspected in patients who have been symptomatic for a short period of time, who are 60 years or older, and who have lost a considerable amount of weight. In these patients, an upper endoscopy with endoscopic ultrasound and a CT scan of the abdomen and chest may help in clarifying the diagnosis.

5. *Ambulatory pH monitoring.* This test is important to differentiate GERD from achalasia, to determine if reflux is present in patients after failed pneumatic dilatation and in young patients after Heller myotomy. Postoperative reflux should be treated with acid reducing medications even in the absence of symptoms. It is essential to review the tracing to distinguish between true reflux and reflux due to esophageal stasis and fermentation.

B. Laparoscopic Heller Myotomy and Dor Fundoplication

1. Positioning

Place the patient supine atop a beanbag to create a saddle under the perineum to avoid sliding when in steep reverse Trendelenburg. Pneumatic compression stockings are used for mechanical prophylaxis against deep vein thrombosis. After induction of general endotracheal anesthesia, an

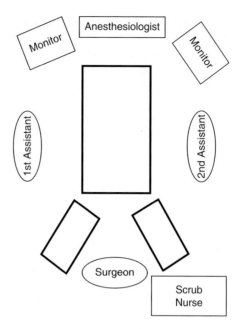

Fig. 11.1. Position of the patient and surgical team in the operating room.

oro-gastric tube is placed to keep the stomach decompressed during the procedure. The tube is removed before starting the myotomy.

The legs are placed in stirrups with knees flexed 20–30°. The surgeon stands between the patient's legs, with an assistant on the patient's left and one on the patient's right side (Fig. 11.1).

2. Placement of the Trocars

Five 10 mm trocars are used for the operation (Fig. 11.2).

a.   Place the first trocar (A) in the midline, 14 cm distal to the xiphoid process, and it is used for the 30° scope. This trocar can also be placed slightly to the left of the midline. This port must be placed with caution since the insertion site is just above the aorta. We recommend initially inflating the abdomen to a pressure of 18 mm Hg to increase the distance between the abdominal wall and the aorta. Subsequently, we use an optical trocar with a zero-degree scope to obtain access. Once this port is

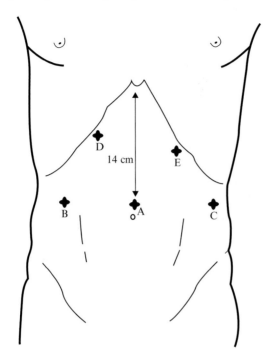

Fig. 11.2. Position of the trocars for laparoscopic Heller myotomy and Dor fundoplication.

placed, the intraperitoneal pressure is reduced to 15 mm Hg and the other trocars are placed under direct vision.

b. Place a second trocar (B) in the right midclavicular line at the same level of the previous trocar, and use it for the insertion of a fan retractor to lift the left lateral segment of the liver to expose the esophagogastric junction. Hold the retractor in place by a self-retaining system fixed to the operating table.

c. Place a third trocar (C) in the left midclavicular line at the same level as the other 2 trocars, and use it for the insertion of a Babcock clamp or for instruments used to divide the short gastric vessels.

d. Place the fourth (D) and fifth (E) trocars under the right and left costal margins so that their axis forms an angle of about 120° with the camera. These ports are used for the dissecting and suturing instruments. If the angle is too narrow, the instruments will cover part of the operating field and hinder the operation.

3. Division of the Gastrohepatic Ligament; Identification of the Right Crus of the Diaphragm; and the Posterior Vagus Nerve

Once the ports are placed, the gastrohepatic ligament is divided. Begin this dissection above the caudate lobe of the liver, where the ligament is thin, and continue toward the diaphragm until the right crus is identified. Then, separate the crus from the right side of the esophagus by blunt dissection, and identify the posterior vagus nerve. Electrocautery must be used with caution during the dissection as monopolar current tends to spread laterally and the posterior vagus nerve may sustain damage even without direct contact. A bipolar instrument is safer.

4. Division of Peritoneum and Phrenoesophageal Membrane Above the Esophagus: Identification of the Left Crus of the Diaphragm and Anterior Vagus Nerve

Transect the peritoneum and phrenoesophageal membrane above the esophagus, and identify the anterior vagus nerve. Leave the nerve attached to the esophageal wall. Separate the left pillar of the crus from the esophagus by blunt dissection. Continue the dissection into the mediastinum, lateral, and anterior to the esophagus, to expose 6–7 cm of the esophagus. No posterior dissection is necessary if a Dor fundoplication is performed after the myotomy.

5. Division of the Short Gastric Vessels

Divide all short gastric vessels all the way to the left pillar of the crus. Bleeding can occur from the short gastric vessels and it is usually caused by excessive traction or by division of a vessel that is not completely coagulated. In addition, take care not to damage the gastric wall with either the electrocautery or by traction applied by graspers or the Babcock clamp.

6. Myotomy

Remove the fat pad to expose the gastroesophageal junction. Take care to preserve the anterior vagus nerve. Use a Babcock clamp to pull the stomach downward and to the left in order to expose the right side of the esophagus. After identifying the course of the anterior vagus nerve, perform the myotomy using a hook cautery in the 11 o'clock position. Begin the myotomy about 3 cm above the gastroesophageal junction, with the goal of entering the submucosal plane at this point. Once the proper plane is identified, extend the myotomy for about 6 cm proximally, and then distally onto the gastric wall for about 2.0–2.5 cm. Thus, the total length of the myotomy is typically about 8–8.5 cm (Fig. 11.3). Gently separate the muscle edges to expose the mucosa for about 30–40% of the circumference. At the beginning of a surgeon's experience, it is useful to use intra-operative endoscopy to confirm the distal extent of the myotomy onto the gastric wall. Once enough experience is gained, this step can be omitted.

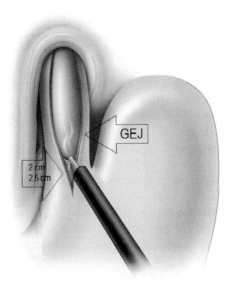

Fig. 11.3. Myotomy. Distal extent onto the gastric wall.

In patients who have had previous treatment with botulinum toxin injection, fibrosis can occur at the level of the gastroesophageal junction leading to loss of the normal anatomic planes. In these cases, the myotomy is technically more difficult and there is an increased risk of mucosal perforation. If a perforation occurs, close it with fine absorbable material (5–0), and test the repair with saline or methylene blue.

Bleeding may also occur during the myotomy, usually from submucosal veins at the level of the gastroesophageal junction. We recommend applying pressure with a sponge rather than using the cautery which can lead to a thermal injury and eventually a perforation.

7. Dor Fundoplication

Gastroesophageal reflux occurs in about 50% of patients if a myotomy alone is performed. A 360° fundoplication, while the most effective operation for GERD, is generally avoided due to the high rate of postoperative dysphagia. A partial fundoplication is the procedure of choice, as it takes into account the lack of esophageal peristalsis.

Our preference is for a partial anterior fundoplication (Dor procedure) because it is simpler to perform as compared to posterior fundoplication, and because it covers the mucosa. This type of fundoplication does not add resistance at the level of the gastroesophageal junction and avoids gastroesophageal reflux in most patients.

The Dor fundoplication is constructed using two rows of sutures. The first row of sutures is on the left side of the esophagus, and has three stitches. The uppermost stitch incorporates the gastric fundus, the muscle layers of the left side of the esophagus, and the left pillar of the crus (Fig. 11.4). The second and the third stitch incorporate the muscle layers of the left side of the esophagus and the gastric wall only (Fig. 11.5). The fundus is then folded over the exposed mucosa so that the greater curvature of the stomach lies next to the right pillar of the crus. The second row of sutures also consists of three stitches. The uppermost stitch incorporates the gastric fundus, the right side of the cut edge of the muscle layers, and the right pillar of the crus. The second and third stitches are placed between the greater curvature of the stomach and the right pillar of the crus (Fig. 11.6).

Finally, two additional stitches are placed between the anterior rim of the esophageal hiatus and the superior aspect of the fundoplication (without incorporating the esophageal wall) to decrease the tension on the right row of sutures (Fig. 11.7).

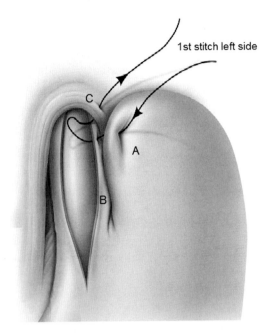

Fig. 11.4. Dor fundoplication, left row of stitches. First stitch. (**a**) fundus; (**b**) esophageal wall; (**c**) left pillar of the crus.

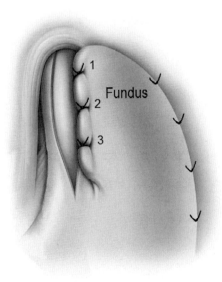

Fig. 11.5. Dor fundoplication, left row of stitches. Second and third stitches.

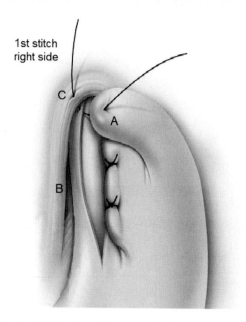

Fig. 11.6 Dor fundoplication, right row of stitches. First stitch. (**a**) fundus; (**b**) esophageal wall; (**c**) right pillar of the crus.

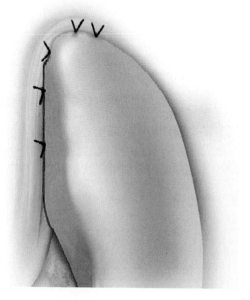

Fig. 11.7. Completed Dor fundoplication.

8. Toupet Fundoplication

A partial posterior fundoplication (Toupet fundoplication) can be used as an alternative to a Dor fundoplication. Each procedure has some advantages: the anterior fundoplication requires less dissection and covers the mucosa; the posterior fundoplication keeps the edges of the myotomy separated and it might be more effective in preventing reflux.

The Society of American Gastrointestinal and Endoscopic Surgeons (SAGES) is now conducting a prospective, randomized, and multicenter study comparing laparoscopic Heller myotomy with Dor fundoplication and laparoscopic Heller myotomy with Toupet fundoplication. End points of the study will include the relief of dysphagia and incidence of postoperative reflux as measured by pH monitoring.

9. Complications

a. **An esophageal leak** may occur during the first 24–36 h after the operation. This is usually secondary to a thermal injury of the esophageal mucosa. Characteristic signs and symptoms include chest or abdominal pain, fever, and a pleural effusion on chest x-ray. The presence and location of the leak are confirmed with an esophagogram. Treatment options depend on the time of diagnosis and on the size and location of the leak. Early, small leaks can be repaired primarily. If the damage is too extensive to permit a primary repair, an esophagectomy should be performed.

b. **Pneumothorax** happens if the pleura is violated during the mediastinal dissection. Since carbon dioxide is rapidly absorbed, the lung usually re-expands quickly. Placement of a chest tube is rarely needed.

c. **Dysphagia** may persist after the operation or can recur after a symptom-free interval. Persistent dysphagia is usually due to a short myotomy or to wrong configuration of the fundoplication. Recurrent dysphagia may be due to scarring in the distal portion of the myotomy, gastroesophageal reflux, or to the fundoplication. In either case, a complete work-up is necessary, and treatment should be individualized on the basis of the specific findings. Pneumatic dilatation or a reoperation may be indicated.

d. **Abnormal gastroesophageal reflux** occurs in 6–33% of patients after the operation. Because most patients are asymptomatic, it is essential to try to evaluate all patients postoperatively with manometry and pH monitoring. This is particularly important for young patients. Reflux should be treated with acid-reducing medications.

10. Postoperative Care

We do not routinely obtain an esophagram before initiating feeding. Patients are fed on postoperative day 1 and instructed to avoid meat and bread for 2 weeks. About 70% of patients are discharged within 23 h and 90% of patients are discharged within 48 h (4). Most patients are able to resume regular activities in 7–14 days.

Selected References

Burpee SE, Mamazza J, Schlachta CM, et al. Objective analysis of gastroesophageal reflux after laparoscopic Heller myotomy: an anti-reflux procedure is required. Surg Endosc. 2005;19:9–14.

Chen Z, Bessell JR, Chew A, Watson DI. Laparoscopic cardiomyotomy for achalasia: clinical outcomes beyond 5 years. J Gastrointest Surg. 2010;14:594–600.

Fisichella PM, Raz D, Palazzo F, Niponmick I, Patti MG. Clinical, radiological and manometric profile in 145 patients with untreated achalasia. World J Surg. 2008;32:1974–9.

Khajanchee YS, Kanneganti S, Leatherwood AEB, et al. Laparoscopic Heller myotomy with Toupet fundoplication. Outcome predictors in 121 consecutive patients. Arch Surg. 2005;140:827–34.

Khandelwal S, Petersen R, Tatum R, et al. Improvement of respiratory symptoms following Heller myotomy for achalasia. J Gastrointest Surg. 2011;15:235–9.

Kjellin AP, Granqvist S, Ramel S, Thor KBA. Laparoscopic myotomy without fundoplication in patients with achalasia. Eur J Surg. 1999;165:1162–6.

Moonka R, Patti MG, Feo CV, et al. Clinical presentation and evaluation of malignant pseudoachalasia. J Gastrointest Surg. 1999;3:456–61.

Oelschlager BK, Chang L, Pellegrini CA. Improved outcome after extended gastric myotomy for achalasia. Arch Surg. 2003;138:490–7.

Patti MG, Arcerito M, Tong J, et al. Importance of preoperative and postoperative pH monitoring in patients with esophageal achalasia. J Gastrointest Surg. 1997;1:505–10.

Patti MG, Fisichella PM, Perretta S, et al. Impact of minimally invasive surgery on the treatment of achalasia. A decade of change. J Am Coll Surg. 2003;196:698–705.

Patti MG, Fisichella PM. Laparoscopic Heller myotomy and Dor fundoplication for esophageal achalasia. How I do it. J Gastrointest Surg. 2008;12:764–6.

Patti MG, Galvani C, Gorodner MV, Tedesco P. Timing of surgical intervention does not influence return of esophageal peristalsis or outcome for patients with achalasia. Surg Endosc. 2005a;19:1188–92.

Patti MG, Gorodner MV, Galvani C, et al. Spectrum of esophageal motility disorders: implications for diagnosis and treatment. Arch Surg. 2005b;140:442–8.

Patti MG, Herbella FA. Fundoplication after laparoscopic Heller myotomy for esophageal achalasia. What type? J Gastrointest Surg. 2010;14:1453–8.

Perrone JM, Frisella MM, Desai KM, Soper NJ. Results of laparoscopic Heller-Toupet for achalasia. Surg Endosc. 2004 Nov;18(11):1565–71.

Petersen RP, Pellegrini CA. Revisional surgery after Heller myotomy for esophageal achalasia. Surg Laparosc Percutan Tech. 2010;5:321–5.

Portale G, Costantini M, Rizzetto C, et al. Long-term outcome of laparoscopic Heller-Dor surgery for esophageal achalasia. Possible detrimental role of previous endoscopic treatment. J Gastrointest Surg. 2005;9:1332–9.

Rebecchi F, Giaccone C, Farinella E, et al. Randomized control trial of laparoscopic Heller myotomy plus Dor fundoplication versus Nissen fundoplication for achalasia. Ann Surg. 2008;248:1023–30.

Richards WO, Torquati A, Holzman MD, et al. Heller myotomy versus Heller myotomy with Dor fundoplication. A prospective randomized double-blind clinical trial. Ann Surg. 2004;240:405–15.

Roll GR, Ma S, Gasper WJ, et al. Excellent outcome of laparoscopic esophagomyotomy for achalasia in patients older than 60 years of age. Surg Endosc. 2010;24:2562–6.

Rosemurgy AS, Morton CA, Rosas M, Albrink M, Roos SB. A single institution's experience with ore than 500 laparoscopic Heller myotomies for achalasia. J Am Coll Surg. 2010;210:637–45.

Smith CD, Stival A, Howell L, Swafford V. Endoscopic therapy for achalasia before Heller myotomy results in worse outcome than Heller myotomy alone. Ann Surg. 2006; 243:579–86.

Sweet MP, Nipomnick I, Gasper WJ, et al. The outcome of laparoscopic Heller myotomy for achalasia is not influenced by the degree of esophageal dilatation. J Gastrointest Surg. 2008;12:159–65.

Tatum RP, Pellegrini CA. How I Do It: Laparoscopic Heller Myotomy with Toupet Fundoplication for Achalasia. J Gastrointest Surg. 2009;13:1120–4.

Topart P, Deschamps C, Taillefer R, Duranceau A. Long-term effect of total fundoplication on the myotomized esophagus. Ann Thorac Surg. 1992;54:1046–51.

Zaninotto G, Constantini M, Rizzetto C, et al. Four hundred laparoscopic myotomies for esophageal achalasia: a single center experience. Ann Surg. 2008;248:986–93.

12. Laparoscopic Paraesophageal Hernia Repair

Nathaniel J. Soper, M.D.

A. Introduction

Laparoscopy is accepted as the standard operative approach for the surgical treatment of gastroesophageal reflux disease (GERD), and it is widely used for the repair of paraesophageal hiatal hernia (PEH). Although technically challenging, this approach provides excellent exposure of the surgical field and adds the known general advantages of laparoscopy in terms of reduced morbidity, more rapid recovery, short hospital stay, and decreased pain medication requirements compared with laparotomy or thoracotomy. These advantages are especially valuable in this patient population, since most PEH patients are elderly and many have significant multiple comorbidities.

The technical difficulty of laparoscopic repair of PEH is greater than that for laparoscopic antireflux surgery (LARS). The inherent difficulties of this operation include a compromised gastric wall (which has been incarcerated chronically in a mediastinal hernia sac), the necessity of excising the hernia sac without damaging critical structures, the difficulty of gaining exposure in a closed abdomen where there is a great laxity of the tissues, and the problem of closing the enlarged hiatus adequately. It is unwise for a laparoscopic surgeon to attempt repair of a PEH before performing 20–50 laparoscopic antireflux operations, the typical "learning curve" for LARS.

A classification system for hiatal hernias is given in Table 12.1.

N.T. Nguyen and C.E.H. Scott-Conner (eds.), *The SAGES Manual: Volume 2 Advanced Laparoscopy and Endoscopy*, DOI 10.1007/978-1-4614-2347-8_12,
© Springer Science+Business Media, LLC 2012

B. Indications for Surgery

Paraesophageal hernias account for only 5% of all hiatal hernias. In all types of PEH (II-IV), the herniated stomach lies besides the thoracic esophagus. When left untreated, PEH may lead to life-threatening complications, which include hemorrhage, strangulation, and volvulus (Table 12.2). If the blood supply is compromised, necrosis and perforation may occur, with mortality rate at this stage of disease approaching 50%. Traditionally, most surgeons believed that all paraesophageal hernias should be corrected electively on diagnosis, irrespective of symptoms, to prevent the development of complications and to avoid the risk of emergency surgery. However, recent evidence suggests that nonoperative management of asymptomatic patients is a reasonable alternative. Surgical repair of PEH is generally recommended for symptomatic patients. However, the operative strategy remains a matter of debate, as there is not a single technique guaranteeing uniform long-term success.

There are several controversies regarding laparoscopic repair of PEHs. These include the necessity of excising the hernia sac, the best technique for closing the diaphragm, the requirement of an antireflux procedure, and the need to perform a gastropexy. The reported recurrence

Table 12.1. Types of hiatal hernia.

I.	Sliding hiatal hernia; migration of the gastroesophageal junction (GEJ) into the thorax
II.	Isolated paraesophageal hernia with the GEJ in its normal anatomic location below the diaphragm; however, the proximal stomach protrudes through the hiatus, "rolling" alongside the distal esophagus
III.	Upward displacement of the GEJ above the diaphragm, with the stomach protruding cephalad adjacent to the esophagus
IV.	Herniation of other viscera through the esophageal hiatus, usually in association with types I to III

Table 12.2. Complications of paraesophageal hernia.

1. Bleeding from associated esophagitis, erosions (Cameron ulcers), or a discrete esophageal ulcer resulting in anemia
2. Gastric volvulus with strangulation is a surgical emergency if the stomach cannot be decompressed. The stomach becomes angulated in its midportion just proximal to the antrum (Fig. 12.1). (**Borchardt's triad:** chest pain, retching but no vomiting, and inability to pass a nasogastric tube.)
3. Incarceration of a paraesophageal hernia. Patients present with abrupt onset of vomiting and pain; may require immediate operative intervention
4. Torsion, obstruction, gangrene, perforation

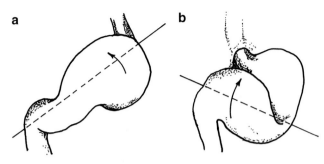

Fig. 12.1. (**a**) Organoaxial rotation. (**b**) Mesentericoaxial rotation.

rate for laparoscopic PEH repair has varied widely. If patients are followed closely, the reported recurrence rates range from 10 to 42%, especially when routine postoperative X-ray contrast studies are performed.

C. Preoperative Evaluation

1. Clinical Presentation

Most patients are symptomatic, but there is no clear correlation between the size of the hiatal hernia and severity of the symptoms.

   a. **Symptoms**
- i. Asymptomatic in a minority of patients
- ii. Vague epigastric or substernal discomfort
- iii. Postprandial fullness, nausea, dysphagia
- iv. Pulmonary complications are common: recurrent pneumonia; chronic atelectasis; dyspnea (pleural space compression by the huge hernia sac)
- v. GERD symptoms (heartburn, regurgitation)
- vi. Chronic anemia

   b. **Diagnostic Evaluation**
- i. **Chest radiograph** often demonstrates a retrocardiac air–fluid level.
- ii. **Barium upper-gastrointestinal series** establishes the diagnosis with greater accuracy and helps distinguish a sliding from a paraesophageal hernia.
- iii. **Upper endoscopy** is used to diagnose complications, such as erosive esophagitis, Cameron's ulcers (erosions of the

gastric mucosa at the site of entry into the hiatus), Barrett esophagus, and/or tumor. A hiatal hernia is confirmed by endoscopy on retroflexed views once inside the stomach.

iv. **Esophageal manometry** for the evaluation of esophageal motility disorders: Measurement of esophageal body peristalsis and lower esophageal sphincter position/length/pressure.

v. **Optional**: gastric emptying test, if significant nausea or postprandial fullness, **24-h pH test** to document GERD.

c. **Medical therapy**. No medical therapy will fix the anatomic abnormality of a hiatal hernia. Symptomatic management of PEH includes the reduction of gastroesophageal reflux, improving esophageal clearance, and reducing acid production. This is achieved in the majority of patients by modifying lifestyle factors, use of acid reduction medication, and enhancing esophageal and gastric motility.

d. **Surgical therapy**

i. A PEH in a symptomatic patient of suitable anesthetic risk is an indication for repair.

ii. Complications of GERD (strictures, ulcers, and bleeding) despite medical treatment (proton pump inhibitors) may also prompt repair. In addition, young patients with PEH and severe or recurrent complications of GERD may prefer to avoid long-term medication use.

iii. Patients with PEH and pulmonary complications (asthma, recurrent aspiration pneumonia, chronic cough, dyspnea, or hoarseness) are also potential surgical candidates.

D. Patient Position and Room Setup

1. Prepare and position the patient as for LARS (see Chap. 10). The operating room personnel and equipment are arranged with the surgeon between the patient's legs, the assistant surgeon on the patient's right, and the camera holder to the left.

2. Place video monitors at either side of the head of the table. These should be viewed easily by all members of the operating team and minimize strain on the core musculature of the operating surgeon.

3. Irrigation, suction, and electrocautery connections come off the head of the table on the patient's right side. Special instruments

include atraumatic endoscopic Babcock graspers, cautery scissors, curved dissectors, clip applier, atraumatic liver retractor, 5-mm needle holders, and ultrasonic coagulating shears.

4. Port arrangement should allow easy access to the hiatus and permit comfortable suturing by placing the optics between the surgeon's hands. Access to the abdominal cavity is achieved by either a closed or open technique superior to the umbilicus and just to the left of midline. The initial laparoscopic camera port should be placed higher on the abdominal wall than for Nissen fundoplications, because the dissection often needs to be performed well up into the mediastinum, and a low port placement renders poor visualization.

5. The initial port is placed 12–15 cm below the xiphoid. Four additional ports are placed under direct vision of the laparoscope. Ports are typically placed in the following locations to optimize visualization, tissue manipulation, and facilitate suturing (Fig. 12.2). A port is placed 3–4 cm inferior and to the right of the xiphoid process for the surgeon's left hand. Subcostal ports are placed in the midclavicular line on the right and left

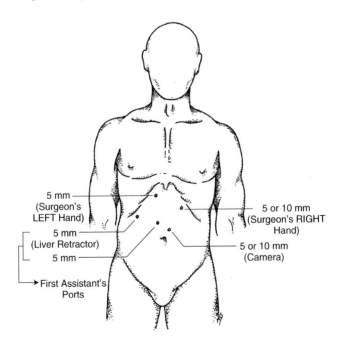

Fig. 12.2. Trocar placement for laparoscopic PEH repair.

sides. The fifth port is placed in the far right lateral subcostal position to insert the liver retractor.

6. With current 5-mm equipment and optics, we generally use only one 10- to 12-mm port, for the surgeon's right hand, to allow insertion of an SH needle through the valve mechanism.

E. Hernia Reduction

1. The surgeon and assistant first reduce as much of the intrathoracic contents of the hiatal hernia sac as much as possible, using atraumatic graspers and careful hand-over-hand technique.

2. Divide the gastrohepatic ligament, beginning just superior to the hepatic branch of the vagus nerve; this dissection is carried up to the medial border of the right crus of the diaphragm (Fig. 12.3).

3. To gain the appropriate plane for dissecting the hernia sac out of the mediastinum, aggressively divide the tissues that form the border between the sac and crural margin. Use the ultrasonic

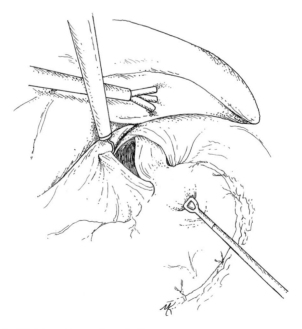

Fig. 12.3. Division of gastrohepatic ligament and exposure of the right crus of the diaphragm.

shears to target the medial border of the right crus of the diaphragm, and divide the endoabdominal and endothoracic fascia layers to create a plane between the right crus and the hernia sac in the supradiaphragmatic mediastinum.

4. Spreading motions of the surgeon's instruments open this plane further and allow the insufflated carbon dioxide to dissect some of the tissues away. Blunt dissection is continued up into the mediastinum while the sac is swept back toward the abdominal cavity. This combination of sharp and blunt dissection is continued until the entire anterior circumference of the crural arch has been freed from the hernia sac (Fig. 12.4). Use long blunt motions to sweep the sac inferiorly, exposing the right lateral border of the esophagus and posterior vagus nerve, as well as the anterior and left side of the esophagus and anterior vagus nerve. In a patient with no previous operations, the tissues usually separate readily. This sequence will divide and reduce the anterior component of the hernia sac, corresponding to the greater abdominal cavity.

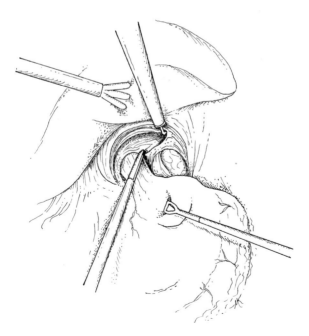

Fig. 12.4. Dissection of the hernia sac away from the right crus.

5. There are usually adhesions of variable density between the sac and the pleura and other mediastinal structures that must be divided with the harmonic shears. Small blood vessels connect the aorta directly to the esophagus posteriorly, which also must be divided.

F. Excision of the Hernia Sac

1. After the dissection of as much of the plane anterior to the esophagus as possible, divide the short gastric vessels. Enter the lesser sac to the left of the stomach, and divide the perifundic tissues up to the base of the left crus of the diaphragm.
2. Divide the endoabdominal and endothoracic fascia posterior to the esophagus at the medial border of the crura until a circumferential dissection has been undertaken and all of the sac has been pulled down beyond the lower esophagus and over the proximal stomach (Figs. 12.5 and 12.6). This sequence will divide and reduce the posterior component of the hernia sac, corresponding to the lesser sac cavity.
3. The sac itself may be allowed to remain attached to the proximal stomach if small, unobtrusive, and well vascularized; otherwise, it can be excised with impunity, while taking care to preserve the vagus nerves and avoid injury to the gastric and esophageal wall.

G. Mobilization of the Esophagus

Mobilize the intrathoracic esophagus as far proximally as possible. Most of the dissection can be done bluntly, but scar tissue or other adhesions may mandate using sharp or harmonic dissection to divide tissues tethering the esophagus. Maintain the vagal trunks in their position adjacent to the esophageal wall and use these as anatomical landmarks to direct the dissection. It is important to achieve adequate esophageal mobilization such that ~3 cm of intraabdominal esophagus is achieved without axial traction being applied.

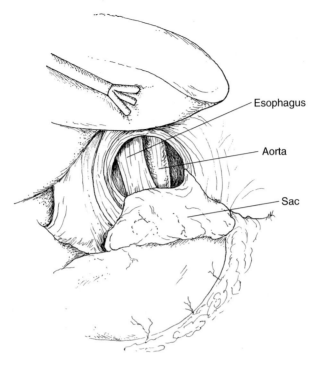

Fig. 12.5. Reduction of the hernia sac into the abdominal cavity away from mediastinal structures.

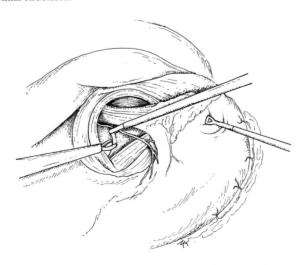

Fig. 12.6. Dissection posterior to the esophagus within the mediastinum.

H. Closure of the Hiatal Defect

1. After the hernia sac has been dissected completely from the mediastinum, there is a space of variable size separating the crura. Because this space is shaped like an inverted teardrop, there is less distance between the right and left crura posterior to the esophagus (near the origin of the crural leaves) than anterior to it. Decreasing the intraabdominal pressure delivered by the insufflator to 8–10 mm Hg may help reduce tension on the diaphragm during crural closure.

2. Approximate the right and left crura, beginning posteriorly and working anteriorly. In closing the crura from their posterior aspect, the esophagus is transposed anteriorly toward the dome of the diaphragm, thereby effectively lengthening it, because the distance between the dome of the diaphragm and the oropharynx is less than that from the oropharynx to the posterior aspect of the diaphragm.

3. We currently use unpledgeted 0- or 2–0 gauge braided polyester sutures for the closure and try to incorporate endoabdominal fascia on the abdominal surface of the crura to minimize tearing of the crural muscle (Fig. 12.7).

4. Place sutures until either the hiatal hernia is completely closed posterior to the esophagus or the esophagus has been moved anteriorly to the point that it appears to be angulated. The crura can almost always be closed primarily. When closed adequately, the crura will be just touching the walls of the empty esophagus.

5. If the hiatal defect is too large to be closed primarily without tension, a bioprosthetic patch may be used.

6. If a space remains between the crura anterior to the esophagus, additional anterior sutures may be placed after the fundoplication has been performed.

7. The routine use of prosthetic material to decrease hernia recurrence is controversial. Polypropylene or PTFE material may erode into the esophagus or stomach. The use of bioprosthetic patches may decrease the early recurrence of hiatal hernias, but may have little impact on long-term outcomes.

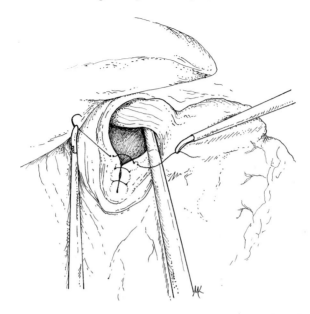

Fig. 12.7. The crural opening is closed with simple, interrupted nonabsorbable suture (0 Ethibond). For large defects, pledgets and/or bioprosthetic mesh may be used.

I. Fundoplication

1. After the hiatal hernia has been repaired, we advocate performing a fundoplication (Fig. 12.8; see also Chap. 10), usually a Nissen fundoplication, to prevent postoperative GERD. Even in the absence of preoperative GERD, the extensive mobilization of the GE junction will likely lead to significant postoperative GERD if this step is not taken.

2. In patients with normal preoperative esophageal motor function, a complete fundoplication is performed, whereas a partial fundoplication is used in patients with poor esophageal motility.

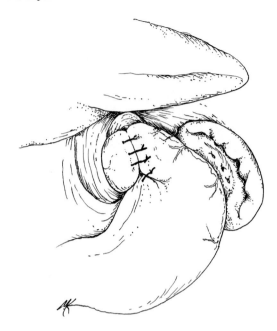

Fig. 12.8. A 2-cm, 360° wrap is created using three interrupted, nonabsorbable sutures with care to avoid the anterior vagus.

J. Gastropexy

1. After the completion of the fundoplication, an anterior gastropexy may be performed. The use of gastropexy is controversial. We reserve gastropexies for patients in whom most of the stomach was in the chest and those with organoaxial volvulus of the stomach. In these situations, anterior gastropexy can either be performed by placing a gastrostomy tube, or the anterior gastric wall can simply be sutured to the posterior abdominal wall.

2. Brown-Mueller **T**-fasteners (Ross Laboratories, Columbus, OH) are ideally suited to perform a simple, fast, and effective anterior gastropexy (Fig. 12.9). Grasp the anterior gastric wall with Babcock forceps at the greater curvature of the antrum of the stomach. Gently pull this portion of the stomach anteriorly to assess whether it reaches the posterior abdominal wall without tension, remembering that the pneumoperitoneum increases this distance.

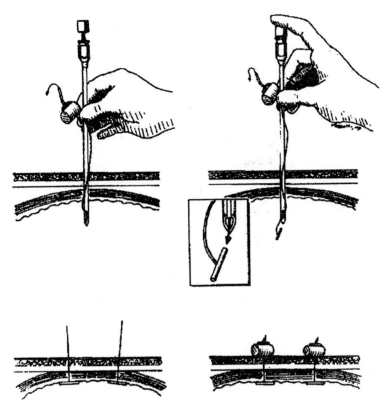

Fig. 12.9. Use of **T**-fasteners for anterior gastropexy.

3. If necessary, reduce the pneumoperitoneum pressure.
4. Lightly score the gastric wall with monopolar electrocautery to stimulate subsequent adhesion formation.
5. Place a **T**-fastener within the slotted needle and pass it percutaneously through the skin of the epigastrium several centimeters inferior to the costal margin. Pass the needle tip into the gastric lumen while elevating the stomach slightly.
6. Next, use the stylet to dislodge the metal bar of the **T**-fastener from the needle, causing the bar to turn sideways and reside within the lumen of the stomach.
7. Place two additional **T**-fasteners in a triangulated configuration with a distance of approximately 2 cm around each **T**-fastener.

8. After these three **T**-fasteners have been placed, slowly exsufflate the abdominal cavity, allowing the carbon dioxide to escape while gently retracting all three **T**-fasteners. In this manner, the stomach is pulled to the anterior abdominal wall under direct vision, preventing interposition of colon or other intraabdominal viscera between the stomach and anterior abdominal wall.

9. The **T**-fasteners are allowed to remain for 2–4 weeks, at which time the nylon suture is cut at the level of the skin, and the metal bar is allowed to pass through the intestinal tract.

K. Postoperative Care

1. A nasogastric tube is not used unless the patient requires gastric decompression for relief of nausea or abdominal distention. Intravenous antiemetics are administered prophylactically.

2. The patients are more frail and elderly and often do not take a full diet as quickly.

3. Clear liquids are given the morning of the first postoperative day and advanced to a soft diet as tolerated.

4. Patients are usually discharged on the first or second postoperative day.

5. Early postoperative contrast studies of the upper GI tract are necessary only in patients with worrisome symptoms—retching, significant chest pain, or significant early dysphagia.

L. Complications

1. Intraoperative pleural injury/capnopneumothorax is the result of inadvertent entry into the pleura during the mediastinal dissection. This event occurs in up to a third of patients undergoing laparoscopic PEH repair, but clinically significant pleural injuries rarely occur, and a chest tube is almost never indicated. The balance between positive airway pressure and pneumoperitoneum pressure may be adjusted if necessary. Dissection close to the esophagus may prevent pleural injury. At the

conclusion of the procedure, suction is applied transhiatally to the mediastinum while administering vital capacity breaths to allow venting of the pneumoperitoneum through the trocar sites. A postoperative chest radiograph is obtained only if the patient experiences respiratory distress.

2. Bleeding from the short gastric vessels is an uncommon complication, which can be managed with the ultrasonic scalpel or a clip.

3. Splenic injury/liver injury during retraction and dissection can occur. An atraumatic liver retractor and gentle, meticulous technique will in general prevent severe hemorrhage. Most bleeding can be stopped by direct pressure or with topical hemostatic agents.

4. Esophageal perforation occurs in less than 1% of cases. Patients with severe periesophageal inflammation are at greater risk for injury given that tissue planes are less clear. Prevention of injury includes circumferentially dissecting the esophagus under direct vision with an angled laparoscope, and not directly grasping the esophagus for retraction. Repair of simple perforations can involve laparoscopic placement of interrupted sutures with coverage by the fundoplication.

Selected References

Diaz S, Brunt LM, Klingensmith ME, Frisella P, Soper NJ. Laparoscopic paraesophageal hernia repair, a challenging operation. Medium-term outcome of 116 patients. J Gastrointest Surg. 2003;7(1):59–67.

Gantert WA, Patti MG, Arcerito M, et al. Laparoscopic repair of paraesophageal hiatal hernias. J Am Coll Surg. 1998;186:428–32.

Hashemi M, Peters JH, DeMeester TR, et al. Laparoscopic repair of large type III hiatal hernia: objective follow-up reveals high recurrence rate. J Am Coll Surg. 2000;190:553–60.

Mattar SG, Bowers SP, Galloway KD, Hunter JG, Smith CD. Long-term outcome of laparoscopic repair of paraesophageal hernia. Surg Endosc. 2002;16:745–9.

Oddsdottir M. Paraesophageal hernia. Surg Clin North Am. 2000;80:1243–52.

Oelschlaeger BK, Pellegrini CA, Hunter JG, et al. Biologic prosthesis reduces recurrences after laparoscopic paraesophageal hernia repair: a multi-center prospective randomized trial. Ann Surg. 2006;244:481–90.

Stylopulos N, Gazzele MS, Rattner DW. Paraesophageal hernias: operation or observation. Ann Surg. 2002;236(4):492–500.

Trus TL, Bax T, Richardson WS, et al. Complications of laparoscopic paraesophageal hernia repair. J Gastrointest Surg. 1997;1(3):1221–28.

Willekes CL, Edoga JK, Frezza EE. Laparoscopic repair of paraesophageal hernia. Ann Surg. 1997;225:31–8.

Wu JS, Dunnegan DL, Soper NJ. Clinical and radiologic assessment of laparoscopic paraesophageal hernia repair. Surg Endosc. 1998;13:497–502.

13. Minimally Invasive Esophagectomy

Ninh T. Nguyen, M.D.
Esteban Varela, M.D.

A. Introduction

The enthusiasm for minimally invasive surgery, which began with the first laparoscopic cholecystectomy, has since expanded to many other areas of abdominal and thoracic surgery. The speed by which acceptance of a new minimally invasive operation evolves is often a reflection of the degree of technical difficulty of the procedure and the frequency of performance of the operation. For example, within only a few years of the first clinical report of laparoscopic cholecystectomy, the number of laparoscopic cholecystectomies performed in the USA exceeded that of open cholecystectomies. In contrast, it took more than 5 years from the first report of laparoscopic Roux-en-Y gastric bypass for the treatment of morbid obesity before widespread dissemination of this complex operation occurred. It was not until 2004 that the number of laparoscopic gastric bypass operations exceeded that of open gastric bypass. Open esophageal resection for benign or malignant disease is another complex gastrointestinal operation, and minimally invasive surgical approaches have been reported since 1992. However, to date, there have been only a few large studies reporting outcomes of minimally invasive esophagectomy (MIE). Although every imaginable technique for MIE has been described in the literature, it is difficult to determine the best minimally invasive approach for esophageal resection due to the limited experience with this complex operation at most centers. We reported on an initial experience of thoracoscopic and laparoscopic esophagectomy performed on 46 consecutive patients with a mean follow-up of 26 months. In a

N.T. Nguyen and C.E.H. Scott-Conner (eds.), *The SAGES Manual: Volume 2*
Advanced Laparoscopy and Endoscopy, DOI 10.1007/978-1-4614-2347-8_13,
© Springer Science+Business Media, LLC 2012

recent series of 104 consecutive patients, we demonstrated MIE to be technically feasible, safe, and associated with a low conversion rate (2.9%), short length of hospital stay (median 8 days), and acceptable morbidity and mortality (2.9%). This chapter describes the indications for surgery, preoperative workup, different minimally invasive surgical approaches, complications, and patient follow-up after MIE.

B. Indications

Indications for esophagectomy include both benign and malignant esophageal and gastric pathology. Benign pathology of the esophagus requiring esophagectomy includes severe recalcitrant esophageal stricture from complication of gastroesophageal reflux, esophageal injury and stricture from lye ingestion, and end-stage achalasia. The most common condition requiring esophagectomy is esophageal cancer at various stages starting with carcinoma in situ to T4 cancer. Additionally, a small number of patients undergo esophagectomy for Barrett's esophagus with high-grade dysplasia. Another major indication for esophagectomy is gastric cardia cancer with involvement of the gastroesophageal junction. In this condition, an Ivor Lewis esophagogastrectomy is often performed to obtain clear proximal and distal margins.

C. Preoperative Evaluation

Standard preoperative workup for patients with esophageal or gastric cardia cancer includes upper endoscopy with biopsy, barium swallow, endoscopic esophageal ultrasound, computed tomography (CT) scan of the chest and abdomen, and positron emission tomography (PET). In selected cases, cardiopulmonary evaluation is performed, including pulmonary function testing and a 2D echocardiogram. If patients are considered to be surgical candidates after these evaluations, they will undergo laparoscopic staging and placement of a jejunostomy feeding catheter approximately 2–10 days prior to resection. At the time of laparoscopic staging, patients undergo placement of a 10-F jejunostomy catheter and gastric ischemic conditioning with division of the left gastric pedicle using a linear stapler.

D. Surgical Approaches

1. Thoracoscopic and Laparoscopic Esophagectomy with Cervical Anastomosis

Routine upper endoscopy is performed in the operating room immediately prior to surgical resection to determine the upper and lower extent of the cancer. The operation is typically conducted in three stages.

a. First Stage

i.   Place the patient in the left lateral decubitus position. Single-lung ventilation with collapse of the right lung is used to enable exposure.

ii.   Introduce four thoracic trocars into the right chest. Carbon-dioxide insufflation is not used during thoracoscopy.

iii. Retract the lung anteriorly.

iv.   Divide the mediastinal pleura overlying the esophagus to expose the intrathoracic esophagus and the azygous vein. Divide the azygos vein with a linear stapler.

v.   Pass a Penrose drain around the esophagus to facilitate esophageal retraction.

vi.   Circumferentially mobilize the esophagus from the esophageal hiatus up to the thoracic inlet.

vii. Dissect paraesophageal lymph nodes and maintain these nodes en bloc with the surgical specimen. Perform a subcarinal lymph node dissection.

viii. Insert a 28-F chest tube at the 12-mm trocar site for postoperative drainage and have the anesthesiologist reinflate the right lung.

b. Second Stage

i.   Reposition the patient supine.

ii.   Insert five abdominal ports. A 12-mm trocar is placed in the left midclavicular line, below the umbilicus. Another 12-mm trocar is placed in the midline above the umbilicus. A 5-mm trocar is placed in the right subcostal region with another 5-mm trocar placed in the right anterior axillary line, below the costal margin. Lastly, a 5-mm trocar is placed in the left anterior axillary line, below the costal margin.

iii.   Mobilize the greater curvature of the stomach, preserving the right gastroepiploic vessels.

iv.   If not divided at the time of laparoscopic staging, isolate and divide the left gastric vessels with a linear stapler.

v.   Resect lymph nodes along the celiac axis en bloc with the surgical specimen.

vi.   We do not perform pyloroplasty since changing our technique to construction of a tubular gastric conduit.

vii.   Construct the gastric conduit by dividing the stomach, starting on the lesser curvature and finishing at the angle of His.

viii. Temporarily suture the tip of the gastric conduit to the esophageal specimen for later retraction.

c. Third Stage

i.   Create a horizontal incision on the left neck, one fingerbreadth above the suprasternal notch.

ii.   Mobilize the cervical esophagus to communicate with the dissection plane achieved in the right chest.

iii.   Deliver the entire esophageal specimen with the attached gastric conduit up through the cervical incision.

iv.   Construct an esophagogastric anastomosis either with a 21-mm circular stapler or the two-layer hand-sewn technique.

2. Laparoscopic and Thoracoscopic Ivor Lewis Resection

This approach consists of laparoscopic construction of the gastric conduit and thoracoscopic esophageal resection with thoracic removal of the surgical specimen and construction of a high intrathoracic esophagogastric anastomosis. This is currently our preferred approach for MIE.

a. First Stage

i.   Position the patient supine.

ii.   Place five abdominal ports as described in the above section.

iii.   Mobilize the greater curvature of the stomach by dividing the short gastric vessels.

iv.   Divide the left gastric vessels with a linear stapler.

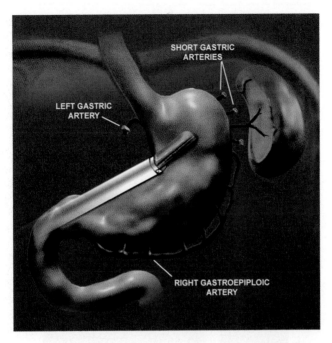

Fig. 13.1. Laparoscopic construction of a gastric conduit (reprinted with permission from Nguyen NT, et al. Minimally invasive esophagectomy: lessons learned from 104 operations. Ann Surg. 2008;248(6):1081–91).

v.   Construct the gastric conduit. During this construction, the green stapler load is often used for the first application along the lesser curvature of the stomach, and then blue stapler loads are used as the stomach thins out toward the angle of His (Fig. 13.1).

vi. Temporarily attach the tip of the gastric conduit to the surgical specimen with interrupted sutures.

vii. Circumferentially mobilize the esophagus for a length of 5–6 cm into the mediastinum.

viii. Pass a Penrose drain around the distal esophagus for retrieval during the thoracic portion of the operation (Fig. 13.2).

ix. Finally, the proximal jejunum is sutured to the peritoneum of the abdominal wall. A 10-F jejunostomy catheter is placed into the jejunum using the Seldinger technique. A Witzel tunnel is performed around the entrance of the catheter.

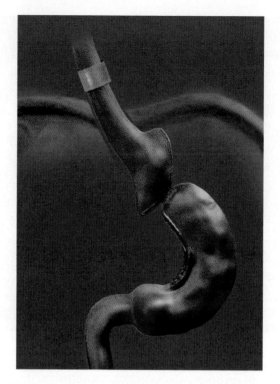

Fig. 13.2. The tip of the gastric conduit is temporarily sutured to the surgical specimen in preparation for gastric pull-up. A Penrose drain is positioned around the esophagus in the mediastinum for retrieval in the thorax (reprinted with permission from Nguyen et al. Nguyen NT, et al. Minimally invasive esophagectomy: lessons learned from 104 operations. Ann Surg. 2008;248(6):1081–91).

b. Second Stage

    i.   Reposition the patient to the left lateral decubitus position with single-lung ventilation to collapse the right lung.

    ii. Introduce four thoracic trocars into the right chest (Fig. 13.3).

    iii. Retract the right lung anteriorly for exposure of the mediastinal esophagus.

    iv. Divide the mediastinal pleura overlying the esophagus.

    v. Locate the previously placed Penrose drain and use it to retract and mobilize the esophagus from the esophageal hiatus up to the level of the azygous vein (Fig. 13.4).

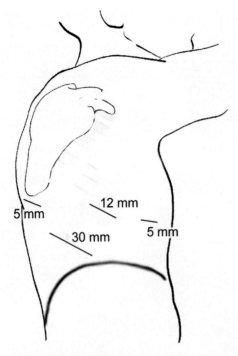

5 mm

12 mm

30 mm   5 mm

Fig. 13.3. Trocar position for thoracoscopic esophagectomy (reprinted with permission from Nguyen NT, et al. Minimally invasive esophagectomy: lessons learned from 104 operations. Ann Surg. 2008;248(6):1081–91).

vi.   Isolate and divide the azygous vein with a linear stapler (Fig. 13.5).

vii. Pull the esophageal specimen and the attached gastric conduit into the right thoracic cavity.

viii. Divide the esophagus at the level of the azygous vein (Fig. 13.6).

ix.   Place the specimen into a protective bag and remove it through a 4-cm thoracic incision without rib resection.

x.   Create the esophagogastric anastomosis with the linear stapler, hand-sewn or circular stapler technique.

xi.   For the circular stapler technique, place the 25-mm anvil transthoracically into the esophageal stump and secure it with a purse-string suture (Fig. 13.7).

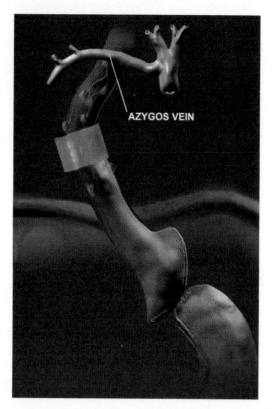

AZYGOS VEIN

Fig. 13.4. Thoracoscopic esophageal mobilization using the Penrose drain to retract the esophagus (reprinted with permission from Nguyen NT, et al. Minimally invasive esophagectomy: lessons learned from 104 operations. Ann Surg. 2008;248(6):1081–91).

xii.   Make a gastrotomy at the tip of the gastric conduit and the place the 25-mm circular stapler transthoracically into the gastric conduit to create a stapled esophagogastric anastomosis (Fig. 13.8). A nasogastric tube is placed under direct visualization into the gastric conduit.

xiii.   Staple the gastrotomy closed with a linear stapler (Fig. 13.9).

xiv.   Place a 28-F chest tube and a Jackson Pratt drain in the pleural cavity for postoperative chest drainage (Fig. 13.10) and allow the right lung to re-expand.

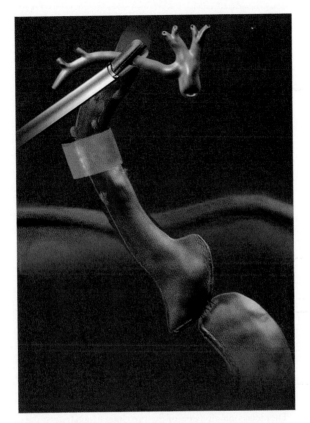

Fig. 13.5. Thoracoscopic division of the azygous vein (reprinted with permission from Nguyen NT, et al. Minimally invasive esophagectomy: lessons learned from 104 operations. Ann Surg. 2008;248(6):1081–91).

E. Postoperative Care and Follow-up

a. Extubate the patient in the operating room prior to transfer to the ICU for cardiorespiratory monitoring.

b. Provide postoperative analgesia by patient-controlled analgesia.

c. Perform a Gastrografin contrast study on postoperative days 3–6.

d. Remove the chest and nasogastric tubes when the contrast study demonstrates an intact anastomosis.

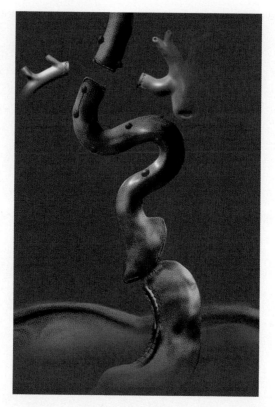

Fig. 13.6. Thoracoscopic division of the proximal esophagus at the level of the azygous vein using a linear stapler (reprinted with permission from Nguyen NT, et al. Minimally invasive esophagectomy: lessons learned from 104 operations. Ann Surg. 2008;248(6):1081–91).

e. Discharge the patient home with the right-chest Jackson Pratt drain in place, for removal at the first clinic visit.

f. Supplemental jejunostomy tube feedings are given for 2–3 weeks and the tube is removed thereafter.

g. Patients are seen for follow-up at 3-month intervals for a year and yearly thereafter.

h. CT scans of the chest and abdomen are performed yearly after surgery for patients with cancer.

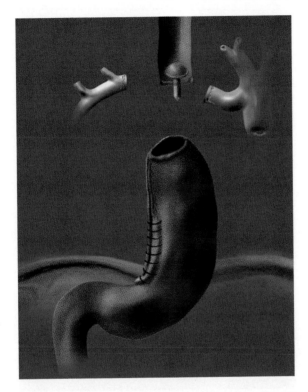

Fig. 13.7. The anvil is placed within the esophageal stump and a gastrotomy is performed at the tip of the gastric conduit (reprinted with permission from Nguyen NT, et al. Minimally invasive esophagectomy: lessons learned from 104 operations. Ann Surg. 2008;248(6):1081–91).

F. Complications

1. Intraoperative Complications

Intraoperative complications during MIE are divided into complications during thoracoscopy or complications during laparoscopy. Complications during thoracoscopy may include bleeding during transection of the azygous vein and potential injury to the pulmonary parenchyma, the pulmonary hilum (particularly the inferior pulmonary vein), or the trachea and bronchus. Complications during laparoscopy include bleeding during division of the left gastric vessels and short gastric vessels, and

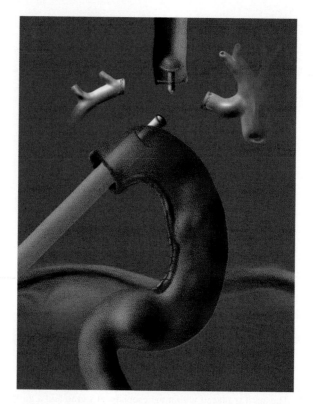

Fig. 13.8. The 25-mm circular stapler is placed transthoracically into the gastric conduit in preparation for construction of the esophagogastric anastomosis (reprinted with permission from Nguyen NT, et al. Minimally invasive esophagectomy: lessons learned from 104 operations. Ann Surg. 2008;248(6):1081–91).

inadvertent devascularization of the gastric conduit with interruption of the right gastroepiploic vessels.

2. Early Postoperative Complications

Early complications include postoperative bleeding, atelectasis, respiratory failure, prolonged chest tube air leak, pneumonia, chylothorax, arrhythmia, myocardial infarction, deep venous thrombosis, hoarseness, urinary retention, anastomotic leak, or gastric conduit

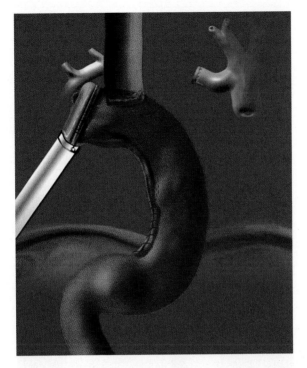

Fig. 13.9. The tip of the gastric conduit is closed with a linear stapler (reprinted with permission from Nguyen NT, et al. Minimally invasive esophagectomy: lessons learned from 104 operations. Ann Surg. 2008;248(6):1081–91).

staple-line failure. Leak is one of the most serious complications after esophagectomy, particularly if it is in the chest. In the neck, anastomotic leaks often can be treated by opening the neck wound and local wound care; however, even leak in the neck can track into the chest, resulting in the development of an empyema. Management of a thoracic leak depends on site and extent of the defect. The options for treatment include placement of a T-tube drain through the gastrointestinal opening with wide drainage of the pleural cavity and, more recently, endoscopic stenting. If a large staple-line dehiscence is encountered, proximal esophageal diversion may be necessary.

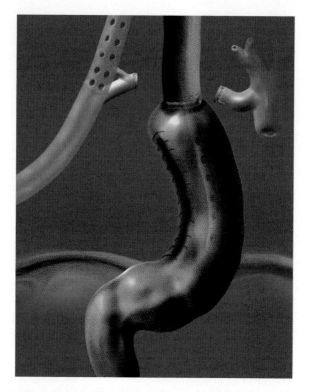

Fig. 13.10. Final intraoperative view showing a reinforced gastric conduit staple line. A nasogastric tube is positioned within the gastric conduit and a chest tube is placed in the pleural space for postoperative drainage (reprinted with permission from Nguyen NT, et al. Minimally invasive esophagectomy: lessons learned from 104 operations. Ann Surg. 2008;248(6):1081–91).

3. Late Complications

Late complications include mostly anastomotic stricture and, occasionally, delayed gastric emptying. The preferred treatment of anastomotic stricture is endoscopic balloon dilation. Delayed gastric emptying is uncommon but can occur even after a pyloroplasty. Treatment consists of endoscopic dilation and/or Botox injection of the pylorus.

G. Outcomes

The largest MIE study to date was reported by Luketich and colleagues from the University of Pittsburgh Medical Center. They reported on outcomes of 222 patients who underwent MIE. Conversion to open procedure was required in 7.2% of cases. The median intensive care unit stay was 1 day with a median hospital stay of 7 days. The operative mortality was 1.4% and the anastomotic leak rate was 11.7%. In a report of 104 MIE operations, we reported a conversion rate of 2.9%. The median intensive care stay was 2 days and the median hospital stay was 8 days. The incidence of leak was 9.6% with an in-hospital mortality of 2.9%. The mean number of lymph nodes retrieved was 13.8 nodes. At a mean follow-up of 54 months, the Kaplan–Meier 5-year survival for stages 0 and I, II, II, and IV were 96, 69, 20, and 0%, respectively.

Selected References

Kawahara K, Maekawa T, Okabayashi K, et al. Video-assisted thoracoscopic esophagectomy for esophageal cancer. Surg Endosc. 1999;13:218–23.

Luketich JD, Alvelo-Rivera M, Buenaventura PO, et al. Minimally invasive esophagectomy: outcomes in 222 patients. Ann Surg. 2003;238:486–95.

Nguyen NT, Follette DM, Wolfe BM, Schneider PD, Roberts P, Goodnight Jr JE. Comparison of minimally invasive esophagectomy with transthoracic and transhiatal esophagectomy. Arch Surg. 2000;135:920–5.

Nguyen NT, Roberts P, Follette DM, et al. Thoracoscopic and laparoscopic esophagectomy for benign and malignant disease: lessons learned from 46 consecutive procedures. J Am Coll Surg. 2003;197:902–13.

Nguyen NT, Longoria M, Sabio A, et al. Preoperative laparoscopic ligation of the left gastric vessels in preparation for esophagectomy. Ann Thorac Surg. 2006a;81:2318–20.

Nguyen NT, Longoria M, Chang K, et al. Thoracolaparoscopic modification of the Ivor Lewis esophagogastrectomy. J Gastrointest Surg. 2006b;10:450–4.

Nguyen NT, Hinojosa MW, Smith BR, Chang KJ, Gray J, Hoyt D. Minimally invasive esophagectomy: lessons learned from 104 operations. Ann Surg. 2008;248(6):1081–91.

Varela E, Reavis KM, Hinojosa MW, Nguyen NT. Laparoscopic gastric ischemic conditioning prior to esophagogastrectomy: technique and review. Surg Innov. 2008;15(2):132–5.

14. Robotic Esophageal Surgery

Brendan Marr, M.D.
W. Scott Melvin, M.D.

A. Introduction

Surgical procedures of the esophagus provide a challenging dissection. A mucosa-lined muscular tube lacking a serosa, the esophagus traverses three compartments of the body as it makes its way from the pharynx to the stomach. Access to the esophagus has proven somewhat difficult requiring thoracotomy in some procedures, as well as blind dissection in others. It lies in close proximity to the great vessels and takes much of its blood supply directly from the aorta. Furthermore, the esophagus is bounded by fascia anteriorly and posteriorly as well as confined distally by the diaphragmatic crura. Operations on the esophagus are frequently associated with high morbidity and mortality rates. Historically, several open techniques have been described for esophageal procedures. These procedures eventually gave way to minimally invasive techniques. Minimally invasive procedures provide shorter operative times, decreased blood loss, and shorter length of stay. The minimally invasive procedures also result in fewer pulmonary complications for postoperative patients.

The first laparoscopic transhiatal esophagectomy was reported by De Paula et al. in 1995. However, minimally invasive esophageal procedures can be technically challenging and have a steep learning curve. This precipitated a strong interest in the application of the surgical robotic technology to esophageal procedures. While the surgical robot was quick to catch on for prostatectomy, it has not been as rapidly adapted to other surgical fields. The anatomic considerations of the esophagus lend itself quite well to robotic dissections. Robotic assisted minimally invasive surgery allows for precise dissection and manipulation in a confined operating space. Our chapter examines the application to and feasibility of surgical robotic technology to various esophageal surgical procedures,

N.T. Nguyen and C.E.H. Scott-Conner (eds.), *The SAGES Manual: Volume 2*   221
Advanced Laparoscopy and Endoscopy, DOI 10.1007/978-1-4614-2347-8_14,
© Springer Science+Business Media, LLC 2012

including transthoracic and transhiatal esophagectomy, myotomy for achalasia, and benign resection of localized esophageal mass.

B. The Advantages of Robotic Esophageal Surgery

Robotic surgery holds several advantages over conventional laparoscopy. These advantages are most valuable when operating in a confined or restricted area, for which esophageal surgery certainly qualifies.

1. Among the advantages is improved visualization. Conventional laparoscopy provides two dimensional viewing. The surgical robot uses two separate lenses to provide true three dimensional vision. Furthermore, the surgical robot provides magnification of 5–15× which is greater than conventional laparoscopy. The visualization advantages are particularly beneficial when dissecting the esophagus which has structures like the thoracic duct and vagus nerves in very close proximity.

2. Another advantage is the elimination of tremor. In minimally invasive esophageal surgery, this phenomenon can be exacerbated because of the distance from the operating port to the tissue being dissected. The fulcrum, or pivot point, of the port is closer to the operator's hand than it is to the tip of the instrument, magnifying the tremor effect. This is eliminated with the surgical robot.

3. Furthermore, the confined area in which the esophagus is located makes dissection with the fixed tips of conventional laparoscopic instruments a challenge. The surgical robot has tips which angulate at multiple angles making dissection and suturing much easier. These instruments imitate the human wrist, but have an even greater range of motion.

C. Robotic Esophageal Procedures

1. **Esophagectomy**. Robotic esophagectomy has been performed through both transabdominal and transthoracic approaches. Although first utilized by Melvin et al. in 2002, the first robotic-assisted esophagectomy was described by Horgan et al. in 2003.

In that report, a 56-year-old male with history of Barrett's esophagus had a positive endoscopic biopsy for adenocarcinoma. The patient underwent robotic-assisted resection of the esophagus. The procedure was performed transabdominally consisting of a cervical esophagogastrostomy with gastric conduit. Total operative time was 246 min. The robotic portion was 52 min. Estimated blood loss was less than 50 ml. The final pathology revealed a well-differentiated T1N0M0 adenocarcinoma with negative margins. The authors concluded that the robotic procedure was most appropriate for patients diagnosed at an early stage. Interestingly, the authors also noted that one of the advantages the surgical robot provided was a 7.5 cm increased instrument length affording greater proximal dissection.

Kernstine and colleagues described the first combined transthoracic and transabdominal robotic esophagectomy in 2004. The procedure was performed on a 59-year-old male with ulcerated esophageal adenocarcinoma. The patient was preoperatively judged to have T3N0 disease. A two-stage operation was performed in which the patient was placed in a nearly prone position for the transthoracic stage then supine for the transabdominal stage. An esophagogastrostomy was completed through a separate cervical incision after fashioning a gastric conduit. The resection included the esophagus and adjacent thoracic duct, as well as the periesophageal and peritracheal nodes. Total operative time was 11 h. The robotic portion was 4 h 20 min. Estimated blood loss was 900 ml.

Since these initial case reports, several series have subsequently been published. In 2005 Bodner et al. reported a robotic-assisted transthoracic esophagectomy successfully performed on three patients with squamous cell and adenocarcinoma. The median operative time was 173 min with 147 min of time spent at the robotic console. It should be noted that this time applies only to the thoracic portion of the case and does not include the cervical or abdominal portions which were performed open. Average number of lymph nodes harvested was 12.

van Hillegersberg et al. (2006) reported transthoracic robotic esophagectomy in 21 patients of which 18 were performed successfully. Three of these procedures were converted to open for extensive adhesions, bulky adhesive tumor, and bleeding. Similar to the prior study the robot was used for the thoracic portion of the case while the cervical and abdominal portions were performed open. Total median operative time was 450 min with 180 min for the thoracic portion. Median estimated blood loss was 400 ml. Median lymph nodes harvested was 20.

In 2007, Galvani and colleagues presented a study of successful robotically assisted esophagectomy in 18 patients utilizing transhiatal technique. The majority (50%) of these cases were performed for high grade dysplasia; however, 12% had adenocarcinoma in situ, 28% had T1N0M0 lesions, 5% had T2N0M0 lesions, and 5% had T3N0M0 lesions. Total median operative time was 267 min and average estimated blood loss was 54 ml. The average number of lymph nodes harvested was 14.

Also in 2007, Kernstine et al. published a series of completely robotic three field esophagectomies. Their study consisted of 14 patients, 12 with cancer (4 squamous and 8 adenocarcinoma) and 2 cases of high grade dysplasia. The participants were divided into three groups with varying portions of the operation performed robotically. Eight of the patients had a complete three field robotic esophagectomy. Total mean operative time was 666 min. Average estimated blood loss was 400 ml. Average number of lymph nodes obtained was 18.

Kim et al. published a series of 21 patients in 2010 that underwent transthoracic robotic esophagectomy. These patients were in prone position as the authors felt it facilitated mediastinal dissection and minimized lung injury. The vast majority (95.2%) had a diagnosis of squamous cell carcinoma with one patient with adenocarcinoma. In all patients, the thoracic portion of the case was completed robotically. The abdominal portion of the case was performed robotically in four patients. Esophagogastrostomy with gastric conduit was performed through a cervical incision. Total median operative time was 410 min of which 108 min were robotic. Average estimated blood loss was 150 ml. Average number of lymph nodes harvested was 11.6 mediastinal and 21.1 abdominal.

All the studies noted were similar in that they had no 30-day mortality with the exception of the Van Hillegersberg series that had a single mortality due to tracheo-neo-esophageal fistula requiring pneumonectomy. Average number of lymph nodes obtained ranged from 12 to 38. Average estimated blood loss ranged from 50 to 900 ml. Rate of anastomotic leak ranged from 2 to 6%. These figures compare favorably to the outcomes achieved in open and laparoscopic studies. It should be noted however that there have been no comparative trials of robotic-assisted esophagectomy, the available studies are small, and there exists considerable heterogeneity in techniques. However, the available data suggests that robotic-assisted esophagectomy when compared to other techniques is safe and feasible.

2. **Esophageal Myotomy for Achalasia**. The basic principles of esophageal myotomy for achalasia have not changed since Heller's initial description in 1913. What has changed is the way surgeons gain access to perform the procedure with the first minimally invasive Heller myotomy being described in the 1990s. The minimally invasive approach demonstrated comparable outcomes with decreased morbidity, shorter length of stay, and decreased postoperative pain.

The operation can fail however, with potential complications, including failure to divide all the circular muscular fibers, esophageal perforation, and general progression of the disease. The surgical robot with its improved magnification, visualization and enhanced motor control has been successfully used for esophageal myotomy with the first procedure described in 2001.

The initial report of robotic esophageal myotomy was performed on a 76-year-old female with a 10-year history of achalasia. The procedure was done through four operative ports. An incision was made through the esophageal musculature and carried caudally for 8 cm. The incision was then extended on to the stomach for 1.5 cm. The underlying mucosa was freed for approximately 50% of the total circumference. A posterior toupet fundoplication was fashioned. The daVinci surgical robot was used for the dissection, myotomy, and intracorporeal knot-tying portions of the procedure. The total operative time was 160 min. The patient was discharged from the hospital the following day.

In 2006, Galvani et al. published a series of 54 patients who underwent robotic-assisted Heller myotomy. Of these 54 patients, 26 had undergone previous endoscopic treatment, including 17 patients who had pneumatic dilatation, 4 patients who had Botox injection, and 5 patients who had both. The operation itself was fairly similar to the initial report with the exception of the use of an anterior Dor fundoplication. The average operative time, including robot setup time, was 162 min. Average blood loss was 24 ml. None of the procedures were converted to open or conventional laparoscopy. Average length of stay was 1.5 days. The patients did very well with 91% of patients considering their postoperative swallowing status to be good or excellent.

A comparative study between robotically assisted and conventional Heller myotomy was published in 2005. The study was a multicenter retrospective review in which 121 patients were divided into two groups, those who received robotic myotomy and those who underwent conventional laparoscopic procedures. Interestingly, the rate of esophageal mucosal perforation in the laparoscopic group was 16% while in the robotic group no perforations occurred. This result is balanced by the fact that the two groups of patients were operated on at different institutions by different surgeons. However, it is the first study to suggest that the robot confers an operative advantage in Heller myotomies.

The potential advantage of decreased incidence of esophageal perforation was reinforced by a study by Melvin et al. in 2005. The authors completed robotic Heller myotomies on 104 patients at three institutions. No esophageal mucosal perforations were observed.

A study released in 2007 by Huffman et al. evaluated 61 patients undergoing minimally invasive Heller myotomy by a single surgeon. These patients were divided into two groups in a nonrandomized fashion. Thirty-seven patients had laparoscopic and twenty-four had robotic myotomies. The study examined quality of life scores in both groups pre- and postoperatively using two instruments, the Short Form Health Status Questionnaire (SF-36) and the gastroesophageal reflux disease activity index (GRACI). The results showed improved scores in both groups with the robotic group results mildly superior. The study also examined the rate of esophageal perforation and found an 8% rate in the laparoscopic group and no events in the robotic group.

In general, esophageal perforation during Heller myotomy occurs as a technical failure during the dissection and division of the muscle fibers overlying the esophageal mucosa. If the perforation is recognized intraoperatively and repaired immediately the outcome is generally good. However, a delayed diagnosis can be devastating and possibly fatal. The reduction in risk of this complication is a substantial advantage. The robotic Heller myotomy demonstrates this advantage in multiple studies.

3. **Resection of Benign Esophageal Mass**. The role of the surgical robot in the treatment of esophageal malignancy has been described in the previous section, however, the esophagus is also subject to benign lesions as well. Leiomyomas comprise up to 80% of these lesions. Most esophageal leiomyomas present in the middle to lower one third of the esophagus and most remain asymptomatic. However, when patients do experience symptoms they are most likely to complain of dysphasia and atypical chest pain.

The esophageal leiomyoma is a well-circumscribed mass located within the esophageal wall arising from the smooth muscle. The overlying mucosa is intact. Malignant transformation is rare, however enucleation of these masses is recommended for confirmation. Endoscopic biopsy should be avoided because scarring and adhesion makes future enucleation difficult. Biopsies also tend to be nondiagnostic because of the submucosal location of the tumor.

Robotic leiomyoma enucleation has been described in several case studies. Resection of an esophageal leiomyoma involves making a myotomy for removal of the lesion while leaving the mucosa intact. While some surgeons leave the myotomy unrepaired, many prefer to close the myotomy to prevent mucosal bulging and possible diverticula formation. One of the great advantages of the robot is the ease of intracorporeal suturing especially in this confined space.

Robotic surgical technology has also been described in the resection of an esophageal cyst. In this procedure, a 2.6 cm cyst was removed using a robotically assisted thorascopic approach. There is also one report of an esophageal diverticulum being excised robotically. Again the primary advantage of the robot was the ease of suturing, as the defect was close in a two-layer repair.

D. Summary

Esophageal surgery remains a challenging endeavor for most surgeons. The anatomy of the esophagus with its close proximity to vital structures and location in a confined area make dissection and suturing difficult. The last two decades have witnessed major advances in the field of esophageal surgery. The introduction of minimally invasive techniques to the field have resulted in decreased morbidity, shorter hospital stays, less postoperative pain, and fewer complications. Robotic technology has added several advantages, including improved visualization and magnification, elimination of tremor, and increased articulation of instruments. The application of robotic technology to esophageal surgery has been slowly progressing. A variety of procedures have been safely performed. In most cases, the robotic approach to esophageal surgery has shown comparable outcomes to conventional laparoscopic and open techniques. In the cases of Heller myotomy, the robot demonstrates a significant advantage in the form of decreased incidence of esophageal perforation. With regard to oncologic outcomes from esophagectomy, the robotic technique has demonstrated equivalence. The number of lymph nodes harvested and positive surgical margins are comparable to conventional laparoscopic and open techniques. Finally, the surgical robot has been safely used for a variety of resections of benign esophageal masses and a diverticulum.

The future of robotic esophageal surgery remains uncertain. Although its safety has been demonstrated, the increased cost, set-up time and additional training of surgeons and operating room staff have hampered it widespread use. Prospective randomized control trials with larger numbers of patients showing an identifiable benefit will ultimately be required for robotic esophageal surgery to gain wider acceptance.

Selected References

Bodner JC, Zitt M, Ott H, et al. Robotic-assisted thoracoscopic surgery (RATS) for benign and malignant esophageal tumors. Ann Thorac Surg. 2005;80:1202–6.

Boone J, Draaisma WA, Schipper ME, Broeders IA, Rinkes IH, van Hillegersberg R. Robot-assisted thoracoscopic esophagectomy for a giant upper esophageal leiomyoma. Dis Esophagus. 2008;21(1):90–3.

Csendes A, Braghetto I, Henriquez A, Cortes C. Late results of a prospective randomised study comparing forceful dilatation and oesophagomyotomy in patients with achalasia. Gut. 1989;30:299–304.

DePaula AL, Hashiba K, Ferreira EA, de Paula RA, Grecco E. Laparoscopic transhiatal esophagectomy with esophagogastroplasty. Surg Laparosc Endosc. 1995;5(1):1–5.

DeUgarte DA, Teitelbaum D, Hirschl RB, Geiger JD. Robotic extirpation of complex massive esophageal leiomyoma. J Laparoendosc Adv Surg Tech A. 2008;18(2):286–9.

Elli E, Espat NJ, Berger R, Jacobsen G, Knoblock L, Horgan S. Robotic-assisted thoracoscopic resection of esophageal leiomyoma. Surg Endosc. 2004;18:713–6.

Fernando HC, Erdem CC, Daly B, Shemin RJ. Robotic assisted thoracic surgery for resection of an esophageal cyst. Dis Esophagus. 2006;19(6):509–11.

Galvani C, Gorodner MV, Moser F, Baptista M, Donahue P, Horgan S. Laparoscopic Heller myotomy for achalasia facilitated by robotic assistance. Surg Endosc. 2006;20: 1105–12.

Galvani CA, Gorodner MV, Moser F, et al. Robotically assisted laparoscopic transhiatal esophagectomy. Surg Endosc. 2008;22:188–95.

Horgan S, Berger RA, Elli EF, Espat NJ. Robotic-assisted minimally invasive transhiatal esophagectomy. Am Surg. 2003;69:624–6.

Horgan S, Galvani C, Gorodner MV, Omelanczuck P, Elli F, Moser F, et al. Robotic-assisted Heller myotomy versus laparoscopic Heller myotomy for the treatment of esophageal achalasia: multicenter study. J Gastrointest Surg. 2005;9:1020–30.

Huffmanm LC, Pandalai PK, Boulton BJ, James L, Starnes SL, Reed MF, Howington JA, Nussbaum MS. Robotic Heller myotomy: a safe operation with higher postoperative quality-of-life indices. Surgery. 2007;142(4):613–8.

Kernstine KH, DeArmond DT, Karimi M, et al. The robotic, 2-stage, 3-field esophago-lymphadenectomy. J Thorac Cardiovasc Surg. 2004;127:1847–9.

Kernstine KH, DeArmond DT, Shamoun DM, et al. The first series of completely robotic esophagectomies with three-field lymphadenectomy: initial experience. Surg Endosc. 2007;21:2285–92.

Kim DJ, Hyung WJ, Lee CY, et al. Thoracoscopic esophagectomy for esophageal cancer: feasibility and safety of robotic assistance in the prone position. J Thorac Cardiovasc Surg. 2010;139:53e1–9e1.

Melvin WS, Needleman BJ, Krause K, Wolf RK, Michler RE, Ellison EC. Computer-assisted robotic Heller myotomy: initial case report. J Laparoendosc Adv Surg Tech. 2001;11:251–3.

Melvin WS, Needleman BJ, Krause KR, Schneider C, Wolf RK, Michler E, Ellison EC. Computer-enhanced robotic telesurgery. Surg Endosc. 2002;16:1790–2.

Melvin WS, Dundon JM, Talamini M, Horgan S. Computer enhanced robotic telesurgery minimizes esophageal perforation during Heller myotomy. Surgery. 2005;138: 553–9.

Shimi S, Nathanson LK, Cuschieri A. Laparoscopic cardiomyotomy for achalasia. J R Coll Surg Edinb. 1991;36:152–4.

van Hillegersberg R, Boone J, Draaisma WA, et al. First experience with robot-assisted thoracoscopic esophagolymphadenectomy for esophageal cancer. Surg Endosc. 2006;20:1435–9.

15. Laparoscopic or Endoscopic Management of Esophageal Diverticula

Garth R. Jacobsen, M.D.
Mark A. Talamini, M.D.

A. Introduction

Diverticula are outpouchings or sacs which protrude from the bowel lumen. They may be found anywhere in the gastrointestinal tract. Diverticula are classified as true or false. True diverticula involve all layers of the wall. False diverticula typically contain only the mucosa and submucosa. Most esophageal diverticula are false. The etiology of false diverticula of the esophagus is pulsion. Pulsion diverticula arise in areas subjected to abnormally high intraluminal pressure which exerts undue tension upon the wall of the esophagus. This causes herniation of the mucosa and submucosa through the muscular wall. Diverticula may also form when traction on the wall of the esophagus pulls out on the wall, deforming the lumen and forming a true diverticulum. Esophageal diverticula are categorized and treated based on their location within the esophagus, and whether or not they are true or false diverticula. Herein, we focus on the laparoscopic or endoscopic management of Zenker's, mid-esophageal and epiphrenic diverticula.

B. Zenker's Diverticulum

1. **Pathophysiology and Indications for treatment:**
   a. Inappropriately termed an esophageal diverticulum, a Zenker's diverticulum is anatomically a false diverticulum of the hypopharynx. Ludlow first described this entity in 1769, but it was Zenker whom first correlated an increased

N.T. Nguyen and C.E.H. Scott-Conner (eds.), *The SAGES Manual: Volume 2   231
Advanced Laparoscopy and Endoscopy*, DOI 10.1007/978-1-4614-2347-8_15,
© Springer Science+Business Media, LLC 2012

intrapharyngeal pressure with the development of the diverticulum. Zenker's diverticula are pulsion diverticula that protrude through Killian's triangle. Killian's triangle is an anatomic area of weakness which lies between the inferior pharyngeal constrictor muscle and the cricopharyngeus on the dorsal wall of the most caudal part of the hypopharynx. Most agree that Zenker's diverticula are secondary to poor or uncoordinated relaxation of the cricopharyngeus muscle. This generates a proximal high pressure zone resulting in the development of the diverticulum. A definitive cause for this loss of coordination has not been elucidated but it is likely related to a primary neurologic or myogenic disorder. Some have postulated that reflux may play a role, but this is yet to be proven. Zenker's diverticula are rare, with the true incidence estimated at 2 per 100,000 people. The most common patients are middle aged males. Symptoms are variable and range from regurgitation, chronic cough, and aspiration, to complaints of weight loss, globus, and halitosis. There seems to be a direct correlation of diverticular size to degree of symptoms. The diagnosis is established with contrast enhanced radiographic evaluation, as Zenker's diverticula may be missed during endoscopic evaluation. Care must be taken to obtain multiple views of the area in question so as to not miss a small diverticulum hidden by a column of contrast.

b.   Given the safety and efficacy of today's current management techniques and risk of complications, such as aspiration and pneumonia, almost all patients are considered candidates for surgery.

2.   **Operative Considerations and Technique**

a.   The management of Zenker's diverticula has changed dramatically over the last two decades. The standard operations of the past included open neck exploration with resection or suspension of the diverticulum, and may or may not have included myotomy. Increased understanding of the disease process, along with progression of technology, has led to increasingly minimally invasive approaches. Most of today's operations center upon transoral endoscopic division of the common wall between the lumen of the diverticulum and the esophagus in effect joining the two. This allows for rapid drainage of the diverticulum into the upper esophagus.

The common wall is composed of the esophageal and diverticular mucosa and submucosa separated by the cricopharyngeus muscle. This is visualized as a cricopharyngeal bar on endoscopy. Many techniques have been described for dividing this bar, including sharp dissection, cautery, a variety of lasers, and more recently ultrasonic dissection. All have been relatively successful, but most have reports of esophageal leak and mediastinitis due to inadequate sealing of the mucosa. The most common contemporary technique, and the one most utilized at our institution involves the use of cutting stapler, which seals both the mucosa and submucosa and divides the muscle.

b.   The operation is carried out under general anesthesia. Position the patient supine with the neck carefully extended. Place a roll beneath the shoulder blades to elevate the esophagus and facilitate in-line passage of the rigid endoscope. The surgeon stands at the head of the bed and the monitor is placed at the foot. Our current technique involves the use of the use of a rigid bivalved endoscope, the Weerda scope (Karl Storz, Tuttlingen, Germany) as seen in Fig. 15.1. We highly suggest collaboration with an ear nose and throat surgeon if unfamiliar with the utilization of this

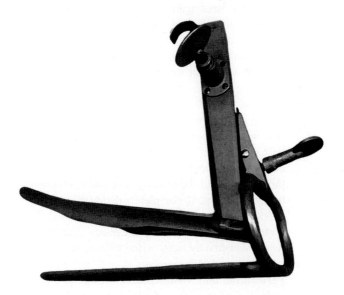

Fig. 15.1.   Weerda scope (Karl Storz, Tuttlingen, Germany).

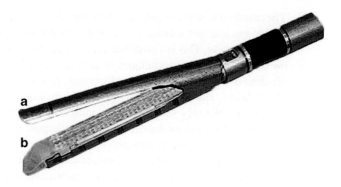

Fig. 15.2. Endoscopic stapler, notice the excess portion of the anvil (**a**), and staple cartridge (**b**). These are areas in which no staples are fired, and the cutting blade does not divide making a complete myotomy impossible without modification.

scope, as the exposure of the diverticulum, the lumen of the esophagus, and the cricopharyngeal bar is critical to the success of the procedure. Protect the maxillary teeth (or gums in the edentulous patient) before inserting the scope. The rigid platform is then held in place by means of a static support. An optical scope is attached to a camera and light source and then introduced into the fixed bivalved scope. Assess the field again, and aspirate any foreign material from the diverticulum. Some have advocated placing one or more stay sutures on the common wall in order to aid in positioning of the stapler. This may be potentially useful in small pouches, but we do not routinely employ this tactic. Next, use an endoscopic linear cutting stapler to divide the common wall. Position this stapler so that the anvil is placed in the diverticulum lumen. It may take as little as one, but occasionally several firings of a 35 mm cartridge with a vascular (2.5 mm) load. As seen in Fig. 15.2, standard endoscopic staplers do not staple or divide through the full length of the cartridge and anvil. This makes it virtually impossible to completely divide the common wall. It is possible to remove the distal tip of the anvil, though this is difficult and may not be necessary given the excellent results reported by many without doing so.

3. Complications and Management:

a. **Perforation and Mediastinitis.** Mosher first described an endoscopic approach to Zenker's diverticulum in 1917 and quickly abandoned it secondary to an increased incidence of mediastinitis. The stapled, laser, ultrasonic and a myriad of other approaches seek to seal the cut edges of the mucosa to decrease the possibility of this occurring. Indeed the stapled approach has been the safest in this regard, and mediastinitis is rare.

b. **Other complications** such as thermal injury to the recurrent laryngeal nerve, various mucosal injuries and perforations, bleeding, dental injury, and death have been described. Just as importantly, recurrence of symptoms may be a factor especially if the myotomy is incomplete. Adequate exposure can be difficult if not impossible in up to one third of patients resulting in at best an aborted case and at worse an esophageal perforation.

c. **Prevention and Management.** Obtaining good exposure is of utmost importance in avoidance of the above complications. A recent study identified a neck length shorter than 7.2 cm, a hyomental distance of less than 5.0 cm, and a BMI greater than 27 as having a significantly negative effect on performing a stapled diverticulotomy. Patients in whom adequate exposure cannot be obtained with a rigid operating platform may be candidates for flexible endoscopic methods of myotomy if the endoscopist has the prerequisite skills and equipment. The surgeon may also resort to an open procedure. Perforations are treated at the very least by making the patient nil per os and administering broad spectrum antibiotics, however they may need either percutaneous or open drainage and possibly esophageal repair. We advocate a water soluble contrast study in all patients prior to the resumption of feeding, and patients are vigorously monitored overnight for signs and symptoms of perforation.

C. Mid-Esophageal Diverticula

1. Pathophysiology and indications for treatment
   a. Mid-esophageal diverticula are usually located within 5–7 cm of the tracheal bifurcation. They can be classified as being either true diverticula or false pulsion diverticula.

True diverticula at the level of the carina are the most common esophageal diverticula in Japan. These diverticula are small (1–2 cm) and mostly asymptomatic. They result from traction upon the mid-esophagus secondary to lymphadenitis and are often seen in patients with a history of tuberculosis. These diverticula are generally not operated upon, though there have been reports of carcinoma developing within them, mandating surveillance. In Europe and America, mid-esophageal diverticula are the rarest of esophageal diverticulum and are increasingly identified to be associated with an underlying esophageal motility disorder. Mid-esophageal diverticula should always be evaluated by a contrast-enhanced radiologic evaluation. This aids in operative planning as well as establishing the diagnosis. In any patient with dysphagia, endoscopy is mandatory to rule out malignancy as a concomitant cause of dysphagia. Esophageal manometry while not absolutely necessary may elucidate an underlying esophageal motility disorder and allow for optimization of management, whether pharmaceutical or surgical.

b.   Most esophageal diverticula are asymptomatic until they become very large and subsequent spillover of the diverticula leads to regurgitation of these contents. A history of related aspiration should prompt consideration for surgical resection. It must be noted however that symptoms of chest pain and dysphagia are almost always solely related to either reflux or an underlying esophageal motility disorder. Combining a myotomy with resection not only decreases the risk of postoperative esophageal leak, and chances of recurrence, but may provide symptomatic relief of the underlying motility disorder.

2.   Operative Considerations and Technique

a.   The traditional approach for exposure of the mid-esophagus has been through a right sided thoracotomy. Advances in technology and surgeon experience now allow minimally invasive approaches to mid-esophageal lesions, such as benign and malignant tumors, and esophageal diverticula.

b.   The patient is given DVT prophylaxis as indicated and appropriate antibiotic coverage. The video endoscopic approach to mid-esophageal diverticula is through the right chest. Patients are intubated with a double lumen

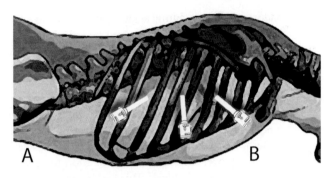

Fig. 15.3. Port positioning for prone video assisted thoracoscopic diverticulectomy Positioning of sand bags at A and B.

endotracheal tube. Care is taken that they do not aspirate, especially if the diverticulum is large. It is not always necessary to deflate the lung, but preparation in the form of a dual lumen tube will pay off should the need arise. The patient is then placed in the prone position with right arm extended above the head with sand bags placed beneath the hips and chest (Fig. 15.3). A Veress needle is used to insufflate the chest cavity to 5 mm Hg. Obtain access to the chest with the first trocar at the seventh intercostal margin—this can be a 5 mm trocar if a 5 mm scope is to be used, otherwise a larger trocar will be needed. Next, perform esophagoscopy with a standard gastroscope. Use the gastroscope to help visualize the diverticulum and to clean out debris. The next two ports triangulate upon the diverticulum and are usually placed in the fifth and ninth intercostal spaces, respectively. The fifth interspace trocar may be 5 mm in nature, the ninth interspace trocar should be large enough to accommodate an endoscopic stapler. Begin the operation by incising the pleura overlying the diverticulum for the length of the esophagus. This is most readily accomplished utilizing endoscopic shears. Encircle the esophagus with a Penrose drain to aid in esophageal manipulation and retraction. Completely mobilize the diverticulum with a combination of blunt and sharp dissection. Both the diverticulum and esophagus must be fully mobilized prior to proceeding to resection and myotomy. After completely mobilizing the diverticulum, obtain an articulating endoscopic linear cutting stapler with a vascular (2.5 mm) load is obtained. The stapler must be articulating in order to achieve a parallel course for staple firings. Under direct endoscopic visualization transect the base of the diverticulum utilizing one or more firings of the stapler with care not to significantly narrow the esophageal lumen. Our preference is to use endoscopic guidance, though a 52 french bougie can be inserted prior to stapled transection for calibration. Next, approximate the longitudinal muscle of the esophagus over the staple line in an effort to decrease the risk of postoperative leak. This can be interrupted or running absorbable suture. Then, perform an esophageal myotomy by splitting the longitudinal muscular fibers and carefully lysing the circular muscle of the esophagus with care to preserve the underlying mucosa. This is done as close to 180° opposite to the staple line as possible, with the proximal point being well above the mouth of the diverticulum and the distal point determined by the underlying esophageal motility disorder identified on preoperative manometry. If there has not been a preoperative manometry, continue the dissection inferiorly at least a few centimeters if not more. Again, reapproximate the longitudinal muscle to aid in prevention of postoperative mucosal herniation and formation of subsequent diverticulum. Finally, use the endoscope to perform an underwater insufflation test to check for a potential leak. Place the diverticulum in a retrieval bag and remove it. Place a thoracostomy tube through the largest trocar, and close the wounds.

3.   Complications and Management:

    a.   The worldwide experience in the thoracoscopic resection of mid-body esophageal diverticulum is small owing to the rare nature of disease. Perhaps the most vexing of complications is esophageal leak. Reapproximating (oversewing) the longitudinal muscle layer over the staple line may help prevent leaks. Failure to perform an adequate distal myotomy may place undue pressure upon the staple line, predisposing to leak. In addition to the intraoperative leak test, it is essential to perform contrast evaluation before feeding. Early identification of a leak, should it occur, is key to obtaining a satisfactory patient outcome.

b. Management of a leak after esophageal diverticulum resection is similar to that of any mid-esophageal perforation. The patient is made nil per os and given broad spectrum antibiotics. This is accompanied by wide drainage of the affected area and control of the systemic septic response. There are increasing reports of managing esophageal perforations with endoscopic stenting though this should be considered investigational unless utilized by those equipped with the resources, knowledge, and experience to deploy such techniques. Patients may require thoracotomy and repair, including buttress with and autogenous tissue flap, and in the worst cases proximal diversion and distal decompression.

D. Epiphrenic Diverticula

1. Pathophysiology and indications for treatment

a. Epiphrenic diverticula are pulsion diverticula of the distal esophageal body. They arise in the distal 10–12 cm and comprise mucosa and submucosa. Their true nature as pulsion diverticula was defined by Belsey and Effler in the mid part of the last century. In Europe and America, they are second to Zenker's diverticula in incidence. There is uniform agreement that virtually 100% of all epiphrenic diverticula are accompanied by an underlying esophageal motility disorder. The most frequently associated esophageal motility disorders are achalasia and diffuse esophageal spasm, followed by nutcracker esophagus and a hypertensive lower esophageal sphincter. This was confirmed in a recent study by Nehra et al. in which patients underwent ambulatory manometry. In their study, all patients with epiphrenic diverticula who did not have an underlying motility disorder on static manometry demonstrated diffuse esophageal spasm at prolonged ambulatory monitoring. Symptoms of epiphrenic diverticula can be extraesophageal, such as asthma, laryngitis, nocturnal cough, and pneumonia. All are at least partially related to reflux and regurgitation. Esophageal symptoms, such as dysphagia, chest pain, and weight loss, can also accompany epiphrenic diverticula, but are usually related to the

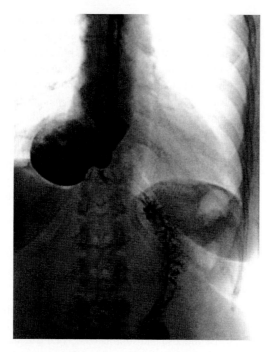

Fig. 15.4. Barium-enhanced radiograph of an epiphrenic diverticulum.

underlying motility disorder. The diagnosis is established utilizing contrast radiography and endoscopy (Fig. 15.4). Endoscopy again is essential should dysphagia be a component of the patient's symptom complex, and can also be used to appropriately place a manometry catheter if the surgeon wishes. Manometry is not absolutely essential because all patients have an underlying motility disorder, but may be useful to ascertain the length and proximal/distal extent of the most effective myotomy.

b.   A careful history should be obtained in all patients who are being considered for resection of an epiphrenic diverticulum. Only those who are symptomatic should be treated, given the inherent risk of esophageal leak which accompanies resection. That is, patients should be symptomatic from their diverticulum, not simply from their underlying motility disorder. Complications related to reflux or regurgitation of diverticulum contents, such as aspiration pneumonias should be treated and then patients should be offered surgery, if they can tolerate the operation. A recent investigation found that 20% of patients with diverticular symptoms who were conservatively managed aspirated at some time during the monitoring period with a 50% mortality.

2. Operative Considerations and technique

a. The traditional approach to the distal esophagus is through the left chest by way of a left thoracotomy. With current laparoscopic techniques and equipment, the experienced foregut surgeon can easily gain access to the distal 10 cm of the esophagus laparoscopically. This clearly includes a decreased morbidity and mortality rate, less pain, shorter hospital stay, and shorter recovery time than those undergoing thoracotomy.

b. The patient is given DVT prophylaxis as indicated and appropriate antibiotic coverage. Position the patient supine on the operating room table with a beanbag underneath them. General anesthesia is induced while taking appropriate precautions to avoid aspiration, again, especially if the diverticulum is large. We prefer to then place the patient in a low lying modified lithotomy position, though supine and split leg positions can be equally effective. The trocar positioning is identical to that of a laparoscopic fundoplication or Heller myotomy. We prefer to access the abdomen with an optical view 5 mm trocar just superior to the margin of the ribs and slightly to the left of midline. Insert the next two ports with an aim to triangulate upon the hiatus, with the left being large enough to accommodate a linear cutting stapler. Place a 5 mm assistant port inferior to the left costal margin, as lateral as possible (Fig. 15.5). Then, place the patient in steep reverse Trendelenburg position. Make a small incision in the epigastrium and deploy the Nathanson liver retractor. Perform endoscopy is now undertaken and clean out the diverticulum. Dissect the crura, exposing enough of each posterior crus to do a posterior crural repair if necessary. Completely mobilize the distal esophagus. We use an ultrasonic dissector for the majority of the dissection and begin by taking down the first few short gastric vessels to allow for mobilization of the fundus and exposure of the left crus. The gastrohepatic ligament is then taken down and the right crus exposed. This is followed by

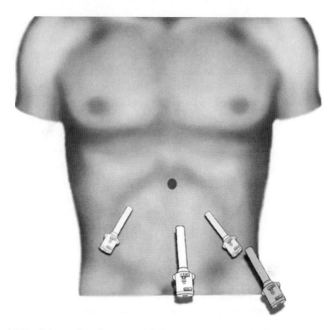

Fig. 15.5. Schematic of trocar and liver retractor positioning for epiphrenic diverticulectomy.

anterior mobilization of the esophagus with care to identify and preserve the vagus nerve. If significant, the anterior fat pad can be taken down to facilitate later myotomy. Place a Penrose drain circumferentially around the esophagus for retraction. While the assistant provides retraction via the Penrose, mobilize the esophagus and expose the diverticulum. There may be considerable inflammation at the level of the diverticulum and care must be taken during this portion of the dissection. Once the diverticulum has been fully mobilized, transect it at its base utilizing an endoscopic reticulating linear cutting stapler with a vascular (2.5 mm) load. One or more sequential firings may be needed. Take care not to narrow the lumen of the distal esophagus. This can be avoided by utilizing a 50–56 french bougie or maintaining direct endoscopic visualization. Place the diverticulum in a specimen bag and remove it from the abdomen. Plicate the longitudinal muscle of the esophagus over the underlying staple line for reinforcement as described above. Perform an underwater leak test with the aid of endoscopic insufflation. Attention is then turned to completing the myotomy. This is done on the contralateral side of the esophagus, starting above the level of the diverticulum neck and extending distally. Given the high incidence of achalasia in these patients, we prefer to carry the myotomy onto the proximal 2 cm of the stomach. Next, if necessary, perform a posterior crural repair with interrupted silk sutures. Fashion a partial fundoplication either anterior or posterior (Dor or Toupet). We prefer a Dor fundoplication as it nicely covers the mucosa of the myotomy and has provided an excellent antireflux barrier in conjunction with a Heller myotomy.

3. Complications and Management

    a. The most common intraoperative complication is pneumothorax, especially if the diverticulum is inflamed and adherent to the pleura. Postoperatively esophageal leak is of the greatest concern. A recent collection of reported case series in the management of epiphrenic diverticulum have demonstrated it to be safe and effective in 85 reported patients. This was contrasted to 147 patients reported as managed via an open thoracotomy. Mortality in the minimally invasive group was 1 vs. 6% in the open. There was still a significant leak rate of 14%. In one case series, 23% of patients developed a leak following a routine application of a 360° fundoplication. The overall success rate in this collection of studies was 83–100% and there was only one reported recurrence.

    b. **Intraoperative pneumothorax** can usually be managed by simple closure of the pleura with either sutures or locking clips followed by rapid absorption of the CO_2 and resolution. In the unlikely event of a concomitant injury to the pulmonary parenchyma followed by air leak, a thoracostomy tube will be necessary.

    c. In regards to **postoperative leak**, prevention starts at the time of operation. It is important to reapproximate the longitudinal fibers of the esophagus over the staple line. The choice of fundoplication and completeness of the myotomy are also factors. Incomplete myotomies have been implicated in postoperative staple line disruptions with the thought that distal obstruction leads to perforation. Likewise, in a reported series of 360° fundoplications mentioned earlier there was an inordinately high leak rate. Most authors agree on a partial fundoplication, but there is no consensus as to the superiority of an anterior or posterior partial wrap. Leaks are managed with early identification and the steps outlined earlier.

Selected References

Bloom JD, Bleier BS, Mirza N, Chalian AA, Thaler ER. Factors predicting endoscopic exposure of Zenker's diverticulum. Ann Otol Rhinol Laryngol. 2010;119(11): 736–41.

Del Genio A, Rossetti G, Maffetton V, et al. Laparoscopic approach in the treatment of epiphrenic diverticula: long-term results. Surg Endosc. 2004;18(5):741–5.

Jamieson GG. Other esophageal motility disorders and diverticula. In: Soper NJ, editor. Mastery of endoscopic and laparoscopic surgery. Third Editionth ed. Philadelphia, PA: Lipincott Williams & Williams; 2009. p. 142–7.

Kilic A, Schuchert MJ, Awais O, Luketich JD, Landreneau RJ. Surgical management of epiphrenic diverticula in the minimally invasive era. JSLS. 2009;13(2):160–4.

Melman L, Quinlan J, Robertson B, et al. Esophageal manometric characteristics and outcomes for laparoscopic esophageal diverticulectomy, myotomy, and partial fundoplication for epiphrenic diverticula. Surg Endosc. 2009;23(6):1337–41.

Nehra D, Lord RV, DeMeester TR, et al. Physiologic basis for the treatment of epiphrenic diverticulum. Ann Surg. 2002;235(3):346–54.

Palanivelu C, Rangarajan M, Maheshkumaar GS, Senthilkumar R. Minimally invasive surgery combined with peroperative endoscopy for symptomatic middle and lower esophageal diverticula: a single institute's experience. Surg Laparosc Endosc Percutan Tech. 2008a;18(2):133–8.

Palanivelu C, Rangarajan M, Senthilkumar R, Velusamy M. Combined thoracoscopic and endoscopic management of mid-esophageal benign lesions: use of the prone patient position: thoracoscopic surgery for mid-esophageal benign tumors and diverticula. Surg Endosc. 2008b;22(1):250–4.

Rosati R, Fumagalli U, Elmore U, de Pascale S, Massaron S, Peracchia A. Long-term results of minimally invasive surgery for symptomatic epiphrenic diverticulum. Am J Surg. 2011;201(1):132–5.

Soares R, Herbella FA, Prachand VN, Ferguson MK, Patti MG. Epiphrenic diverticulum of the esophagus From pathophysiology to treatment. J Gastrointest Surg. 2010;14(12): 2009–15.

Tedesco P, Fisichella PM, Way LW, Patti MG. Cause and treatment of epiphrenic diverticula. Am J Surg. 2005;190(6):891–4.

Varghese Jr TK, Marshall B, Chang AC, Pickens A, Lau CL, Orringer MB. Surgical treatment of epiphrenic diverticula: a 30-year experience. Ann Thorac Surg. 2007; 84(6):1801–9. discussion 1801–09.

Verhaegen VJ, Feuth T, van den Hoogen FJ, Marres HA, Takes RP. Endoscopic carbon dioxide laser diverticulostomy versus endoscopic staple-assisted diverticulostomy to treat Zenker's diverticulum. Head Neck. 2011;33(2):154–9.

Wasserzug O, Zikk D, Raziel A, Cavel O, Fleece D, Szold A. Endoscopically stapled diverticulostomy for Zenker's diverticulum: results of a multidisciplinary team approach. Surg Endosc. 2010;24(3):637–41.

16. Endolumenal Approaches to Gastroesophageal Reflux Disease

Kevin M. Reavis, M.D., F.A.C.S.
Allan K. Nguyen, B.S.

A. Introduction

Gastroesophageal reflux disease (GERD) develops as a result of the loss of the antireflux barrier created by the lower esophageal sphincter (LES). The lack of this barrier allows gastric contents to reflux into the esophagus causing typical symptoms of heartburn, dysphasia, and regurgitation. If left untreated, GERD may lead to the development of Barrett's esophagus and eventually esophageal adenocarcinoma. The prevalence of GERD in Western nations ranges from 10 to 20% in the general population, and the number of ambulatory visits for GERD in the USA is on the rise.

The medical treatment for GERD is based on antisecretory pharmaceuticals, such as proton-pump inhibitors, histamine$_2$ blockers, and antacids. Unfortunately, some patients do not respond to standard dosage regimens and those who do are required to adhere to lifelong treatment to avoid recurrent symptoms and progression of disease. Patients who receive little to no symptomatic relief or who do not wish to use long-term antisecretory medications can opt for a surgical fundoplication to potentially improve their quality of life. The laparoscopic Nissen fundoplication is the standard surgical treatment for severe GERD with 90–94% overall patient satisfaction and excellent outcomes during long-term follow-up. The main objective of fundoplication is to restore the antireflux barrier by the reconstruction of the LES. However, due to surgical morbidity and common side effects of dysphagia, bloating, flatulence, difficulty belching, and vomiting, patients may be dissuaded from the surgical approach.

In search for an alternative and less invasive approach, numerous attempts to create the ideal endolumenal treatment for GERD have

N.T. Nguyen and C.E.H. Scott-Conner (eds.), *The SAGES Manual: Volume 2 Advanced Laparoscopy and Endoscopy*, DOI 10.1007/978-1-4614-2347-8_16,
© Springer Science+Business Media, LLC 2012

been developed over the last couple of decades. Unfortunately, due to inadequate initial results, failure to objectively treat GERD during long-term follow-up, or overall poor reimbursement, no single endolumenal treatment has enjoyed long-term use. Currently, two endolumenal approaches are clinically available and are described.

1. Transoral incisionless fundoplication (TIF®) performed with the EsophyX® device (Endogastric Solution Inc., Redmond WA, USA) results in the creation of a 270–320° omega-shaped fundoplication.
2. The Stretta® procedure (Mederi Therapeutics Inc., Greenwich CT, USA) utilizes radiofrequency ablation through extended probes into the esophageal musculature to decrease compliance of the LES and creates a physiologic antireflux barrier.

B. Indications for Endolumenal Treatment for GERD

A standard workup of the GERD patient should be followed whether the patient seeks medical, surgical, or endolumenal treatment. Ideally, patients with objective evidence of moderate-to-severe GERD without significant hiatal hernia who wish to avoid long-term medical treatment as well as formal laparoscopic surgical treatment are candidates for endolumenal treatment. The workup includes the following.

1. **Contrast esophagram** evaluates the overall anatomy of the esophagus and stomach, serves as a preoperative "road map," and identifies hiatal hernias (>2 cm hiatal hernia is a contraindication to current endolumenal treatments).
2. **Upper endoscopy** evaluates the esophagogastric mucosa, allows for identification of hiatal hernias, and allows for biopsy of any suspect lesions. The histological results of tissue biopsies can then guide additional treatments.
3. **pH testing** is the current "gold standard" for the diagnosis of GERD. This is necessary to objectively characterize the presence and severity of disease.
4. **Esophageal manometry**: In any patient with a complaint of dysphagia, manometry is important in characterizing relative esophageal motility and allowing for customization of treatment in patients with esophageal dysmotility.

Appropriate candidates for endolumenal treatment include those patients with fairly normal anatomy on esophagram, 24-h pH study results with an elevatated Demeester score (normal being ≤14.7), no evidence of malignancy on endoscopy, and fairly normal esophageal motility.

Relative contraindications to endolumenal treatment include body mass index >35 kg/m^2, Barrett's Esophagus, immediate prior esophageal myotomy, esophageal varices, and major connective tissue disorders.

C. Technique

1. TIF®
   a. Prepare the patient for standard upper endoscopy, placing the patient in the left lateral decubitus position. Test the EsophyX® device (Fig. 16.1) and endoscope on a back table for size compatibility.
   b. Patient should have neck extended with bite block. Tilt bed slightly (head higher) to avoid risk of aspiration.
   c. General anesthesia with nasotracheal or orotracheal intubation.
   d. Perform diagnostic upper endoscopy to reconfirm no obvious evidence of malignancy or other concerning mucosal abnormalities.

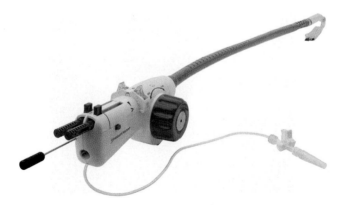

Fig. 16.1. EsophyX® device (reprinted with permission; Endogastric Solutions Inc. image bank).

e. Lubricate the endoscope and EsophyX® device with medical-grade olive oil or similar lubricant. Load the fastener cartridge and the first anterior and posterior polypropylene H-fasteners using the stylet knobs.

f. The EsophyX® device is placed over the endoscope with the endoscope protruding through the device rubber band and well beyond the EsophyX® device. The EsophyX® helical retractor and stylets are locked in retracted position for safety.

g. Introduce the EsophyX® device and endoscope as a unit transorally down through the esophagus into the stomach under direct retroflexed visualization.

h. With the EsophyX® device facing the greater curvature, withdraw the endoscope back to the level of the hinge.

i. Partially flex the EsophyX® device. Advance the endoscope behind the EsophyX® hinge and retroflex the scope as the EsophyX® device is fully flexed into closed position. (Orientation is now as follows: 12 o'clock describes the lesser curvature of the esophagogastric junction. 6 o'clock describes the greater curvature direction located at the Angle of His. 3 o'clock describes the anterior aspect and 9 o'clock describes the posterior aspect) (Fig. 16.2).

j. Advance the helical retractor into the 12 o'clock position and secure the tissue.

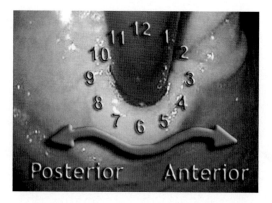

Fig. 16.2. Clock-face orientation of retroflexed view of gastroesophageal junction (reprinted with permission; Endogastric Solutions Inc. image bank).

    k. Partially open the tissue mold at the 6 o'clock position and close it over 2–3 cm of tissue.

    l. Engage the invaginator.

    m. Swing the tissue mold toward 1 o'clock and simultaneously desufflate the stomach.

    n. Lock the tissue mold. Insufflate the stomach and then advance the anterior and posterior stylets and fasteners (via the fastener pushers) in sequential fashion (Fig. 16.3).

    o. Unlock the tissue mold, and reposition and relock it. Deploy two more fasteners and release the tissue invaginator.

    p. Swing the tissue mold around the 12 o'clock position and similarly place a total of four fasteners at the 11 o'clock position.

    q. Release the helical retractor and reengage it at the 6 o'clock position. Reengage the tissue invaginator.

    r. Deploy two fasteners after grasping 3 cm of tissue in the tissue mold at the 8 o'clock position and then at the 4 o'clock position. There is no need for tissue swinging or disinflation during these fastener deployments.

        A total of 12 fasteners are deployed approximately 1–2 cm above the esophageal Z-line. Additional fasteners can be deployed as necessary to develop a 2–3-cm 270–320° omega-shaped esophagogastric wrap.

        The endoscope and EsophyX® device (with stylets and helical retractor locked in retracted position) are then removed. Prior to concluding the procedure, a final upper endoscopy is performed to confirm that an adequate fundoplication has been created and that no perforation or bleeding is present. The patient is extubated and taken to the recovery room prior to going to the ward or home for postoperative care.

2. Stretta®

    a. Prepare for standard upper endoscopy, placing the patient in the left lateral decubitus position.

    b. Patient should have neck extended with bite block. Tilt bed slightly (head higher) to avoid risk of aspiration.

    c. Prepare the patient using standard technique for monopolar electrosurgery.

    d. To ensure proper electrical contact, apply the return electrode pad to a clean and hairless area on the patient's right mid scapular area off the mid line.

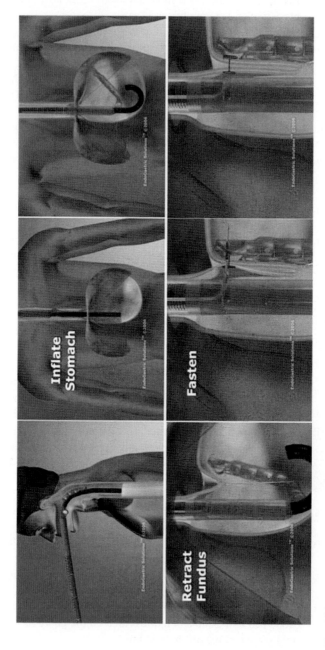

Fig. 16.3. Transoral Incisionless Fundoplication (TIF®) procedure (reprinted with permission; Endogastric Solutions Inc. image bank).

e. Patients most commonly undergo conscious sedation, and monitor patient vitals. A gel anesthetic can be applied in back of patient's throat.
   – Physician may also choose to use general anesthesia.
f. The recommended treatments for Stretta® are 4 antegrade treatment levels in and around the LES, 5 mm apart from each other (two 1-min treatment sites per level at home position and the 45° to right for treatment levels 1–4) and two pull-back treatment levels in the gastric cardia (three 1-min treatment sites per level, home position, 30° to the left and 30° to the right of home for levels 5–6).
g. Perform endoscopic inspection of the esophagus, and measure the distance from Z-line to bite block to confirm the location and depth of the patient's Z-Line (squamo-columnar tissue) versus the fixed oral bite-block. The Z-line serves as the reference landmark for the first four (antegrade) of six total treatment levels. Pass a guide wire through the scope and into the stomach of the patient to pass the Stretta® catheter.
h. From Standby mode, push the Power On/Mode button to advance to Ready mode. Lubricate the catheter (Fig. 16.4)

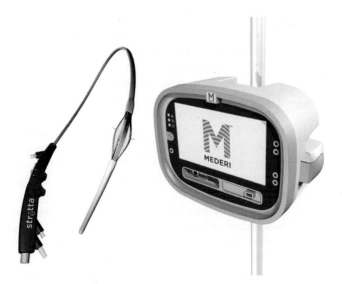

Fig. 16.4. Stretta® device and control box (reprinted with permission; Mederi Therapeutics Inc. image bank).

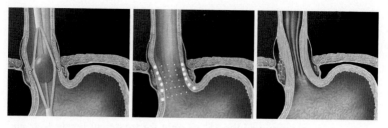

Fig. 16.5. Stretta® procedure (reprinted with permission; Mederi Therapeutics Inc. image bank).

and insert it into the esophagus down to the Z-Line measurement and then retract it to a position 1 cm above the Z-line for treatment level 1.

i. Attach suction to catheter.

j. Attach the pressure release valve (PRV) to the air syringe. Draw 30 ml of air into the syringe and insert it into the insufflation port on the Stretta® catheter until the PRV releases excess air. Once the balloon is inflated, extend the needles into the tissue of the esophagus.

k. ANTEGRADE TREATMENTS (Fig. 16.5): The needles are extended to the full extent, and then retracted to the treatment depth. Impedance readings are monitored on the generator screen. Optimal impedance readings below 200 indicate proper placement of needles. Once proper placement is confirmed, depress the foot pedal once, beginning a 1-min treatment cycle. Once the 1-min cycle is complete, the generator will go into a "Pause" mode to allow for repositioning of the catheter.

l. BETWEEN TREATMENTS: Retract the needles and deflate the balloon. Pull the catheter back up to 25 cm to allow for suction, rotate 45° to the right, and then advance catheter down guide wire to desired depth as measured against the bite block. If resistance is experienced while pulling the catheter back, release suction and then reestablish suction prior to the next treatment. (NOTE: Use the shaft of the catheter as well as the handle to rotate, NOT just the handle.)

m. Reinflate balloon using the PRV to prevent overinflation. The foot pedal is depressed to begin the next 1-min treatment cycle and a second set of lesions is created, establishing the first antegrade ring of eight lesions. Three more rings are created in this manner: 0.5 cm above the Z-line, at the Z-line, and 0.5 cm below the Z-line.

n. Be sure to use the BETWEEN TREATMENT instructions above after each set of lesions are created in the antegrade levels.

o. CARDIA PULL-BACK/RETROGRADE TREATMENTS NOTE: For these treatment levels, do not pull back higher than 2 cm above the Z-line, and do not advance into the stomach lower than 2 cm below the Z-line. Remove PRV and guide wire; they are not needed for the cardia pull-back treatments. For treatment level 5, advance the catheter into the fundus of the stomach, inflate the balloon with 25 mL of air, and slowly pull back the inflated balloon against the hiatus until snug. Extend the needles and deliver the first of three 1-min treatments at this level. At the completion of the first 1-min treatment cycle, retract the needles, advance into the stomach, rotate 30° to the right, pull back until snug, extend needles, and repeat. For the third treatment on this level, rotate catheter 30° to the left of first treatment. For treatment level 6, retract needles and advance the catheter again into the fundus of the stomach. Deflate balloon, then reinflate with 22 mL, and pull back against the hiatus to fit snugly, above treatment level 5. Extend the needles and deliver the first treatment cycle in this level. Following the first treatment cycle, retract the needles, advance into the stomach, rotate 30° to the right, extend needles, and repeat, and then repeat cycle again 30° to the left of first treatment.

p. Following completion of six levels of treatment, deflate the balloon and remove the catheter. An endoscopic inspection of the treatment area should confirm safe delivery and completion of Stretta® therapy.

q. Disconnect Stretta® catheter and dispose of device. Follow shut down procedure outlined in Generator Operator's Manual.

r. The patient is awakened or extubated depending on anesthesia used and taken to the recovery room prior to going to the ward or home for postoperative care.

D. Follow-Up

A liquid diet is commonly prescribed immediately following endolumenal treatments and advanced to regular food as the patient tolerates. Assertive anti-nausea medication is also helpful to avoid stress to the treated area.

Standard post-antireflux surgery follow-up clinic appointments are appropriate with additional evaluations, such as upper endoscopy and/or pH testing being instituted, if patients report recurrent symptoms.

E. Results

1. TIF® has been shown by Cadiere et al. to be safe and effective in humans at 12 months with reports of 85% discontinuation of PPIs and 75% elimination of GERD-related symptoms. This device has been in practice in the USA since 2007 for treatment of moderate-to-severe GERD. One advantage of TIF® over surgical treatment is the application of this procedure in patients who have undergone prior gastric operations, including surgical fundoplication as well as antrectomy (as part of a pancreaticoduodenectomy). This subset of patients offers a potentially hostile environment for standard laparoscopic and open approaches but a straightforward approach for endolumenal treatments. Several initial case series in the USA have been reported with results ranging from dissatisfaction and overt failure in nearly half of patients to more recent objective data showing high-level satisfaction in a majority of patients. Currently, the Randomized EsophyX TIF Versus Sham/Placebo Controlled Trial—The RESPECT Study (Clinical Trials.gov NCT01136980)—is being conducted. This is a multicenter randomized control trial in the USA to objectively determine the effectiveness of TIF with a 6-month follow-up.

2. Stretta® has a relatively long track record of successful clinical outcomes with over 1,400 patients analyzed in over 20 studies. Due to financial considerations, the Stretta® technology was largely unavailable between 2006 and 2008 but has returned and is now clinically available. Studies have shown it to be effective not only in reducing symptoms of GERD and

improving quality of life scores, but objective reduction in esophageal acid exposure and improvements in esophagogastric physiology have also been demonstrated with >12 months' follow-up.

An advantage of the Stretta® technology is its design. Since it has no retracting component, Stretta® can be used in challenging anatomic situations, requires minimal working space, and can be used to treat the LES of patients who have undergone prior gastric bypass or subtotal gastrectomy.

E. Complications

1. Perforation
    a. Cause and prevention: Overassertiveness while placing either the EsophyX® device or Stretta® device can result in esophageal injury. This can be prevented by recognizing resistant anatomy.
    b. Recognition and management: Mucosal injury requires only close observation. Transmural injury requires definitive source control through either laparoscopy/laparotomy or thoracoscopy/thoracotomy or cervical repair of the injured esophageal or gastric segment. Endolumenal stenting of esophageal injuries is a technique under current investigation; however, the appropriate application of this technology is yet to be formalized.
2. Hemorrhage
    a. Cause and prevention: Endolumenal bleeding following TIF® or Stretta® is caused by penetration of submucosal vessels. The avoidance of attempting to treat patients with esophageal varices is imperative.
    b. Recognition and management: Endolumenal bleeding following TIF® can be controlled with direct pressure of the clasped tissue mold for a period of time. Ongoing bleeding following this maneuver or bleeding following Stretta® can usually be controlled through standard endolumenal methods with injection/cautery or placement of clips.
3. Mediastinal/Abdominal Abscess
    a. Cause and prevention: Penetration of the left crus during TIF® or assertive movements with the extended Stretta®

probes can result in microperforation of the esophagogastric fundoplication or LES, respectively, with potential abscess. Recognizing the left crus, applying the tissue invaginator to advance the esophagus during TIF®, and placement of fasteners to the abdominal portion of the esophagus help prevent this complication.

b. Recognition and management: Abscess should be suspected in patients displaying signs of sepsis in the post-procedure period. Radiographic studies provide confirmation. Source control with percutaneous abdominal or thoracic drainage, along with indicated antimicrobial treatment, is usually adequate.

4. Recurrent Symptoms

a. Cause and prevention: Technical error or stress to the operative area allows for recurrence of symptoms. Adequate training and technique and assertive anti-nausea therapy during the post-procedure period reduce the likelihood of recurrent symptoms.

b. Recognition and management: Objective evaluation as performed in the pre-procedure period is warranted to confirm recurrent disease. Reperforming the treatment in appropriate patients is possible with both TIF® and Stretta® technologies.

F. Future Directions

TIF® and Stretta® both appear technically safe in well-selected patients, including those with prior esophageal and gastric surgeries. Long-term effectiveness with regards to both technologies is being evaluated with ongoing investigations. Given the current enthusiasm for increasingly less invasive surgical techniques, the inertia for endolumenal therapies continues to grow. In addition to the two techniques discussed in this chapter, other endolumenal therapies for GERD have initiated trials in Europe and the USA. These therapies pursue similar fundoplication or LES reconstruction using simpler techniques with fewer steps. As all endolumenal approaches to GERD evolve, objective evaluation for symptom resolution and reduced esophageal acid exposure with improved esophagogastric physiology will remain constant.

Selected References

Allgood PC, Bachmann M, et al. Medical or surgical treatment for chronic gastrooesopha-geal reflux? A systematic review of published evidence of effectiveness. Eur J Surg. 2000;166:713–21.

Banerjee A, Melvin WS, Naber SJ, Perry KA. Radiofrequency Energy Delivery to the Lower Esophageal Sphincter Reduces Esophageal Acid Exposure and Improves GERD Symptoms: a Meta-Analysis. Presented at the Society for Surgery of the Alimentary Tract, Chicago IL, May 2011.

Bell RC, Freeman KD. Clinical and pH-metric outcomes of transoral esophagogastric fun-doplication for the treatment of gastroesophageal reflux disease. Surg Endosc. 2011; 25(6):1975–84.

Bergman S, Mikami DJ, Hazey JW, Roland JC, Dettore R, Melvin WS. Endoluminal fun-doplication with Esophyx: the initial North American experience. Surg Innov. 2008; 15:166–70.

Cadiere GB, Buset M, Muls V, Rajan A, et al. Antireflux transoral incisionless fundoplica-tion using EsophyX: 12-month results of a prospective multicenter study. World J Surg. 2008a;32:1676–88.

Cadiere GB, Rajan A, Germay O, Himpens J. Endolumenal fundoplication by a transoral device for the treatment of GERD: a feasibility study. Surg Endosc. 2008b;22: 333–42.

Cadiere GB, Van Sante N, Graves JE, Gawlicka AK, Rajan A. Two-year results of a feasi-bility study on antireflux transoral incisionless fundoplication using EsophyX. Surg Endosc. 2009;23:957–64.

Coelho JC, Wiederkehr JC, Campos AC, et al. Conversions and complications of laparoscopic treatment of gastroesophageal reflux disease. J Am Coll Surg. 1999;189:356–61.

Dallemagne B, Weerts J, Markiewicz S, et al. Clinical results of laparoscopic fundoplica-tion at ten years after surgery. Surg Endosc. 2006;20:159–65.

Demeester TR, Johnson LF, Joseph GJ. el al. Patterns of gastroesophageal reflux in health and disease. Ann Surg. 1976;184:459–70.

Demyttenaere SV, Bergman S, Pham T, Anderson J, Dettorre R, Melvin WS, et al. Transoral incisionless fundoplication for gastroesophageal reflux disease in an unselected patient population. Surg Endosc. 2010;24:854–8.

Dent J. Landmarks in the understanding and treatment of reflux disease. J Gastroenterol Hepatol. 2009;24 Suppl 3:S5–14.

Dent J, El-Serag HB, Wallander MA, Johansson S. Epidemiology of gastrooesophageal reflux disease: a systematic review. Gut. 2005;54:710–7.

Fock KM, Poh CH. Gastroesophageal Reflux Disease. J Gastroenterol. 2010;45:808–15.

Friedenberg FK, Hanlon A, Vanar V, et al. Trends in gastroesophageal reflux disease as measured by the National Ambulatory Medical Care Survey. Dig Dis Sci. 2010;55: 1911–7.

Hoppo T, Immanuel A, Shuchert M, Dubrava Z, et al. Transoral Incisionless Fundoplication 2.0 Procedure Using EsophyX for Gastroesophageal Reflux Disease. J Gastrointest Surg. 2010;14(12):1895–901.

Hunter JG, Trus TL, Branum GD, Waring JP, Wood WC. A physiologic approach to laparoscopic fundoplication for gastroesophageal reflux disease. Ann Surg. 1996;223: 673–87.

Kamolz T, Granderath FA, Bammer T, et al. Dysphagia and quality of life after laparoscopic Nissen fundoplication in patients with and without prosthetic reinforcement of the hiatal crura. Surg Endosc. 2002;16:572–7.

Lafullarde T, Watson DI, Jamieson GG, Myers JC, Game PA, Devitt PG. Laparoscopic Nissen fundoplication: five-year results and beyond. Arch Surg. 2001;136:180–4.

Locke III GR, Talley NJ, Fett SL, Zinsmeister AR, Melton III LJ. Prevalence and clinical spectrum of gastroesophageal reflux: a population-based study in Olmsted County, Minnesota. Gastroenterology. 1997;112:1448–56.

Lundell L. Complications after anti-reflux surgery. Best Pract Res Clin Gastroenterol. 2004;18:935–45.

Lundell L, Miettinen P, Myrvold HE, et al. Seven-year follow-up of a randomized clinical trial comparing proton-pump inhibition with surgical therapy for reflux oesophagitis. Br J Surg. 2007;94:198–203.

Mahon D, Rhodes M, Decadt B, Hindmarsh A, Lowndes R, Beckingham I, Koo B, Newcombe RG. Randomized clinical trial of laparoscopic Nissen fundoplication compared with proton-pump inhibitors for treatment of chronic gastrooesophageal reflux. Br J Surg. 2005;92:695–9.

Mederi Therapeutics Inc. Instructions For Use. 2011.

Medigus SRS Endoscope http://www.medigus.com/.

Nguyen A, Vo T, Nguyen X, Smith BR, Reavis KM. Transoral Incisionless Fundoplication: Initial Experience in Patients Referred to an Integrated Academic Institution. Presented at the Southern California Chapter of the American College of Surgeons. 2011.

Hays RD, Sherbourne CD, Mazel RM. The RAND 36-Item Health Survey 1.0. Health Econ. 1993;2:217–27.

Terry M, Smith CD, Branum GD, Galloway K, Waring JP, Hunter JG. Outcomes of laparoscopic fundoplication for gastroesophageal refluxdisease and paraesophageal hernia. wSurg Endosc. 2001;15:691–9.

17. Endoscopic Resection for Barrett's Esophagus with Dysplasia

John G. Lee, M.D.

A. Introduction

Barrett's esophagus is defined as endoscopically visible metaplastic transformation of the distal esophageal squamous epithelium into specialized intestinal epithelium. Endoscopy shows Barrett's esophagus as salmon pink mucosa in contrast to the grayish white color of the normal squamous esophageal tissue. It displaces the squamocolumnar junction proximal to the gastroesophageal junction, either in finger-like projections or circumferentially. The second part of the definition for Barrett's esophagus in the USA requires demonstration of intestinal metaplasia with the presence of goblet cells on biopsy. Not all patients with salmon pink mucosa have intestinal metaplasia nor do all patients with intestinal metaplasia on biopsy have endoscopically visible salmon pink mucosa. Both components must be presented to fulfill the accepted definition of Barrett's esophagus in the USA.

B. Background

1. Barrett's esophagus is a complication of gastroesophageal reflux.
2. Barrett's esophagus is most commonly found in Caucasian males >50 years old with long standing heartburn symptoms.
3. Short segment Barrett's esophagus is defined as <3 cm.
4. Barrett's esophagus is often acid insensitive so patients may initially deny heartburn symptoms.
5. Barrett's esophagus is found in 10–15% of patients undergoing endoscopy for reflux.

N.T. Nguyen and C.E.H. Scott-Conner (eds.), *The SAGES Manual: Volume 2 Advanced Laparoscopy and Endoscopy*, DOI 10.1007/978-1-4614-2347-8_17,
© Springer Science+Business Media, LLC 2012

    a.   Incidence of Barrett's in the USA is 3.6/100,000 Caucasian males.

    b.   The prevalence of Barrett's esophagus in the general population was 1.6% in Sweden with a third being long segment disease.

6.   Barrett's esophagus is a premalignant condition.

    a.   The annual risk of developing esophageal adenocarcinoma is estimated to be 0.4–0.5%/year for Barrett's esophagus.

    b.   Cancer risk is 30- to 125-fold higher in Barrett's esophagus.

    c.   Cancer incidence in high grade dysplasia (HGD) is 6.58/100 patient-years.

    d.   5–10% of patients with Barrett's esophagus can develop cancer without intervention.

    e.   Recent Mayo study showed 12.8% of patients with HGD who underwent esophagectomy between 1994 and 2004 had incidental cancer.

C. Diagnosis of Barrett's Esophagus

1.   Diagnosis requires both endoscopic visualization of the specialized columnar epithelium and histological confirmation of intestinal metaplasia.

2.   The usual protocol is to biopsy any suspicious mucosal lesion and to take four quadrant biopsies every 1- to 2-cm intervals, preferably using jumbo biopsy forceps.

3.   Alternative biopsy protocols used include

    a.   Chromoendoscopy—not helpful on recent meta-analysis.

    b.   Narrow band imaging—predicts HGD and is sensitive but not specific for Barrett's esophagus.

4.   Diagnosis of dysplasia

    a.   The American College of Gastroenterology recommends that an expert pathologist confirm the diagnosis of dysplasia.

    b.   Surveillance intervals

        i.   HGD—treat or survey every 3 months.

        ii.   Low grade dysplasia (LGD)—every 6 months; after two consecutive negative studies every 3 years.

        iii.   No dysplasia—every 3 years.

D. Treatment

1. There is no known medical therapy.
2. Recommended only for patients with HGD.
3. Esophagectomy is the traditional treatment for HGD.
   a. Morbidity and mortality are 37 and 1% and may be higher in
      i. Low volume centers (<20 cases/year)
      ii. Known cancer
4. Endoscopic therapy
   a. Ablation and lifelong acid suppression is required to regrow and maintain the normal squamous epithelium.
      i. Examine nodular Barrett's with endoscopic ultrasound (EUS) to rule out cancer then resect using endoscopic mucosal resection (EMR) or endoscopic submucosal dissection (ESD).
      ii. Flat Barrett's does not require EUS and is best treated with radiofrequency ablation.
      iii. Laser, argon plasma coagulation, electrocoagulation, and photodynamic therapy are not used anymore.
   b. Endoscopic mucosal resection
      i. Determine the lateral margins of the lesion
         – Magnification, chromoendoscopy, narrow band imaging or other techniques may be helpful
         – Mark the boarders using a snare tip and brief burst of cautery
      ii. Lift the lesion using
         – Salin injection
            i. Mix with methylene blue to highlight the lesion and epinephrine for hemostasis.
            ii. Inject distally first to prevent the lesion from pushed away from the endoscopic view.
            iii. Stop injecting and redirect the needle if a bleb is not seen immediately with injection.
            iv. Avoid injecting through the lesion to prevent spreading unrecognized cancer.
            v. Inject enough to clearly lift the entire lesion (usually 10–15 ml for a 1 cm lesion).
         – Suction then banding as done during variceal therapy if the lesion is small enough to fit inside the banding cap (<1 cm)

   iii. Cut by
- Suctioning into a cap and snare, Fig. 17.1
  - i. Use appropriate size (available from 13 to 19 mm diameter) and shaped (straight or oblique tip) cap
  - ii. Tape the cap so it does not dislodge during removal of the endoscope
  - iii. Use dedicated EMR crescent snare (regular snare will not work)
    1. Suction normal mucosa into the cap while slowing opening the snare to fit it around the rim of the cap then release suction
    2. Redirect the endoscope to the lesion and suction into cap and tighten the snare
    3. Release suction, check to make sure the entire lesion has been captured then cut
    4. Inspect the resected site for residual lesion, perforation or bleeding; it should look blue from the injection not yellow or red
    5. Suction the specimen into the cap then remove the endoscope
    6. Consider fixing the specimen on a cork board with pins to orient it for the pathologist
       a. Repeat EMR for any residual lesion
          - i. Reinject as needed
          - ii. Use a new snare for each EMR
          - iii. Use the initial markings to make sure all of the lesion has been removed
- Stiff monofilament snare
  - i. Bury the tip of the snare distal to the lesion then open slowly while pressing down to capture the lesion
  - ii. Cut as above
- Lifted into the open snare using grasping forceps and a double channel endoscope
  - i. Open a conventional snare then feed the grasping forceps through the open snare

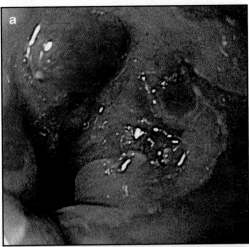

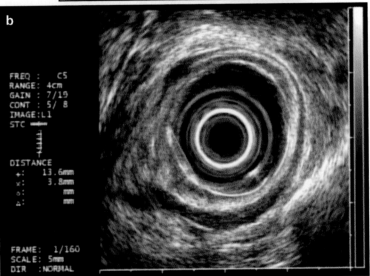

Fig. 17.1 (**a**) Barrett's esophagus with dysplastic nodule. (**b**) EUS shows 14 mm×4 mm mucosal nodule with intact submucosa. (**c**) Cap EMR showing nodule captured with snare. Note bluish saline cushion surrounding the nodule. (**d**) Esophagus after EMR shows large mucosal defect. (**e**) EMR specimen showing the bluish saline cushion.

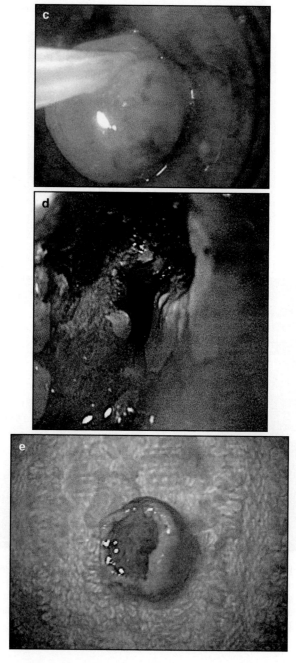

Fig. 17.1 (continued)

    1. Grasp and slowly pull up the lesion into the open snare and resect as above

  iv. Results of EMR
- Requires high degree of endoscopic skill
- A European trial eradicated Barrett's esophagus in 80.5% of 169 patients with median of 3 cm of Barrett's esophagus.
  - i. Patients underwent a median of two sessions, each with median of four piecemeal EMR
  - ii. 61% required argon plasma coagulation
  - iii. Half had symptomatic strictures from the treatments and 3% required surgery.
  - iv. Treatment eradicated dysplasia or cancer in 97.6% and all Barrett's tissue in 85.2%.
    - 1. Eradication persisted in 95.3 and 80.5% of cases at median follow up of 32 months.
- Successful therapy requires ablation of all Barrett's
  - i. In one study neoplasia recurred significantly more in patients who did not undergo ablation.
    - 1. Neoplasia was only found in patients with incomplete ablation.

  v. EMR can be used to remove short segment Barrett's esophagus but is difficult and impractical for long segment Barrett's

  vi. EMR is best for treating nodular Barrett's with ablation of the surrounding Barrett's done using other methods.

 c. ESD—performed by first raising a bleb then using a needle knife to free hand dissect the lesion.
- i. No theoretical limit to the maximal size of the lesion removable.
- ii. Dissection performed to the muscularis propria, which is deeper than EMR.
- iii. Provides clear lateral and deep margins.
- iv. Most ESD devices are not available in the USA.
- v. Very time consuming and difficult in the esophagus and not routinely available in the USA.

5. Selection of patient for treatment

a. The American College of Gastroenterology and the Society of Thoracic Surgeons both recommend EMR or endoscopic ablation or resection for HGD

   i. HGD has 30% risk of cancer development (class II a recommendation based on level B evidence).

   ii. Possible multifocal dysplasia and prevention of future dysplasia require ablation of any surrounding non-dysplastic Barrett's.

   iii. Treatment of LGD or nondysplastic Barrett's may be performed at patient request, or as part of a research protocol, or depending on the clinical scenario.

b. Endoscopic ablation

   i. Radiofrequency (HALO, Barrx Medical Inc, Sunnyvale, CA) is easier, faster, and more effective than EMR for treating underlying nondysplastic Barrett's.

   ii. Radiofrequency ablation is effective treatment for flat HGD and LGD when used with EMR of any nodular lesions.

     − The HALO balloon catheter ablates 3 cm of the esophagus circumferentially

     − The HALO focal ablation device is used for smaller segments

     − The HALO devices only cause mucosal damage without deeper injury using a precise amount of energy (usually 12 J and 40 W/cm^2)

   iii. Clinical results.

     − The US multicenter sham controlled trial

       i. Ablation was significantly better at eradicating Barrett's esophagus (77.4 vs. 2.3%, $P<0.001$), LGD (90.5 vs. 22.7%, $P<0.001$), and HGD (81 vs. 19%, $P<0.001$).

       ii. Ablation significantly reduced esophageal cancer (1.2 vs. 9.3%, $P=0.045$) and disease progression (3.6 vs. 16.3%, $P=0.03$) during the 12-month follow-up period.

       iii. The treatment took median of 36 min under intravenous sedation; 84 patients treated mean of 3.5 sessions.

       iv. Two patients were hospitalized for pain control and one had bleeding treated endoscopically.

      v. Six percent developed esophageal strictures requiring endoscopic dilation.
- EMR only versus EMR plus radiofrequency
  - i. Two were comparable at ablation of dysplasia (100 vs. 96%, respectively) and Barrett's (92 vs. 96%, respectively).
  - ii. EMR resulted in more strictures (88 vs. 14%, $P<0.001$) and severe (24 vs. 0%, $P=0.02$) and moderate (72 vs. 18%, $P=0$) complications.

    iv. Therefore, use EMR to remove nodules followed by radiofrequency ablation of the remaining Barrett's esophagus in 6–8 weeks until all Barrett's esophagus had been eradicated, Fig. 17.2.

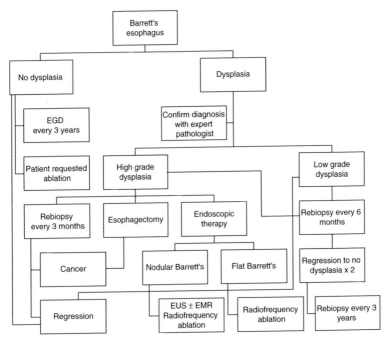

Fig. 17.2 Algorithm for management of patients with Barrett's esophagus.

E. Conclusion

Effective treatment now exists for patients with Barrett's esophagus using EMR to remove any nodular lesion followed by radiofrequency ablation of surrounding Barrett's esophagus. This treatment is cost-effective at significantly decreasing the cancer risk in patients with Barrett's esophagus.

Selected References

de Jonge PJ, van Blankenstein M, Looman CW, et al. Risk of malignant progression in patients with Barrett's oesophagus: a Dutch Nationwide Cohort Study. Gut. 2010; 59(8):1030–6.

Ell C, May A, Gossner L, et al. Endoscopic mucosal resection of early cancer and high-grade dysplasia in Barrett's esophagus. Gastroenterology. 2000;118(4):670–7.

Fernando HC, Murthy SC, Hofstetter W, et al. The Society of Thoracic Surgeons practice guideline series: guidelines for the management of Barrett's esophagus with high-grade dysplasia. Ann Thorac Surg. 2009;87(6):1993–2002.

Fleischer DE, Odze R, Overholt BF, et al. The case for endoscopic treatment of non-dysplastic and low-grade dysplastic Barrett's esophagus. Dig Dis Sci. 2010;55(7): 1918–31.

Inadomi JM, Somsouk M, Madanick RD, et al. A cost-utility analysis of ablative therapy for Barrett's esophagus. Gastroenterology. 2009;136(7):2101–2114.e1-6.

Larghi A, Lightdale CJ, Ross AS, et al. Long-term follow-up of complete Barrett's eradication endoscopic mucosal resection (CBE-EMR) for the treatment of high grade dysplasia and intramucosal carcinoma. Endoscopy. 2007;39(12):1086–91.

Mannath J, Subramanian V, Hawkey CJ, et al. Narrow band imaging for characterization of high grade dysplasia and specialized intestinal metaplasia in Barrett's esophagus: a meta-analysis. Endoscopy. 2010;42(5):351–9.

Ngamruengphong S, Sharma VK, Das A. Diagnostic yield of methylene blue chromoendoscopy for detecting specialized intestinal metaplasia and dysplasia in Barrett's esophagus: a meta-analysis. Gastrointest Endosc. 2009;69(6):1021–8.

Pech O, Behrens A, May A, et al. Long-term results and risk factor analysis for recurrence after curative endoscopic therapy in 349 patients with high-grade intraepithelial neoplasia and mucosal adenocarcinoma in Barrett's oesophagus. Gut. 2008;57(9): 1200–6.

Pech O, May A, Rabenstein T, et al. Endoscopic resection of early oesophageal cancer. Gut. 2007;56(11):1625–34.

Pouw RE, Seewald S, Gondrie J, et al. Stepwise radical endoscopic resection for eradication of Barrett's oesophagus with early neoplasia in a cohort of 169 patients. Gut. 2010;59:1169–77.

Prasad GA, Wang KK, Buttar NS, et al. Long-term survival following endoscopic and surgical treatment of high-grade dysplasia in Barrett's esophagus. Gastroenterology. 2007;132(4):1226–33.

Rastogi A, Puli S, El-Serag HB, et al. Incidence of esophageal adenocarcinoma in patients with Barrett's esophagus and high-grade dysplasia: a meta-analysis. Gastrointest Endosc. 2008;67(3):394–8.

Rees JR, Lao-Sirieix P, Wong A, et al. Treatment for Barrett's oesophagus. Cochrane Database Syst Rev. 2010;1:CD004060.

Shaheen NJ, Sharma P, Overholt BF, et al. Radiofrequency ablation in Barrett's esophagus with dysplasia. N Engl J Med. 2009;360(22):2277–88.

Society for Surgery of the Alimentary Tract. SSAT patient care guidelines. Management of Barrett's esophagus. J Gastrointest Surg. 2007;11(9):1213–5.

Van Vilsteren FG, Pouw RE, Seewald S, et al. Stewise radical endoscopic resection versus radiofrequency ablation for Barrett's oesophagus with high-grade dysplasia or early cancer: a multicentre randomised trial. Gut. 2011;60(6):765–73.

Wang KK, Sampliner RE. Practice Parameters Committee of the American College of Gastroenterology. Updated guidelines 2008 for the diagnosis, surveillance and therapy of Barrett's esophagus. Am J Gastroenterol. 2008;103(3):788–97.

Wani S, Puli SR, Shaheen NJ, et al. Esophageal adenocarcinoma in Barrett's esophagus after endoscopic ablative therapy: a meta-analysis and systematic review. Am J Gastroenterol. 2009;104(2):502–13.

Yousef F, Cardwell C, Cantwell MM, et al. The incidence of esophageal cancer and high-grade dysplasia in Barrett's esophagus: a systematic review and meta-analysis. Am J Epidemiol. 2008;168(3):237–49.

18. Endoscopic Ablative Therapy

Erin W. Gilbert, M.D.
John G. Hunter, M.D.

A. Description

In medicine, the term "ablation" refers to the complete removal or destruction of a piece of biological tissue usually with an operation or other invasive procedure. In patients with Barrett's esophagus (BE), this refers to the obliteration of specialized intestinal metaplastic (SIM) epithelium characterized by the presence of mucin-filled goblet cells as seen in the small intestine. The malignant progression from SIM to esophageal adenocarcinoma (EAC) has been well described; thus, interventions to ablate the premalignant lesion in order to decrease the likelihood of developing EAC seem logical. The current medical and surgical interventions for BE fail to routinely promote complete eradication of SIM. At best, they may prevent progression of the disease and there only indirect evidence that they reduce the risk of EAC. In randomized controlled trials, ablative therapies far outperform medical and surgical treatments at resolving BE, with complete eradication rates of between 75 and 98%.

The current accepted application of endoscopic ablative therapy is for the treatment of flat high-grade dysplasia (HGD) (see Fig. 18.1). Patients with discrete visible lesions should undergo endoscopic mucosal resection prior to ablative therapy. The specimen retrieved can provide an assessment of radial as well as deep margins and can be more accurate than endoscopic ultrasound at differentiating intramucosal from submucosal carcinoma. The risk of lymph node involvement in intramucosal (T_{is} and T1a according to the seventh edition of the American Joint Committee on Cancer [AJCC]) carcinomas is low at 0–1.3% thus these patients may be successfully treated endoscopically without undergoing esophagectomy and its associated morbidity. In contrast, patients with adenocarcinoma that extends to the submucosa (T1b AJCC) should not

N.T. Nguyen and C.E.H. Scott-Conner (eds.), *The SAGES Manual: Volume 2*   273
Advanced Laparoscopy and Endoscopy, DOI 10.1007/978-1-4614-2347-8_18,
© Springer Science+Business Media, LLC 2012

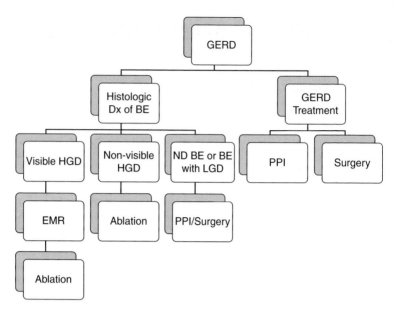

Fig. 18.1. Algorithm for the management of BE and dysplasia. *BE* Barrett's esophagus, *HGD* high-grade dysplasia, *ND* nondysplastic, *LGD* low-grade dysplasia, *PPI* proton pump inhibitor, *EMR* endoscopic mucosal resection (reprinted with permission from Fleischer DE, et al. The case for endoscopic treatment of non-dysplastic and low-grade dysplastic Barrett's esophagus. Dig Dis Sci. 2010;55:1918–31).

undergo focal ablative therapy as lymph node involvement can be present in as many as 45%.

Radiofrequency ablation (RFA) utilizes radiofrequency energy delivered via electrodes 250 µm apart arranged by alternating polarity. A high-powered short burst of radiofrequency energy is applied to the columnar epithelium via direct contact with the electrodes. Depth of tissue destruction is determined by electrode pattern, field geometry, and the intensity of energy delivered. Two doses of energy applied at 300 W and 10–12 J/cm² have been found to provide a controlled ablation depth of 500–1,000 µm effectively removing full-thickness metaplastic epithelium without damaging the underlying submucosa (see Fig. 18.2). Delivery of the ablative energy occurs in less than 1 s. Two systems are available for clinical use. The first is a 360°-circumferential ablation device consisting of a sizing balloon catheter and 3-cm-long balloon ablation catheters of varying sizes (see Fig. 18.3). The second consists of an endoscope mounted 90° focal ablation device (see Fig. 18.4). Both systems require a radiofrequency generator as a power source (see Fig. 18.5).

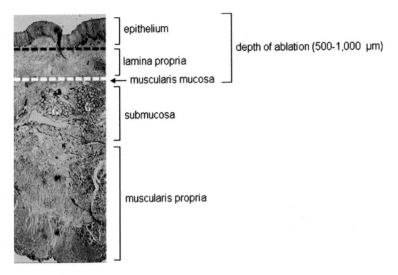

Fig. 18.2. Depth of radiofrequency ablation (reproduced with permission of BÂRRX Medical, Inc).

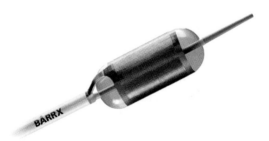

Fig. 18.3. 360°-ablation catheter (reproduced with permission of BÂRRX Medical, Inc).

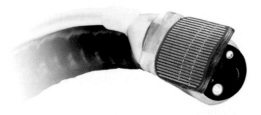

Fig. 18.4. 90°-endoscopic mounted electrode (reproduced with permission of BÂRRX Medical, Inc).

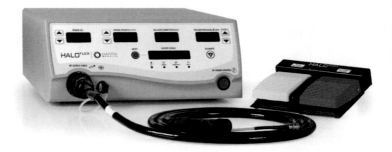

Fig. 18.5.   Energy generator (reproduced with permission of BÂRRX Medical, Inc).

Following ablative therapy, a neosquamous epithelium develops in the treatment area. It is recommended that primary treatment should involve the 360°-ablation device with the goal of ablating all SIM. If only focal treatment is utilized with the 90°-device, as the patient is at risk of developing cancer in the remaining field of BE.

B. Indications

1.   Treatment of HGD within BE without visible lesions.
2.   Treatment of HGD in BE 6–8 weeks following mucosal resection of a visible lesion. (Any visible mucosal lesion should be endoscopically resected with EMR prior to ablation to detect inpatients occult adenocarcinoma).
3.   Eradication of BE with confirmed low-grade dysplasia without visible lesions or esophageal inflammation may be considered on a case by case basis not an absolute indication.

   Treatment of BE with LGD avoids the possibility of leaving behind untreated HGD secondary to sampling error.
4.   Endoscopic ablation of nondysplastic BE is still considered investigational. The low risk of progression to cancer in this condition requires that between 25 and 100 patients would need to be treated to benefit one patient.

C. Patient Preparation, Position, and Setup

1.   Patients must undergo a repeat high-resolution endoscopy with four-quadrant biopsies every 1–2 cm within 2 months prior to the procedure to exclude EAC.

2. Any diagnosis of dysplasia should be confirmed by two experienced pathologists prior to treatment. In cases of early EAC, EUS and CT of the chest/abdomen should be considered to rule out more advanced disease. EMR may provide histological proof of intramucosal cancer if a target lesion is present.

3. Obtain informed written consent concentrating on expected benefits, possible risks, and the experience of the operator.

4. All ablative procedures should be performed in conjunction with at least daily proton pump inhibitor (PPI) therapy. Prior to the procedure, titrate PPI therapy to adequately control GERD symptoms and to heal all erosive esophagitis.

5. Do not permit the patient to eat or drink 6–8 h prior to the procedure.

6. Place the patient comfortably in the left lateral position.

7. Apply monitoring devices to the patient (non-invasive blood pressure monitor, electrocardiography, pulse oximetry) and establish intravenous access.

8. Remove dentures and place a bite block.

D. Performing the Procedure: 360° Ablation Technique (Figs. 18.6 and 18.7)

1. Before begins the procedure, confirm the correct patient, procedure to be performed and that all necessary equipment is readily available and fully functional.

2. Perform a white-light EGD as previously described in the text. Verify that there is no visible abnormality of the mucosa that may be too thick for adequate ablation.

3. Irrigate the esophagus with 1% N-acetylcysteine mixed with water to clear the esophagus of excess mucous.

4. Identify the LES (the top of the gastric folds in a nondistended esophagus) and the most proximal extent of BE (including islands of BE) and note the distance from bite block to each of these landmarks.

5. When the initial EGD assessment has been completed, insert the guide wire (Amplatz extra stiff 0.035 in.; Denmark, Cook Europe) and remove the endoscope.

6. Introduce the 22-mm×4-cm noncompliant sizing catheter balloon over the guide wire and position it 5 cm above the most proximal extent of BE. In this position, the distal end of the

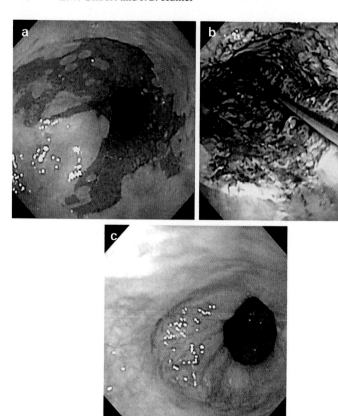

Fig. 18.6. Endoscopic view of 360°-RFA ablation. (**a**) 4 cm of BE. (**b**) Immediately following 360°-balloon RFA. (**c**) The same patient at 12-month follow-up endoscopy. Biopsy specimens confirm no histological evidence of BE (reprinted with permission from Sharma et al. Balloon-based, circumferential endoscopic radiofrequency ablation of Barrett & Apos Esophagus: 1-year follow-up of 100 patients (with video). Gastrointestinal endoscopy. 2007).

> balloon is 1 cm above the BE. This step is generally performed "blind" using the centimeter-scale markings on the sizing balloon catheter for reference.

7.   Sizing is accomplished by activating the appropriate foot pedal of the generator which automatically inflates the balloon (to a standard 4 psi) while displaying and recording the inner esophageal diameter.

8.   Repeat the sizing balloon measurement every 1 cm until an increase in diameter is seen, indicating that the balloon has reached the gastric cardia.

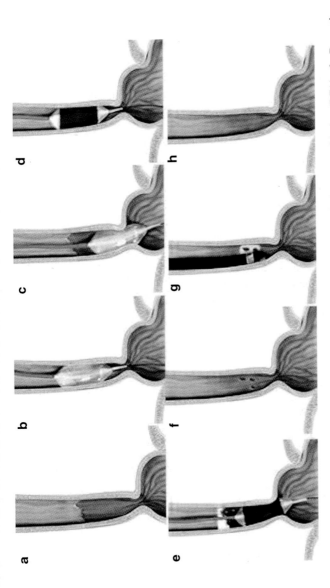

Fig. 18.7. A schematic illustration of primary circumferential and secondary focal radiofrequency ablation (RFA) of a Barrett's esophagus. (**a**) Barrett's esophagus. (**b**) Advancing the sizing balloon. (**c**) Measuring inner esophageal diameter with sizing balloon. (**d**) Advancement of ablation balloon catheter. (**e**) Ablating with balloon catheter. (**f**) Residual BE at 8–12 weeks. (**g**) Focal ablation with 90°-electrode. (**h**) Complete eradication of BE (reproduced with permission of http://www.endosurgery.eu).

9. Remove the sizing balloon catheter leaving the guide wire in place.

10. Choose an appropriately sized ablation catheter smaller than the smallest measured inner diameter and introduce it over the guide wire followed by the endoscope. Available sizes are 22-, 25-, 28-, 31-, and 34-mm outer diameters.

11. Under direct visualization, position the proximal margin of the electrode 1 cm above the most proximal extent of measured BE. Inflate the balloon and initiate ablation via the appropriate foot pedal (Fig. 18.6).

12. Move from the proximal to distal extent of BE in 3-cm intervals allowing for approximately 5 mm of overlap with the prior area of ablation until all areas have been treated.

13. The esophagus must be cleaned of coagulated tissue before commencing the second pass ablation. This may be achieved with a forceful spraying of water or with a soft endoscopic cap to mechanically dislodge coagulum. Adequate cleaning between ablations increases the efficacy of the procedure from 90 to 95%.

14. The ablation catheter should also be cleared of any adherent coagulum using moist gauze.

15. Repeat the ablation procedure described above treating the entire area of BE a second time.

E. Performing the Procedure: 90° Focal Ablation Technique (Fig. 18.7)

1. Attach the 90°-electrode to the tip of the endoscope at the 12 o'clock position.

2. When introducing the endoscope into the laryngeal cavity with electrode in place, angle the endoscope downward allowing the leading edge of the electrode to pass behind the arytenoids and enter the proximal esophagus.

3. Position residual BE at the 12 o'clock position.

4. Deflect the endoscope with electrode upward, ensuring close approximation of the electrode with the mucosa.

5. When in good position, activate ablative energy and reactivate immediately following the first ablation with the electrode in the same position. This results in double ablation of the BE.

6.   After all BE has been doubly ablated, remove residual epithe-
     lium with forceful sprays of water or by using the end of the
     electrode to gently mechanically dislodge coagulum.

F. Post-procedure Care

1.   Patients are to receive high-dose PPI therapy for 2 weeks fol-
     lowing treatment and are to be maintained on at least daily PPI
     therapy thereafter. This is to ensure optimal healing and to min-
     imize patient discomfort following treatment. In addition,
     patients can be supplemented with an H2 blocker at night and
     sucralfate suspension five times daily for 2 weeks following
     ablative therapy.
2.   Patients are restricted to a liquid diet for 24 h, and then a soft
     diet for 1 week. They should also avoid liquids and foods that
     are acidic or hot in temperature for 1 week.
3.   Patients may require liquid acetaminophen with or without
     codeine, antiemetics, and an antacid/viscous lidocaine mixture
     for pain control as needed. Nonsteroidal anti-inflammatory
     drugs (NSAIDs) are not advised.

G. Follow-Up

1.   Every 2–3 months following ablation therapy, patients should
     undergo repeat endoscopy with repeat 360° ablation for any
     residual circumferential BE 2 cm or greater or for diffuse
     areas of BE islands greater than 2 cm until no residual BE
     remains. Irregular Z-lines and scattered residual islands or
     small tongues of BE should be treated with focal (90°) abla-
     tive therapy. It may be difficult to achieve complete ablation if
     there is ongoing GERD. In these situations, fundoplication
     may most effectively stop all GERD, improving the success of
     RFA ablation.
2.   Once complete eradication of Barrett's epithelium is achieved,
     endoscopic surveillance should be continued with repeat endos-
     copy in 6 months and yearly thereafter.

H. Technical Considerations

1. **Difficulty introducing 90°-electrode**: With the 90°-electrode at the 12 o'clock position, advance a biopsy forceps behind the arytenoids and into the proximal esophagus. Deflect the endoscope downward so that the leading edge of the electrode is touching the biopsy forceps. Gently advance the endoscope using the biopsy forceps as a guide.

2. **Difficulty advancing the sizing balloon catheter over the guide wire**: In cases of localized narrowing and difficult balloon introduction, this step may be performed with endoscopic visualization to assure atraumatic advancement of the balloon catheter.

3. **Difficulty fitting the 360 ablation balloon** within the flared portion of the gastroesophageal junction (GEJ) may leave focal areas of BE untreated. Apply gentle traction on the balloon while in the GEJ to achieve a more uniform ablation.

4. Applying suction while ablating may improve electrode apposition and efficacy of ablation.

5. RFA does not interfere with the ability to perform future endoscopic mucosal resection if required.

6. In frail patients with long-segment BE, consider limiting the extent of circumferential ablation to 6 cm or less per session.

I. Complications

1. **Chest pain**: Patients will almost universally complain of chest pain following the procedure. Most will have resolution of this chest pain within 24 h.

2. **Fever**: Mild fever is rare and can usually be treated conservatively with acetaminophen and observation. In cases of a high fever and a high suspicion of severe complication, further workup may be necessary.

3. **Perforation**: This adverse event is a potential risk with the 360°-balloon catheter which can be avoided with careful size selection and gentle introduction of balloon catheters.

4. **Stricture**: The rate of stricture with or without dysphagia is 0–6% and is amenable to treatment with endoscopic balloon dilation (1–3 sessions).

5. **Bleeding**: Bleeding is rare. The risk is increased with concurrent use of antiplatelet agents. It is usually amenable to endoscopic treatment.

6. **Failure to eradicate BE**: RFA results in 72–83% eradication of BE and 89–92% eradication of dysplasia in per protocol analysis. At 12 months, 77–98% have complete eradication of BE and 98–100% have complete eradication of dysplasia. Response rates are inversely proportional to baseline length of BE and multiple ablative sessions may be required to reach complete eradication of BE (Fig. 18.8).

7. The complete response rate of BE following complete endoscopic eradication remains as high as 92% at 5-year follow-up.

8. **Recurrence**: The rate of post-RFA subsquamous intestinal metaplasia is low (<5%) and lower than pre-procedure rate (25%); however, long term follow-up data are limited.

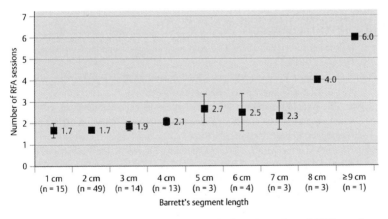

Fig. 18.8. Association of baseline length of BE and number of RFA sessions (mean ± SEM) required to achieve complete eradication of BE (reprinted with permission from Lyday et al. Radiofrequency ablation of Barett's esophagus: Outcomes of 429 patients from a multicenter community practice registry. Endoscopy 2010, Vol. 42, p. 272).

Selected References

Barbour AP, Jones M, Brown I, et al. Risk stratification for early esophageal adenocarcinoma: analysis of lymphatic spread and prognostic factors. Ann Surg Oncol. 2010;17: 2494–502.

Edge SB, Byrd DR, Compton CC, Fritz AG, Greene FL, Tritti A, editors. AJCC cancer staging manual. 7th ed. New York: Springer; 2009.

Fernando HC, Murthy SC, Hofstetter W, et al. The society of thoracic surgeons practice guideline series: guidelines for the management of barrett's esophagus with high-grade dysplasia. Ann Thorac Surg. 2009;87:1993–2002.

Fleischer DE, Odze R, Overholt BF, et al. The case for endoscopic treatment of non-dysplastic and low-grade dysplastic barrett's esophagus. Dig Dis Sci. 2010a;55: 1918–31.

Fleischer DE, Overholt BF, Sharma VK, et al. Endoscopic radiofrequency ablation for barrett's esophagus: 5-year outcomes from a prospective multicenter trial. Endoscopy. 2010b;42:781–9.

Gondrie JJ, Pouw RE, Sondermeijer CM, et al. Effective treatment of early barrett's neoplasia with stepwise circumferential and focal ablation using the HALO system. Endoscopy. 2008a;40:370–9.

Lyday WD, Corbett FS, Kuperman DA, et al. Radiofrequency ablation of barrett's esophagus: outcomes of 429 patients from a multicenter community practice registry. Endoscopy. 2010;42:272–8.

Pouw RE, Sharma VK, Bergman JJ, Fleischer DE. Radiofrequency ablation for total barrett's eradication: a description of the endoscopic technique, its clinical results and future prospects. Endoscopy. 2008;40:1033–40.

Pouw RE, Wirths K, Eisendrath P, et al. Efficacy of radiofrequency ablation combined with endoscopic resection for barrett's esophagus with early neoplasia. Clin Gastroenterol Hepatol. 2010;8:23–9.

Shaheen NJ, Sharma P, Overholt BF, et al. Radiofrequency ablation in barrett's esophagus with dysplasia. N Engl J Med. 2009;360:2277–88.

Sharma VK, Wang KK, Overholt BF, et al. Balloon-based, circumferential, endoscopic radiofrequency ablation of barrett's esophagus: 1-year follow-up of 100 patients. Gastrointest Endosc. 2007;65:185–95.

Stein HJ, Feith M, Bruecher BL, Naehrig J, Sarbia M, Siewert JR. Early esophageal cancer: pattern of lymphatic spread and prognostic factors for long-term survival after surgical resection. Ann Surg. 2005;242:566–73.

Part III

Laparoscopic Gastric Surgery: Advanced Procedures

19. Laparoscopic Surgery for Gastric Cancer[*]

Alfred Cuschieri, M.D., D.Sc., F.R.C.S., F.A.C.S., F.R.S., F.Med.SC

A. Introduction

Since its introduction by Kitano for early gastric cancer in 1994 and by Azagra in 1993 for advanced disease, the uptake of laparoscopic surgery for gastric cancer has steadily grown as a result of increasing experience and enabling energized technologies facilitating dissection and efficient hemostasis. In many centers, the laparoscopic approach is still mainly used for early gastric cancer (limited to the mucosa/superficial submucosa), most commonly for distal disease, for which distal gastrectomy with $D_{1A,B}$ lymph node clearance dissection is performed. Thus, in Japan, laparoscopic distal gastrectomy (LDG) accounted for 70% of all resections for cancer in 2005. However, in some of the high-volume hospitals, laparoscopic D_2 gastrectomy is being adopted in preference to open surgery for advanced gastric cancer with good results either by the direct manual laparoscopic approach (total or laparoscopically assisted) or by the Da Vinci robotic operating system.

Irrespective of the approach used, the indications and the extent of gastric resection remain unchanged from the Japanese Gastric Cancer Association Treatment Guidelines (see references). Overall, the uptake of the laparoscopic approach has been slow, and even in Japan published data from surveys in 2005 indicate that the laparoscopic approach was used for resection of gastric cancer in only 15% of cases. Although there are no recent data on the uptake in Western countries, it is likely, judged by the publication of several retrospective series, that the laparoscopic

---

[*]AJCC Cancer Staging Manual, Seventh Edition (2010) published by Springer Science and Business Media, LLC, http://www.springerlink.com.

approach has gained increasing popularity in the past 5 years because of its documented benefits to the short-term outcome of patients over traditional open surgery without compromise of both the safety and oncologic outcomes. This chapter deals mainly with laparoscopic surgery for gastric cancer, but the same techniques are applicable to resection of other pathologies, including gastrointestinal stromal tumors (for which the laparoscopic approach is ideal).

B. Approaches

There are four techniques used for laparoscopic resections for gastric cancer.

1. **Laparoscopically assisted gastrectomy** is favored in Japan. It uses a minilaparotomy for restoration of the continuity of the gastrointestinal tract after the resection. The advantages include ease of execution of the anastomosis, reduced operative time, and, in some cases, avoiding the use of staplers.
2. **Hand-assisted gastrectomy** (favored by the author) uses some form of hand port introduced through an appropriately placed longitudinal or transverse minilaparotomy (6.0–8.0 cm) usually to the right of the midline from the start of the operation. In our experience, the internal dominant hand of the operator greatly facilitates the complex dissection required in D_2 resections, provides immediate control of any arterial bleeding, facilitates the reconstruction, and generally reduces the operating time.
3. **Total laparoscopic gastrectomy** is favored by the purists and in theory provides the least minimal access approach as the entire procedure is carried out without the creation of a minilaparotomy, although there is no reported evidence to suggest that it offers any advantage in terms of the postoperative recovery and hospital stay than either the laparoscopically assisted or hand-assisted techniques.
4. **Robotic (Da Vinci) gastrectomy** is the most recent technique. It imparts certain obvious advantages: excellent immersive stereoscopic viewing throughout, surgeon comfort (although the assistant surgeon is disadvantaged), greater precision of surgical manipulations, ease of intracorporeal suturing, etc., all of which reduce the level of difficulty of the execution. But it achieves this at increased costs and places an extra burden on the

assistant surgeon. This extra burden, previously ignored, includes encroachment upon the assistant's workspace by the robotic arms, physical separation from the surgeon (leading to communication problems), and the need to perform certain tasks of the operation which would in non-robotic operations be performed by the surgeon. Thus, the role of the assistant surgeon during robotic surgery has changed from the traditional norm.

C. Patient Selection

1. **Stage of disease**: Selection of the appropriate operation for gastric cancer remains based on preoperative image-based (CT/ MRI) accurate tumor staging.

    The details of the current clinical staging of gastric cancer are given in the AJCC staging manual. Although this clinical staging of patients with gastric cancer can be improved by laparoscopy (with or without contact laparoscopic ultrasound), since this may identify intraperitoneal seeding of tumor deposits in the liver or on peritoneal surfaces, some have argued that the advent of improved preoperative imaging technology (multidetector CT, 3.0 Tesla MRI) has reduced the gain in improved staging by laparoscopy. Even if this viewpoint is dismissed and staging laparoscopy is recommended for all patients undergoing surgery for gastric cancer, there is no consensus on whether the staging should be performed at a prior session or immediately before the proposed gastrectomy.

    As previously mentioned, there is no consensus on whether laparoscopic gastrectomy should be reserved for early gastric cancer (T1 and T2) or be used in patients with advanced disease. In many respects, the decision in the individual Institution is influenced by experience which in turn depends on the case volume.

2. **Surgeon experience**: There is some published evidence that the proficiency gain curve (learning curve) for laparoscopic gastrectomy is steep and that a surgeon must perform approximately 60 cases to reach proficiency. Thus, it makes sense for the initial experience to be gained with the simpler resections, such as laparoscopic D_1 gastrectomy, until proficiency is gained, and then advance to the more complex D_2 resections.

3. **Obesity**: Initially, patients with visceral obesity are best avoided as they can prove difficult. In this respect, a report by Ueda et al. provides useful information. These authors measured the visceral fat (VF) in 30 patients undergoing LADG based on cross-sectional computed tomography at the level of the umbilicus. On the basis of the measured VF, 12 patients had high VF accumulation (≥ 100 cm^2) and 18 <100 m^2. Although subcutaneous fat accumulation did not correlate with operating time or operative blood loss, VF accumulation strongly and significantly correlated with both operating time and operative blood loss. The high VF-accumulation group had a significantly longer operating time and operative blood loss, although the authors observed no significant difference in postoperative morbidity or conversion to open laparotomy between the two groups. These authors recommend that preoperative estimation of VF accumulation should be considered when making a decision to treat early gastric cancer by LADG.

D. Laparoscopic Resections for Gastric Cancer

Irrespective of the approach used, the following resections can and have been performed with results equivalent to open surgery in the short term:

- Laparoscopic distal gastrectomy D1 or D1+B
- D2 laparoscopic proximal gastrectomy
- D2 laparoscopic subtotal gastrectomy
- D2 laparoscopic total gastrectomy

1. Extent of Gastric Resection

The extent of the gastric resection is determined by the size/extent of the tumor and its location within the stomach (distal, middle, and upper third). The extent of resection for advanced disease needs to be such as to provide a 5.0 cm macroscopically free margin from the cancer if this is of the intestinal type and 10.0-cm margins for diffuse cancers.

For advanced distal gastric cancers, subtotal gastrectomy provides equivalent oncologic outcome with reduced morbidity. However, for advanced tumors of the middle and proximal third of the stomach, total gastrectomy is essential.

The required resection margins for T1 lesions are much less and most would agree that 2.0–2.5 cm is adequate in ensuring complete resection with no residual tumor. Thus, distal, proximal, and subtotal gastrectomies are possible depending on the location of the lesion.

2. Extent of Lymphadenectomy

The extent of lymphadenectomy in the surgery for gastric cancer remains controversial in Western countries but not in Japan, where D_2 lymphadenectomy is the routine procedure for advanced gastric cancer. Despite the indifferent results of randomized clinical trials (RCTs) in the West, reported data from Japan seem to vindicate the benefit of D_2 resections. The rationale for D_2 resection is based on the centrifugal pattern of the tiers of regional lymph node involvement in invasive gastric cancer.

The more extensive D_3 lymphadenectomy, which includes the additional clearance of the nodes on the aorta/celiac axis and portal vein, carries a significantly higher morbidity, longer operating time, and greater transfusion requirements, and to date there is no evidence that it provides a survival advantage over D_2 resections. Sano et al. reported results from a prospective multicenter randomized trial conducted in Japan comparing D_2 lymphadenectomy alone versus D_2 lymphadenectomy + para-aortic nodal dissection (PAND). They reported similar morbidity and 5-year overall survival rates (69.2 vs. 70.3%).

There have been two large multicenter RCTs in the West comparing D_1 and D_2 dissection: the Dutch Gastric Cancer Group study and the Medical Research Council (MRC) study in the UK. The Dutch randomized 1,078 patients with invasive gastric cancer; of these, 711 patients had a potentially curative resection (380 in the D_1 and 331 in the D_2 arms). This study documented a higher morbidity (25 vs. 43%) and mortality (4 vs. 10%) in the D_2 arm with similar 5-year survival rates (45% for the D_1 and 47% for the D_2 arms). After a follow-up of 11 years, survival between the two groups was similar (30 vs. 35%).

The British MRC trial used the same, almost identical, protocol and indeed for a while the two trials ran concurrently. In this RCT, 737 patients with advanced gastric cancer were registered, but only 400 satisfied the staging intake criteria. These were randomly assigned to D_1 resection ($n=200$) vs. D_2 resection ($n=200$). The MRC trial showed greater postoperative hospital mortality in the D_2 arm (13 vs. 6.5%; $p=0.04$) and higher postoperative morbidity (46 vs. 28%; $p<0.001$). On subset analysis, both the increased postoperative morbidity and mortality in the D_2 arms were attributed to distal pancreaticosplenectomy and splenectomy, which were at that time recommended by the Japanese Society for gastric cancer. The 5-year survival of patients in MRC this trial was also similar, 35% for D_1 resection and 33% for D_2 resection. Multivariate analysis revealed that clinical stages II and III, old age, male gender, and removal of spleen and pancreas were independently associated with poor survival. The authors concluded that the possibility that D_2 resection without pancreaticosplenectomy could provide a better oncologic outcome than D_1 resection could not be dismissed by the results of the MRC trial. It is important to stress that both splenectomy and distal pancreatectomy are no longer considered integral components of D_2 resections and perhaps the exclusion of distal pancreatectomy and spleen preservation has been the most import consequence to surgery for advanced gastric cancer emanating from the MRC study.

Equally important in the author's opinion is the substantive improvement in staging, perioperative care, and experience in high-volume centers in the West with laparoscopic D_2 resections such that conclusions based on the results of the Dutch and British multicenter RCTs performed more than 30 years ago "that D_2 gastrectomy imparts no survival advantage over D_1 resection and is attended by higher postoperative morbidity" are no longer tenable as shown by several subsequent retrospective series. The survival benefit is greatest for T_3 cancers. There is certainly no valid reason why in experienced and competent hands laparoscopic D_2 gastrectomy should not be recommended in modern surgical practice. The findings of even the best RCTs for life-threatening disorders exemplified by cancer may be overtaken by progress in all aspects of patient management: investigational, supportive, and therapeutic.

E. Reported Benefits of Laparoscopic Gastrectomy for Invasive Cancer

Based largely on retrospective, case-controlled, and a few prospective studies (collectively providing level II evidence), several benefits have been consistently reported for the laparoscopic gastric resections irrespective of approach and nature of the operations (D_1 or D_2). These can be outlined as follows:

- Reduced related wound pain
- Lower surgical stress (levels of WBC, CRP, and IL-6)
- Reduced blood loss
- Better retention of pulmonary function (measured by forced vital capacity)
- Earlier passage of flatus
- Earlier resumption of oral food
- Earlier postoperative ambulation
- Earlier hospital discharge

The series reported by Adachi et al. in 2000 was among the first to document the benefits to patient care of the laparoscopic approach in the surgical treatment of gastric cancer: reduced wound pain, reduced operative blood loss, earlier hospital discharge, fewer postoperative complications, and reduced surgical stress (lower elevations of WBC count, C-reactive protein, and interleukin-6). This was followed a year later by the series reported by Shimizu et al., which confirmed most of these benefits but stressed that the laparoscopic approach required a longer operation time.

In a randomized controlled trial comparing laparoscopic versus open distal gastrectomy, Kitano et al. confirmed that for this resection the laparoscopic approach caused less pain during the 1st to the 3rd postoperative day and earlier ambulation. LDG was also accompanied by improved preservation of pulmonary function (forced vital capacity) on the 3rd postoperative day, earlier time to passage of flatus. However, this RCT showed no significant differences in the postoperative morbidity, analgesic usage, time to oral feeding, and hospital discharge.

A case-controlled study based on a prospective gastric cancer database compared 30 consecutive patients undergoing laparoscopic subtotal gastrectomy for gastric cancer with 30 patients undergoing open subtotal gastrectomy. Controls were matched for stage, age, and gender via a statistically generated selection of all gastrectomies performed during the time period. Tumor site and histology were similar between the two groups. The median operative time for the laparoscopic approach was 270 min (range, 150–485 min) compared with 126 min (range, 85–205 min) for the open group ($p < 0.01$). Median hospital stay after laparoscopic gastrectomy was 5 days (range, 2–26 days), compared with 7 days (range, 5–30 days) in the open group ($p = 0.01$). Postoperative pain (measured by the number of days of i.v. narcotic use) was significantly lower for laparoscopic patients (median=3 days, range 0–11 days) compared with 4 days, range 1–13 days for the open patients ($p<0.01$). Although there was a trend for a decrease in the postoperative early complications in the laparoscopic group, the difference was not significant. However, significantly higher rate of late complications was observed in the open group ($p=0.03$). The short-term recurrence-free survival and clearance margins were similar between the two groups as was the number of lymph node harvest.

Peng et al. reported on a meta-analysis involving 218 patients of laparoscopy-assisted distal gastrectomy (LADG) and conventional open distal gastrectomy for early gastric cancer. This confirmed a lower estimated blood loss (weighted mean difference (WMD)=−121.86; 95% CI=−145.61, −98.11; $p<0.001$), earlier postoperative passage of flatus (WMD=−0.95; 95% CI: −1.09, −0.81; $p<0.001$), and shorter hospital stay (WMD=−2.27; 95%CI: −3.47, −1.06; $p=0.0002$), but longer operating time (WMD=58.71; 95% CI: 52.69, 64.74; $p<0.001$) and fewer lymph node harvest (WMD=−3.64; 95% CI: −5.80, −1.47; $p=0.001$). This meta-analysis reported no difference between the two groups in postoperative morbidity (OR=0.57; 95% CI: 0.31, 1.03; $p=0.06$).

A similar meta-analysis of five RCTs on LADG reported by Ohtani et al. involving 326 patients (164 treated with LADG and 162 with open distal gastrectomy) reported significant differences in favor of LADG in the volume of intraoperative blood loss, hospital stay, frequency of analgesic administration, and postoperative morbidity. However, this meta-analysis showed no difference in the resumption of oral intake, rate of tumor recurrence, and mortality. The operative time was significantly longer in LADG and the average number of lymph node harvest was less.

Kitano et al. reported the long-term oncologic outcome (at 10 years) of 116 patients after LDG. The series was composed largely of early gastric cancers (88 mucosal and 36 submucosal) with only 3 T2 cancers and histological node involved was only present in 7 patients (6%), all being located in group 1. Thus, although no recurrence was observed during the mean follow-up time of 60 months, this series was heavily biased to the treatment of early cancer. Nevertheless, the study confirmed that laparoscopic gastrectomy provided equivalent long-term outcome to open surgery in patients treated for early disease.

A recent report from a single institution, on the 10-year experience, attempted to address the oncologic appropriateness of laparoscopic gastrectomy. This study, however, excluded patients undergoing laparoscopic surgery who required conversion to open surgery. The patients included in the study ($n=391$) fulfilled the oncologic requirement of current treatment guidelines. The mean proximal and distal margins were 3.73 ± 2.11 cm and 5.31 ± 3.26 cm for the laparoscopic and open resections, respectively. An average of 22 lymph nodes were harvested for the entire cohort (21.7 ± 12.1). This would be considered suboptimal by Japanese standards. However, the lymph node harvest was similar for the two surgical approaches. The proximal margin in the open surgical cases was 1.0 cm longer than that in laparoscopic group (4.99 ± 2.59 cm vs. 4.06 ± 1.87 cm; $p=0.038$), but the distal margins were similar (6.94 ± 3.52 cm vs. 7.24 ± 4.64 cm).

F. Practical Considerations in Laparoscopic Surgery for Gastric Cancer

At the author's institution, all laparoscopic operations for gastric cancer are carried with miniheparin prophylaxis started 24 h before surgery. Antibiotic prophylaxis (cephalosporin) is also administered as a single intravenous injection after induction of general anesthesia.

1. Position of Patient and Layout of Staff

The anesthetized patient is placed in the supine position with a slight tilt up of head and the table tilted slightly to the right, where the surgeon stands together with the camera person for most of the operation. The scrub nurse and assistant are on the opposite side. Alternatively, the French position may be used with the surgeon standing in between the patient's thighs with the lower limbs supported in the abducted position. Although this position gives the surgeon excellent access to the abdomen, unless a good and atraumatic lower limb support system is available this position can cause venous drainage problems during long operations. The alterative technique used by French surgeons consists of straight leg supports. If the HALS technique is used, the hand-access device is placed through a small (6.0 cm) vertical or transverse incision (Fig. 19.1). The exact placement of the access port is important and depends on the type of gastrectomy (distal, subtotal, total), the principle being that the internal hand must reach but not overlap the operative field. With the HALS approach, the surgeon introduces the nondominant hand inside the inflated abdomen and uses the dominant hand for

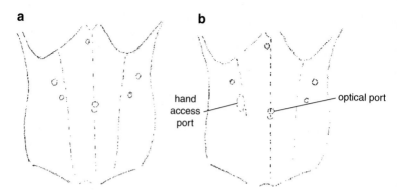

Fig. 19.1. (**a**) Port placement for total and laparoscopically assisted gastrectomy. (**b**) Port placement for HALS gastrectomy. The hand-access device replaces the right pararectal port.

manipulation of instruments/energized dissection devices inserted though the ports. Thus, for gastric resections, the hand port is placed to right of the midline usually at the level of the umbilicus.

One of the essential requirements for laparoscopic gastric resection is complete deflation of the stomach by nasogastric suction.

2. Port Placement

This is influenced by the technique used. In total or laparoscopically assisted technique, usually five ports are needed, the size depending on the diameter of the instruments being used (Fig. 19.2a). There is no set port position in the author's experience, and a sensible initial three ports are inserted: optical at or near the umbilicus (preferably 10 mm 30° optic) and two 5-mm ports along the right and left semilunar lines (pararectal). The other two are then placed in the subxiophoid region and laterally in the right upper quadrant. Sometimes, an extra port on the left upper quadrant may be needed for retraction.

The HALS technique impacts on both the number and position of the ports used. It is best to regard the hand-access port as the equivalent of the right pararectal port, and indeed sometimes instruments are introduced through the device after the surgeon withdraws the internal assisting hand. The use of an extra-long telescope is helpful in avoiding encroachment between the workspace of the surgeon and the camera person. This optical port is placed on the left side of the hand-access device (Fig. 19.1b).

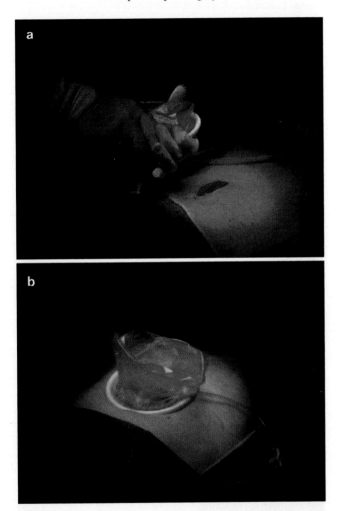

Fig. 19.2. Access port for HALS gastrectomy. (**a**) A wound for insertion of Omniport. (**b**) A Ominport inserted before insertion of hand followed by inflation of cuff.

3. Essential Instruments for Gastric Resections

There is no doubt that energized devices, such as ultrasonic dissectors and Ligasure impedance-controlled system, have greatly facilitated all advanced laparoscopic operation. However, the author still considers electrosurgical hook dissection as being superior for precise dissection of the nodal masses around the arteries in D_2 gastrectomies (Fig. 19.3a, b);

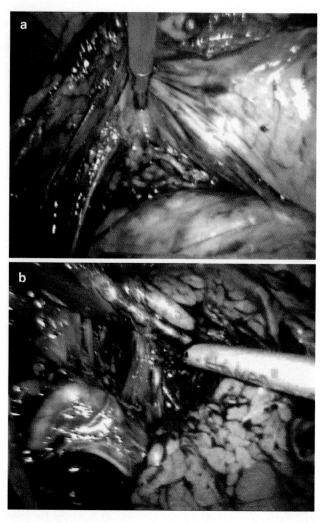

Fig. 19.3. (**a**). Clearance of nodes on the right gastroepiploic and gastroduode-nal arteries. (**b**) Complete D_2 node dissection carried out with the electrosurgical hook knife. The tip of the instrument is on the origin of the celiac axis from the aorta.

but for opening up surgical planes, a division of ligaments, short gastric vessels, etc., both ultrasonic and Ligasure-energized devices are far more efficient and safer (Fig. 19.4). In D_2 resections, the author prefers flush ligation (by external slip knots or intracorporeal knot tying) of the left gastric artery at its origin from the celiac axis to ensure complete node

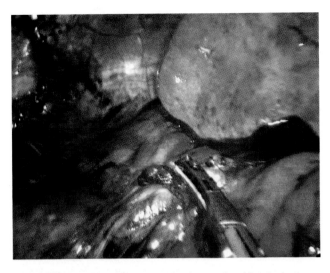

Fig. 19.4. Ligasure division of the short gastric vessels with splenic preservation.

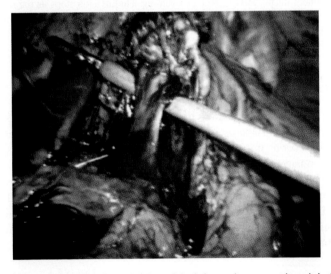

Fig. 19.5. Author prefers flush ligation of the left gastric artery at its origin from celiac axis to ensure complete nodal clearance using either external slip knots or by intracorporeal knot tying.

clearance (Fig. 19.5). Another essential instrument for laparoscopic gastric resection is a good suction/irrigation system. The author has also a preference for the use of distally curved coaxial instruments introduced through flexible port (Fig. 19.6).

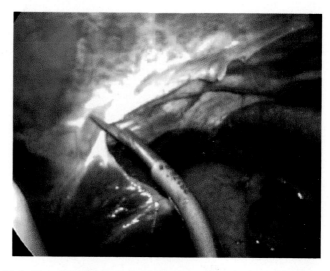

Fig. 19.6. Use of distally curved coaxial scissors for division of the left triangular ligament during HALS total gastrectomy. The division stops as the inferior phrenic vein is reached. The finger of the surgeon's internal hand is seen in the bottom left corner of the image.

4. Reconstruction

In distal resections, the choice is between open through a small minilaparotomy (laparoscopically assisted) or total using either stapling techniques or by intracorporeal hand suturing. Intracorporeal hand suturing is considerably facilitated in HALS distal resection. The most common reconstruction after LDG is by a Polya method (Billroth type II), although some prefer gastroduodenal hand-sutured anastomosis (Billroth type I). For more extensive gastric resections (total or subtotal), internal stapling is most commonly used for restoration of continuity of the upper GI tract, usually by a Roux-en-Y anastomosis.

5. Postoperative Care

Unless the patient has significant comorbidities, postoperative care can be safely managed in a surgical ward setting equipped with high-dependency care facilities. Prophylactic nasogastric suction is not needed in all patients, irrespective of the extent of the gastric resection.

Ambulation is encouraged and is generally possible on the second postoperative day. The period of ileus should not exceed 5 days and resumption of oral light diet is possible in the majority of patients, except after total gastrectomy with an esophageal anastomosis, in which a contrast study is advisable before resumption of oral intake. Heparin prophylaxis is continued until discharge from hospital.

Selected References

Adachi Y, Shiraishi N, Shiromizu A, et al. Laparoscopy assisted Billroth I gastrectomy compared with conventional open gastrectomy. Arch Surg. 2000;135:806–10.

AJCC Cancer Staging Manual, Seventh Edition (2010) published by Springer Science and Business Media, LLC, http://www.springerlink.com.

Azagra JS, Georgen M, De Simone P, Ibanez-Aguire JL. Minimally invasive surgery for gastric cancer. Surg Endosc. 1999;13:351–7.

Bonenkamp JJ, Hermans J, Sasako M, van de Velde CJ, Welvaart K, Songun I, et al. Dutch gastric cancer group. Extended lymph-node dissection for gastric cancer. N Engl J Med. 1999;340:908–14.

Bonenkamp JJ, Songun I, Hermans J, Sasako M, Welvaart K, Plukker JT, et al. Randomised comparison of morbidity after D1 and D2 dissection for gastric cancer in 996 Dutch patients. Lancet. 1995;345:745–8.

Bozzetti F, Marubini E, Bonfanti G, Miceli R, Piano C, Crose N, et al. Total versus subtotal gastrectomy: surgical morbidity and mortality rates in a multicenter Italian randomized trial. The Italian Gastrointestinal Tumor Study Group. Ann Surg. 1997;226:613–20.

Cuschieri A, Fayers P, Fielding J, Craven J, Bancewicz J, Joypaul V, et al. Postoperative morbidity and mortality after D1 and D2 resections for gastric cancer: preliminary results of the MRC randomised controlled surgical trial. The Surgical Cooperative Group. Lancet. 1996;347:995–9.

Cuschieri A, Weeden S, Fielding J, Bancewicz J, Craven J, Joypaul V, et al. Patient survival after D1 and D2 resections for gastric cancer: long-term results of the MRC randomized surgical trial. Surgical Co-operative Group. Br J Cancer. 1999;79:1522–30.

Dicken BJ, Bigam DL, Cass C, Mackey JR, Joy AA, Hamilton SM. Gastric adenocarcinoma: review and considerations for future directions. Ann Surg. 2005;241: 27–39.

Japanese Gastric Cancer Association. Japanese classification of gastric carcinoma. 2nd English edition. Gastric Cancer 1998;1:10–24.

Kitano S, Iso Y, Moriyama M, et al. Laparoscopy-assisted Billroth I gastrectomy. Surg Laparosc Endosc. 1994;65:146–8.

Kitano S, Shiraishi N, Fujii K et al. A randomized controlled trial comparing open vs. laparoscopy-assisted distal gastrectomy for the treatment of early gastric cancer: An interim report. Surgery 2002;131:S 306–11.

Kitano S, Shiraishi N, Kakisako K, et al. Laparoscopy assisted Billroth-I gastrectomy (LADG) for cancer: Our 10 years' experience. Surg Laparosc Endosc Percutan Tech. 2002b;141:204–7.

Naitoh T, Gagner M, Garcia-Ruiz A, Heniford BT, Ise H, Matsuno S. Hand-assisted laparoscopic digestive surgery provides safety and tactile sensation for malignancy or obesity. Surg Endosc. 1999;13(2):157–60.

Nakamori M, Iwahashi M, Nakamura M, Tabuse K, Mori K, Taniguchi K, Aoki Y, Yamaue H. Laparoscopic resection for gastrointestinal stromal tumors of the stomach. Am J Surg. 2008 Sep; 196(3):425–9. Epub 2008 May 7.

Ohtani H, Tamamori Y, Noguchi K, Azuma T, Fujimoto S, Oba H, Aoki T, Minami M, Hirakawa K. Meta-analysis of Laparoscopy-Assisted and Open Distal Gastrectomy for Gastric Cancer. J Surg Res. 2011;171(2):479–85.

Peng JS, Song H, Yang ZL, Xiang J, Diao DC, Liu ZH. A meta-analysis of laparoscopy-assisted distal gastrectomy (LADG) and conventional open distal gastrectomy for early gastric cancer. Chin J Cancer. 2010;29(4):349–54.

Robot-assisted gastrectomy with lymph node dissection for gastric cancer: lessons learned from an initial 100 consecutive procedures.Song J, Oh SJ, Kang WH, Hyung WJ, Choi SH, Noh SH. Ann Surg. 2009 Jun; 249(6):927–32.

Sano T, Sasako M, Yamamoto S, Nashimoto A, Kurita A, Hiratsuka M, et al. Gastric cancer surgery: morbidity and mortality results from a prospective randomized controlled trial comparing D2 and extended para-aortic lymphadenectomy–Japan Clinical Oncology Group study 9501. J Clin Oncol. 2004;22:2767–73.

Sasaki A, Koeda K, Obuchi T, Nakajima J, Nishizuka S, Terashima M, Wakabayashi G. Tailored laparoscopic resection for suspected gastric gastrointestinal stromal tumors. Surgery. 2010 Apr; 147(4):516–20. Epub 2009 Dec 11.

Shimizu S, Uchiyama A, Mizumoto K, et al. Laparoscopically assisted distal gastrectomy for early gastric cancer. Surg Endosc. 2001;14:27–31.

Strong VE, Devaud N, Allen PJ, Gonen M, Brennan MF, Coit D. Laparoscopic versus open subtotal gastrectomy for adenocarcinoma: a case–control study. Ann Surg Oncol. 2009 Jun; 16(6):1507–13. Epub 2009 Apr 4.

The Japanese Gastric Cancer Association. The gastric cancer treatment guidelines. Tokyo: Kanehara Shuppan Ltd; 2001.

Ueda J, Ichimiya H, Okido M, Kato M. The impact of visceral fat accumulation on laparoscopy-assisted distal gastrectomy for early gastric cancer. J Laparoendosc Adv Surg Tech A. 2009;19(2):157–62.

Zhang X, Tanigawa N, Nomura E, Lee SW. Curability of laparoscopic gastrectomy for gastric cancer was based on a 10 year experience. Gastric Cancer. 2008;11(3): 175–80.

20. Laparoscopic Total Gastrectomy for Cancer

Vivian E. Strong, M.D.

A. Introduction

Since the first laparoscopic gastric resection was reported in 1991 by Fowler et al. for a benign tumor, the application of minimally invasive approaches for benign conditions of the stomach has rapidly gained acceptance. Although laparoscopic approaches are now used routinely for bariatric operations, Nissen fundoplication, hiatal hernia repairs, and Heller myotomies, the acceptance of this technique for malignant tumors has been less rapid. Until just a few years ago, the oncologic equivalency of laparoscopic resection of gastrointestinal stromal tumors of the stomach was still debated. Now, many studies have adequately compared laparoscopic to open approaches for GIST, demonstrating safety, efficacy, and oncologic equivalency. The application of laparoscopic techniques for resection of gastric adenocarcinoma has taken the longest, largely due to the relatively low incidence of gastric cancer in Western countries and the steep learning curve associated with the lymphadenectomy in addition to the gastric resection. Eastern countries, like Japan and South Korea, have led the way in laparoscopic gastrectomy for adenocarcinoma; however, it was not until 1994 when Seigo Kitano from Japan reported on the first laparoscopic distal gastrectomy with D2 lymphadenectomy and not until 1996 that Azagra et al. published the first laparoscopic total gastrectomy with D2 lymphadenectomy for carcinoma. Since that time, many more studies, mostly retrospective and a few prospective randomized, have compared the approach as safe and feasible, although with a steep learning curve that is somewhere between 50 and 60 cases. We reported on an initial experience of laparoscopic gastric resections with D2 lymphadenectomy performed for adenocarcinoma in 30 consecutive patients compared to 30 stage-matched patients undergoing open resections.

N.T. Nguyen and C.E.H. Scott-Conner (eds.), *The SAGES Manual: Volume 2 Advanced Laparoscopy and Endoscopy*, DOI 10.1007/978-1-4614-2347-8_20, © Springer Science+Business Media, LLC 2012

We demonstrated the laparoscopic approach to be technically feasible, safe, and oncologically equivalent with decreased hospital stay, less narcotic use, and fewer long-term complications. This chapter describes the indications for surgery, preoperative workup, minimally invasive surgical approaches, complications, and patient follow-up after laparoscopic gastrectomy.

B. Indications

Indications for gastrectomy for adenocarcinoma include patients with nonmetastatic disease that have a documented pathologic diagnosis of gastric carcinoma that is not amenable to endoscopic mucosal resection (for very early T1a lesions meeting appropriate criteria). Additionally, a small number of patients undergo gastrectomy for high-grade dysplasia, now classified as carcinoma in situ. Another indication for gastrectomy is gastric cardia cancer with involvement of the gastroesophageal junction, for Siewert III type, and some Siewert II type tumors. In this condition, a total gastrectomy is often performed. The indication for a laparoscopic approach is largely based on surgeon skill level and having achieved the appropriate learning curve to perform the procedure. It is advisable to achieve this learning curve via a two attending approach for earlier cases. Relative contraindications may include prior abdominal operations if adhesions are prohibitive and high BMI or bulky tumors with local extension that may make safe dissection difficult. A low threshold to convert should be considered to achieve a safe and oncologically sound operation.

C. Preoperative Evaluation

Standard preoperative workup for patients with gastric carcinoma includes upper endoscopy with biopsy, endoscopic ultrasound, computed tomography (CT) scan of the chest, abdomen, and pelvis, and for locally advanced tumors positron emission tomography (PET). Patients who are considered surgical candidates and have by endoscopic ultrasound uT3 or N-positive tumors should undergo laparoscopic staging with peritoneal fluid cytology to rule out metastatic disease. If washings are negative, these patients usually go on to receive neoadjuvant treatment prior to definitive resection. Patients with uT1 or uT2 and N0 disease go directly to operative resection.

D. Surgical Approaches

1. Laparoscopic Gastrectomy with D2 Lymphadenectomy and Roux-en-Y Reconstruction

The operation is typically conducted as follows:

a. Positioning

    i. Place the patient in the supine position in the split leg position with spreader bars and footpads (Fig. 20.1).

    ii. Introduce five trocars into the lower abdomen, typically four 5-mm ports and one 12-mm port. Carbon dioxide insufflation is used at a pressure of 15 mmHg (Fig. 20.2).

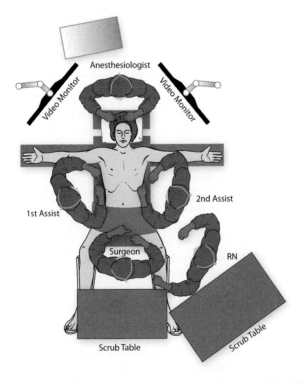

Fig. 20.1. Patient positioning in the operating room (courtesy of the Memorial Sloan-Kettering Cancer Center).

Port Placement

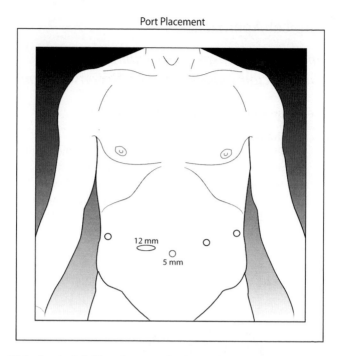

Fig. 20.2. Surgical field and trocar placement for laparoscopic gastrectomy (courtesy of the Memorial Sloan-Kettering Cancer Center).

iii.   Retract the left lobe of the liver with a Nathanson liver retractor placed directly through a 3-mm skin incision in the subxiphoid midline region at the lower edge of the liver and hold in place with a stationary retractor (Fig. 20.3).

iv.   Position the patient in steep reverse Trendelenburg position.

v.   Lift the greater omentum in a cephalad direction to visualize the transverse colon (Fig. 20.4).

vi.   Enter the lesser sac via the top of the transverse colon to visualize the posterior wall of the stomach (Fig. 20.4).

vii.   Retract the posterior wall of the stomach and visualize the omentum from below in order to facilitate a complete omentectomy without injuring the splenic flexure of the colon and taking care to avoid injury to the mesocolon.

viii.   Transect the short gastric vessels allowing for dissection of the splenic hilar as well as the greater curvature lymph node stations.

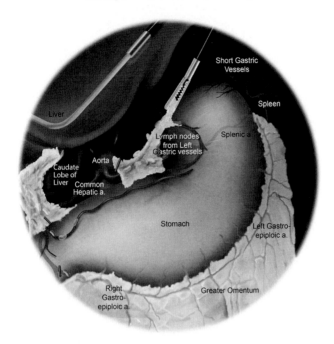

Fig. 20.3. Liver retraction with Nathanson liver retractor (courtesy of the Memorial Sloan-Kettering Cancer Center).

ix. Mobilize the greater curve up to the level of the left crus of the diaphragm.

b. Second Stage

i. Keep the patient in steep reverse Trendelenburg and change the positioning of the camera to view the distal part of the posterior stomach.

ii. Change the direction of the omentectomy to continue complete resection along the transverse colon toward the pylorus of the stomach.

iii. Once the omental attachments are free, the posterior wall of the stomach is visualized and the pancreas is preserved.

iv. Before reaching the pylorus posteriorly, identify the right gastroepiploic vessels and surrounding lymph node bundle (Fig. 20.5).

v. Once the level-6 lymph nodes are completely dissected en bloc toward the stomach, the origin of the gastroepiploic

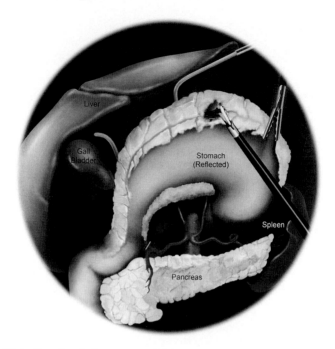

Fig. 20.4. Entering the lesser sac and removal of the greater omentum (courtesy of the Memorial Sloan-Kettering Cancer Center).

vessels is seen. Transect this with endoclips or a vascular stapling device (Fig. 20.5).

vi. This facilitates visualization of the pylorus from a posterior position which is then confirmed by visualization from the anterior position as well.

vii. Free the duodenum of surrounding attachments and small feeding vessels until about 2 cm distal to the pylorus is cleared both inferiorly and superiorly on the duodenum.

viii. Transect the duodenum, taking care to avoid injury to the nearby portal triad, via a blue load stapling device with or without staple line reinforcement.

c. **Third Stage**

i. Next, identify the right gastric artery at its origin. Dissect the associated lymph nodes from level 5 and bring these en bloc with the specimen after ligating the right gastric at its origin, usually with an ultrasonic radiofrequency device (Fig. 20.5).

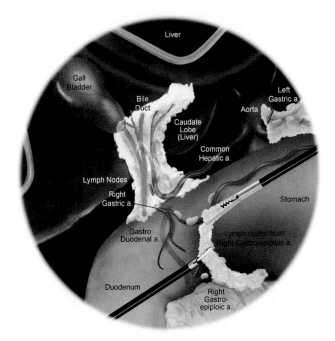

Fig. 20.5. Lymphadenectomy of the right gastroepiploic vessels, right gastric artery, common hepatic lymph nodes, left gastric artery and vein, and pericardial nodes (courtesy of the Memorial Sloan-Kettering Cancer Center).

ii. Mobilize the lesser curvature of the stomach and associated level-3 and -1 lymph nodes in the pericardial region. Take care to check prior to surgery whether an accessory hepatic artery is present.

iii. Identify the left gastric artery and coronary vein and carefully dissect the lymph node bundle here, taking care to avoid injury to the celiac trunk or splenic artery (Fig. 20.5).

iv. Ligate the left gastric vessels via a vascular stapling device or with endoclips (Fig. 20.5).

v. Once the esophageal margin is adequately visualized, use a linear stapling device to transect the esophagus above the gastroesophageal junction (Fig. 20.6).

vi. Place the total gastrectomy specimen with en bloc lymph nodes and omentum in a large bag and remove it through the slightly enlarged right lower quadrant 12-mm port site.

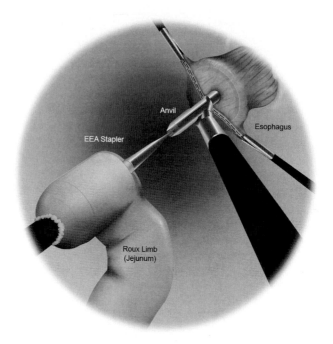

Fig. 20.6. Esophageal transection with linear stapler (courtesy of the Memorial Sloan-Kettering Cancer Center).

vii. Send the specimen to pathology and have frozen sections performed of the proximal margin to ensure a microscopically cancer-free margin.

2. Laparoscopic Reconstruction

Once the margin is confirmed as negative, the reconstruction can begin.

a. First Stage
   i.   Position the patient in Trendelenburg position.
   ii. Identify the ligament of Treitz.
   iii. Measure a point roughly 30 cm distal to the ligament of Treitz that allows for best mobility in an antecolic position up toward the esophageal stump.

iv. Divide the jejunum at this determined point with a blue load stapling device.

v. Prepare the Roux limb by carefully transilluminating the Roux mesentery and dividing vessels that are not needed. Take care to avoid injury to the vascular arch.

vi. Measure 60–65 cm of length along the Roux limb and choose this spot for construction of the jejunojejunostomy.

vii. Align the two antimesenteric limbs of the biliopancreatic limb and Roux limb, make an enterotomy in both limbs of jejunum, fire the 6-cm linear blue load stapler, and close the resultant enterotomy with a running 2–0 silk suture from bottom to top. Additional reinforcing interrupted sutures can be used if needed.

viii. Next, bring the Roux limb up to the esophageal stump and return the patient to steep reverse Trendelenburg position.

ix. An Orvil 25 French EEA circular stapler is then brought on the field. The anvil is attached to the orogastric tube which is then given to the anesthesiologist (Fig. 20.7a, b).

x. The orogastric tube is then placed into the mouth and passed down the esophagus slowly until the tip of the tube is seen pushing against the esophagus anterior to the staple line (Fig. 20.7a, b).

xi. Open the esophagus with an ultrasonic device and bring the tube into the abdomen. Pull it out through the 12-mm port site until the anvil is seen and set in the distal esophageal stump (Fig. 20.7a, b).

xii. Disconnect the orogastric tube from the anvil and the anvil is thus positioned.

xiii. Place the EEA in the Roux limb and launch the spike. Bring the limb up to the anvil and connect the two pieces (Fig. 20.7c).

xiv. Close the stapler device, taking great care to watch the two ends come together and not to pull excessively on the esophageal side. Fire the stapler, open it, and remove the two circular donuts. Confirm that these are intact and send them to pathology as the new proximal margin.

xv. Examine the anastomosis and place interrupted 2–0 silk sutures to reinforce any areas that appear to need this.

xvi. Close the 12-mm port site fascia, remove the liver retractor, desufflate the abdomen, and close the incisions (Fig. 20.8).

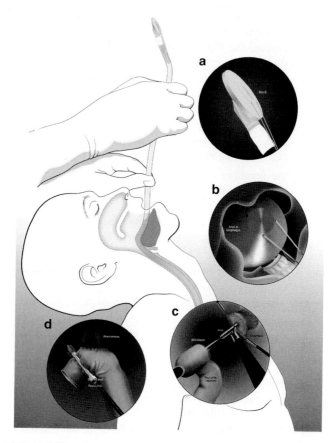

Fig. 20.7. (**a**, **b**) The 25 Fr circular EEA anvil is placed into the oropharynx and positioned in the esophageal stump. (**c**) The anvil is connected with the circular EEA stapler after an enterotomy is created in the Roux limb (courtesy of the Memorial Sloan-Kettering Cancer Center). (**d**) Closure of the enterotomy with a linear stapler.

E. Postoperative Care and Follow-Up

a. Extubate the patient in the operating room prior to transfer to the recovery room. Do not place an orogastric tube.

b. Provide postoperative analgesia by patient-controlled analgesia.

c. The patient may go to the floor after about 4–6 h of stable monitoring in the recovery room.

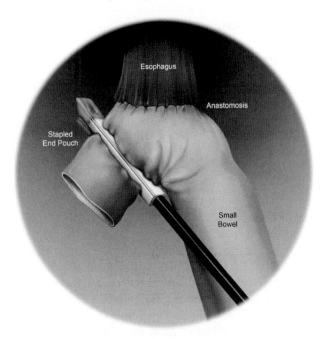

Fig. 20.8. The Roux limb is closed with a linear stapler and shown is the final intraoperative view (courtesy of the Memorial Sloan-Kettering Cancer Center).

d. If stable overnight, the patient may begin taking ice chips the next morning and should begin ambulating and use incentive sprirometer.

e. Postoperative day 2, sips of liquids may be started.

f. Postoperative day 3–5, a postgastrectomy diet may be slowly introduced. A nutritionist will see the patient to discuss dietary recommendations.

g. Patients are seen 1–2 weeks postoperatively.

h. Patients are then seen for follow-up at roughly 3-month intervals for a year, followed by 6-month intervals, and then yearly thereafter.

i. CT scans of the chest, abdomen, and pelvis, alternating with endoscopy, are performed after surgery at 6- to 12-month intervals.

F. Complications

1. Early Postoperative Complications

The main complications that may occur early after operation include postoperative bleeding, atelectasis, pneumonia, wound infection, deep venous thrombosis, and urinary tract infection. The most important early postoperative complications are esophagojejunal anastomotic leak/obstruction, jejunojejunal anastomotic leak/obstruction, or duodenal stump leak. Leak is one of the most serious complications after total gastrectomy, and should be the first complication considered for any deviation of postoperative course. Manifestations to watch for include early fever on postoperative day 2 or 3, tachycardia that is not otherwise well explained, or pain with swallowing in the epigastric region as well as wound infection. Management of a leak depends on the site and clinical stability of the patient. NPO and IV antibiotics with interventional guided radiology drainage are the first steps for otherwise clinically stable patients that have been found to have a leak by Gastrograffin swallow study or CT scan. For patients who are or become clinically unstable, return to the operating room for irrigation and placement of multiple drains in the area of the leak may be necessary. In rare cases of complete anastomotic breakdown, proximal esophageal diversion may be necessary.

2. Late Complications

Late complications include mostly anastomotic stricture. The preferred treatment of anastomotic stricture is endoscopic balloon dilation.

G. Outcomes

The largest published series of laparoscopic gastrectomy in North America come from Memorial Sloan-Kettering Cancer Center and City of Hope. In the Memorial Sloan-Kettering Cancer Center experience, a total of 60 patients were evaluated, including 30 MIG and 30 OG procedures. Median operative time for the laparoscopic approach was 270 min (range 150–485) compared to 126 min (range 85–205) in the open group ($P<0.01$). Hospital length of stay after laparoscopic gastrectomy was

5 days (range 2–26), compared to 7 days (range 5–30) in the open group ($P=0.01$). Postoperative IV narcotic use was shorter for laparoscopic patients, with a median of 3 days (range 0–11) compared to 4 days (range 1–13) in the open group ($P<0.01$). Postoperative late complications were significantly higher for the open group ($P=0.03$). Short-term recurrence-free survival and margin status were similar with adequate lymph node retrieval in both groups.

In the City of Hope experience, a recent review of the gastrectomy experience compared minimally invasive to open gastrectomy. A total of 78 consecutive patients were evaluated, including 30 minimally invasive and 48 open procedures. All laparoscopic patients had negative margin resections and 15 or more lymph nodes in the surgical specimen. There was no difference in the mean number of lymph nodes retrieved by MIG or OG (24 ± 8 vs. 26 ± 15, $P=.66$). MIG procedures were associated with decreased blood loss (200 vs. 383 mL, $P=0.0009$) and length of stay (7 vs. 10 days, $P=0.0009$), but increased operative time (399 vs. 298 min, $P<0.0001$). Overall complication rate following MIG was lower, but statistical significance was not achieved.

These series concluded that laparoscopic gastrectomy for carcinoma is comparable to the open approach with regard to oncologic principles of resection, with equivalent margins and adequate lymph node retrieval, demonstrating technically feasibility and similar short-term recurrence-free survival.

Selected References

Huscher CG, Mingoli A, Sgarzini G, Sansonetti A, Di PM, Recher A, Ponzano C. Laparoscopic versus open subtotal gastrectomy for distal gastric cancer: five-year results of a randomized prospective trial. Ann Surg. 2005;241(2):232–7.

Kim YW, Baik YH, Yun YH, Nam BH, Kim DH, Choi IJ, Bae JM. Improved quality of life outcomes after laparoscopy-assisted distal gastrectomy for early gastric cancer: results of a prospective randomized clinical trial. Ann Surg. 2008;248(5):721–7.

Cunningham D, Allum WH, Stenning SP, Thompson JN, van de Velde CJ, Nicolson M, Scarffe JH, Lofts FJ, Falk SJ, Iveson TJ, Smith DB, Langley RE, et al. Perioperative chemotherapy versus surgery alone for resectable gastroesophageal cancer. N Engl J Med. 2006;355(1):11–20.

Macdonald JS, Smalley SR, Benedetti J, Hundahl SA, Estes NC, Stemmermann GN, Haller DG, Ajani JA, Gunderson LL, Jessup JM, Martenson JA. Chemoradiotherapy after surgery compared with surgery alone for adenocarcinoma of the stomach or gastroesophageal junction. N Engl J Med. 2001;345(10):725–30.

Strong VE, Devaud N, Allen PJ, Gonen M, Brennan MF, Coit D. Laparoscopic versus open subtotal gastrectomy for adenocarcinoma: a case–control study. Ann Surg Oncol. 2009;16(6):1507–13.

Guzman EA, Pigazzi A, Lee B, Soriano PA, Nelson RA, Benjamin PI, Trisal V, Kim J, Ellenhorn JD. Totally laparoscopic gastric resection with extended lymphadenectomy for gastric adenocarcinoma. Ann Surg Oncol. 2009;16(8):2218–23.

21. Laparoscopic Resection of Gastrointestinal Stromal Tumors

Lee L. Swanstrom, M.D., F.A.C.S.

A. Background

1. Pathophysiology of Stromal Cell Tumors

Stromal cell tumors are a class of benign and malignant tumors arising from the muscular layers of the GI tract. The term gastrointestinal stromal cell tumor (GIST) was first used by Mazur and Clark in 1983 to describe mesenchymal tumors specifically derived from the interstitial cells of Cajal. Their genetics have been increasingly well worked out and it is now known that 90% of GIST harbors a tyrosine kinase (KIT) mutation which correlates to their oncologic risk profile and sensitivity to chemotherapy.

2. Epidemiology

GIST tumors are found in around 12/100,000 population, though their numbers have increased with increasing use of upper endoscopy for other reasons. They occur predominately in an older population (mean age 66 years) and have no sexual predilection. The vast majority are small (<5 mm) and incidental findings. Their distribution in the GI tract is listed in Table 21.1.

3. Presentation

Only 70% of GIST are symptomatic. Table 21.2 lists common symptoms associated with GIST. GISTs are frequently found incidentally at endoscopy or on contrast studies, and around 10% are incidental findings at autopsy.

N.T. Nguyen and C.E.H. Scott-Conner (eds.), *The SAGES Manual: Volume 2 Advanced Laparoscopy and Endoscopy*, DOI 10.1007/978-1-4614-2347-8_21, © Springer Science+Business Media, LLC 2012

Table 21.1.   The distribution of GIST in the GI tract.

Location	Incidence (%)
Esophagus	1
Stomach	60
Duodenum	4
Small bowel	30
Colon/appendix	1
Rectum	4

Table 21.2.   When GISTs are associated with symptoms they are fairly nonspecific.

Associated symptoms
Nausea/vomiting
Small bowel obstruction
Abdominal pain
Abdominal distention
Bleeding
Perforation

B.   Indications for Surgery

Small tumors (<2 cm) have a low, but not zero, risk of malignancy and can be watched with either endoscopy or, more accurately, with endoscopic ultrasound (EUS). CT scan can be used for larger tumors but is not the best screening tool as it subjects the patient to radiation and is less accurate than EUS. As these are slow growing tumors, surveillance intervals of 6–12 months are usually adequate.

Surgical excision should be considered for any intramural solid tumor over 2 cm or for a tumor of any size that shows progressive enlargement. Excision is also indicated for any GIST causing symptoms, such as obstruction or bleeding Fig. 21.1. This is very rare for smaller lesions.

1.   Adjuvant Therapies

The recent discovery that Gleevac (Imatinib mesylate) and more recently Sutent (Suitinib malate) are highly effective for GIST tumors has altered the algorithm for their surgical treatment. Large tumors, those that are in areas difficult to resect and those with cellular findings

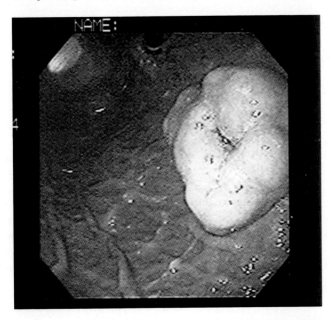

Fig. 21.1. Ulcerated gastric GIST presenting as intermittent GI bleed.

indicating high risk for malignancy (mitotic rate >50 per HPF), can in some cases be down staged by a course of Gleevac or Sutent.

2. Preoperative Evaluation

Preoperative evaluation should always include a full patient evaluation to stratify for the risk of the surgery.

a. An endoscopy and EUS is adequate evaluation for small tumors (<4 cm) which have no ultrasonographic findings suggestive of malignancy (invasion of different layers, inhomogeneity). For larger or suspicious appearing tumors, a CT scan should be added and more recently a PET/CT has shown some usefulness in staging cancers or following neoadjuvant therapy.

b. The question of whether to biopsy or not remains a controversial one. Fine needle biopsies are seldom diagnostic due to the relative acellularity of these tumors. Larger, core-needle biopsies run the risk of disseminating cancer through the wall of the organ. In general, biopsy is not recommended unless a diagnosis would really change the treatment of the patient.

C. Surgical Procedures

1. General Principles

a. Surgery is the mainstay treatment for GIST and remains the only cure.

b. An R0 resection should always be the goal and sometimes necessitates radical resections of adjacent organs.

c. Unlike leiomyomas, simple submucosal enucleation is generally contraindicated as recurrence rates are high. Endoscopic enucleation is occasionally indicated for smaller tumors with low risk factors and in critical areas. Full-thickness resection is indicated and 5 mm clear margins are considered adequate.

d. If metastatic disease is encountered at surgery, the primary lesion should still be removed if it is safe and straightforward to do.

e. Lymphadenectomy has not been shown to be advantageous.

The surgical approach varies according to the location of the lesion. Proximal and mid esophageal lesions are approached transthoracically either by thoracoscopy or by thoracotomy. A key decision to be made is whether the excision will be simple local excision or a radical resection for cancer.

2. Esophagus

Esophageal lesions are ideally approached thoracoscopically and if there is no overt indication that the lesion is malignant, local resection, and primary closure is indicated and will be curative in most cases. For malignant lesions, a total esophagectomy is indicated with a gastric pull-up and intrathoracic or cervical anastamosis. As this indication is no different than esophagectomy for esophageal cancer the technique of open or minimally invasive esophagectomy is not covered here and the reader is referred to Chap. 22.

a. Perform thoracoscopic local resection for proximal or mid lesions with the patient in the traditional lateral decubitus position, or even, better with the patient prone. In the prone position, the surgery can often be done with only three ports as gravity retracts the deflated lung away from the operative field, four are usually needed in the lateral decubitus position.

b. Access is almost always through the right chest even for left-oriented lesions as the heart and aorta are in the way from the left. Valveless thoracoports can be used—and somewhat broaden the selection of instruments—however, their use requires placement of a double lumen endotracheal tube and single lung ventilation. We prefer to use standard laparoscopic ports, a 10 mm and two or three 5 mm and use low pressure (10 mmHg) CO_2 insufflation to drop the lung. This has the advantage of flattening the diaphragm and displacing the mediastinum medially which further expands the functional operating space.

c. Pass a flexible endoscope into the esophagus to help localize the tumor. Place an intralesional suture is placed for retraction and mark an area 3–5 mm around the lesion (Fig. 21.2).

d. On occasion, with very small tumors (<2 cm) a linear endoscopic stapler with a blue load can be positioned transversely under the lesion and fired to perform a non-narrowing full thickness resection. Otherwise, perform a freehand resection with

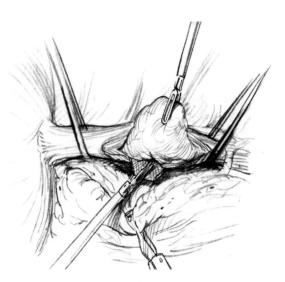

Fig. 21.2. Thoracoscopic approach via the right chest allows for excellent access to mid-esophageal tumors.

grossly clear margins. Close the resulting defect transversely over a 52 French bougie with a 3–0 absorbable monofilament suture.

3. Stomach

GISTs of the stomach are by far the most common. The rules for resection are the same for the rest of the GI tract—full-thickness resection with negative margins of any width. This can be more difficult if the tumor is near the gastroesophageal junction or pylorus.

a. **Gastric body**: GISTs in the body of the stomach are relatively easily excised using an endoscopic linear stapler, providing excision and closure with one maneuver. Concomitant upper endoscopy is necessary to localize the tumor and to ensure stapler placement with adequate margins. Position the patient with legs split and use suitable antibiotic and DVT prophylaxis. Place five ports in the upper abdomen in a pattern similar to that used for a Nissen or gastrectomy. Perform gastric mobilization only so far as is needed to gain wide access to the lesion: minimal if anterior, greater curve for left side or posterior lesions and lesser curve for lesions along the right gastric wall. Ultrasonic coagulation is useful for mobilization. Keep the dissection very close to the gastric wall to preserve the epiploic artery or the vagal branches running parallel to the lesser curve. Perform translumination with the flexible endoscope and mark margins marked with cautery on the serosa. It can be helpful to place a stitch into the tumor to serve as a retractor. Place an endoscopic linear stapler with a thick-tissue cartridge under the lesion and fired multiple times.

b. **Posterior gastric wall**: Another option for lesions in the posterior gastric wall is transgastric laparoscopy. Insufflate the stomach with CO_2 using a flexible endoscope and, using a PEG technique, place a 5 mm laparoscopic port with a balloon tip directly into the distal stomach. Place two more ports in the same fashion configured to access the GIST. The tumor can either be lifted with a grasper or a traction suture placed through it and an endoscopic stapler placed under it for a full thickness resection. Depending on the size of the tumor, remove it through the 12 mm port or through the esophagus using the flexible endoscope. Lesions greater than 2 cm will require placing the tumor in a specimen retrieval bag, pulling the ports out of the stomach and into the peritoneal cavity and enlarging a port site for removal. Suture the gastrotomy closed laparoscopically.

c. **Peripyloric lesions**: GIST of the distal stomach or the proximal duodenum can require the disruption of the pyloric ring in order to achieve margins. Because of the thickness of the pyloric muscle we prefer to do a freehand resection. Once again, with endoscopic help, the oncologic margins are marked. Perform freehand excision using the harmonic shears or a concentrated monopolar device. Perform the reconstruction as a Heinecke-Mikulicz pyloroplasty, i.e., a transverse, non-narrowing closures.

d. **Gastric cardia tumors**: lesions adjacent to the lower esophageal sphincter (LES) are also best resected using a freehand method (Fig. 21.3). If the LES is involved reconstruction can be complex and care needs to taken to avoid narrowing the distal

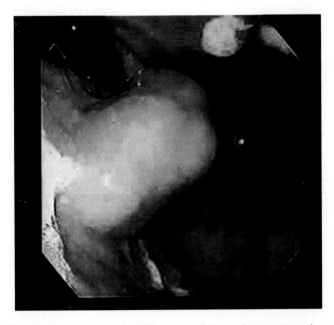

Fig. 21.3. Lesions involving the GEJ may require complex reconstructions after resection.

esophagus. A partial or complete fundoplication will prevent iatrogenic reflux disease and also can be created to cover the repair. Endoscopic enucleation of small tumors (<2 cm) is occasionally the best option for tumors located just at the LES to obviate the need and risks of major reconstruction in this area. The easiest method is simple cap endoscopic mucosal resection (EMR). Careful endoscopic follow-up is indicated after enucleation as there is an increased risk of local recurrence.

4. Intestine

Intestinal stromal cell tumors are rare but are perhaps the easiest to treat surgically as they are usually benign and can easily be resected with good oncologic margins (Fig. 21.4). Establish a typical 4-port access in the right abdomen. Run the small bowel starting at the ligament of Treitz until the lesion is identified. Establish 5-cm margins and divide the bowel with a stapler. Wide mesenteric resection is not needed unless there is obvious adenopathy. Perform a standard anastomosis. Bag and remove the specimen through a widened port site.

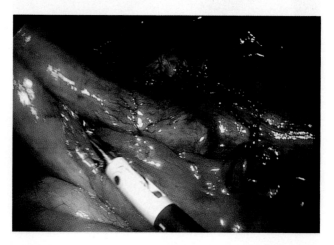

Fig. 21.4. GIST of the small bowel are frequently pedunculated and easily resected.

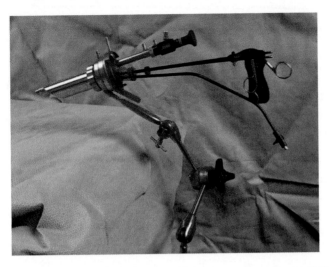

Fig. 21.5. A TEM device is ideal for full thickness resection of rectal GIST.

5. *Rectal*

Truly giant rectal GIST may require a formal laparoscopic rectal resection but this is rare. More typically small-to moderate-sized tumors are found, often incidentally, on colonoscopy. Local full thickness resection is somewhat difficult laparoscopically and requires extensive colon/rectum mobilization. A better approach is transanal excision using transanal endoscopic microsurgery (TEM) (Fig. 21.5). Using TEM, the rectum is insufflated with CO_2, the tumor localized and margins marked with cautery. Full-thickness resection is performed with a monopolar needle electrode and the resulting defect is sutured closed with the TEM instrumentation. IF TEM instruments are not available, there are reports of multiport access devices designed for single port being placed in the anal canal. With these, the rectum is insufflated and standard laparoscopic tools are used for the endoluminal resection and subsequent closure.

D. Outcomes Data

Overall survival following a diagnosis of GIST is not great—only a 69% 5-year disease free survival (DFS) for gastric tumors, and 43% for nongastric GIST, has been reported in North America. The most significant prognostic factors that correlate with shorter DFS in both gastric GISTs and nongastric GISTs were primary tumor size >5 cm and >10 cm and a mitotic index >5 in 50 HPF and >10 in 50 HPF, respectively. Overall survival following surgical resection of GIST is more favorable, with 5-year DFS rates of 92-96% for stage IA tumors, 90-94% for stage IB tumors, 50-65% for stage II tumors, and 22-25% for stage III tumors. For incomplete (R1, R2) resections, adjuvant treatment with Gleevac or Sutent can significantly prolong survival, sometimes for years. Local recurrence occurs 5-15% of the time and repeat surgery can occasionally be effective at achieving a cure as lymph node spread is rare.

E. Follow-Up Protocols

After surgery careful follow-up is needed as GIST can recur locally. Annual endoscopy and a CT scan are indicated for the first 5 years following curative resections. Metastatic disease treated with adjuvant chemotherapy should be closely followed with CT as changing or adjusting the chemotherapy can salvage a significant number of patients and be life prolonging. PET scans have been described as effective in GISTs undergoing multimodal therapy.

Selected Readings

Chang SC, Ke TW, Chiang HC, Wu C, Chen WT. Laparoscopic excision is an alternative method for rectal gastrointestinal stromal tumor. Surg Laparosc Endosc Percutan Tech. 2010;20(4):284–7.

Fan R, Zhong J, Wang ZT, Yu LF, Tang YH, Hu WG, Zhu YB. Prognostic factors and outcome of resected patients with gastrointestinal stromal tumors of small intestine. Med Oncol. 2011;28(1):185–8.

Learn PA, Sicklick JK, DeMatteo RP. Randomized clinical trials in gastrointestinal stromal tumors. Surg Oncol Clin N Am. 2010;19(1):101–13.

Ma JJ, Hu WG, Zang L, Yan XW, Lu AG, Wang ML, Li JW, Feng B, Zhong J, Zheng MH. Laparoscopic gastric resection approaches for gastrointestinal stromal tumors of stomach. Surg Laparosc Endosc Percutan Tech. 2011;21(2):101–5.

Reichardt P, Hogendoorn PC, Tamborini E, et al. Gastrointestinal stromal tumors I: pathology, pathobiology, primary therapy, and surgical issues. Semin Oncol. 2009; 36(4):290–301.

Rubin JL, Sanon M, Taylor DC, Coombs J, Bollu V, Sirulnik L. Epidemiology, survival, and costs of localized gastrointestinal stromal tumors. Int J Gen Med. 2011;4:121–30.

Rutkowski P, Wozniak A, Dębiec-Rychter M, et al. Clinical utility of the new American joint committee on cancer staging system for gastrointestinal stromal tumors: current overall survival after primary tumor resection. Cancer. 2011;117(21):4916–24. doi:10.1002/cncr.26079.

Part IV
Solid Organs

22. Laparoscopic Distal Pancreatectomy

Jayleen Grams, M.D., Ph.D.
Barry Salky, M.D.

A. Indications

1. **Laparoscopic distal pancreatectomy with splenectomy** is indicated for benign diseases or tumors, tumors of low-grade malignant potential, or carcinomas occurring in the neck, body, or tail of the pancreas. Conditions in which this operation is used include:
   a. Cysts
   b. Chronic pancreatitis
   c. Disconnected duct after trauma
   d. Cystadenoma
   e. IPMN
   f. Neuroendocrine tumors
   g. Adenocarcinoma or cystadenocarcinoma
      Postsplenectomy vaccines against *Haemophilus influenzae*, *Meningococcus*, and *Streptococcus* are given at least 2 weeks prior to splenectomy.

2. In benign diseases or tumors with low malignant potential, **laparoscopic distal pancreatectomy with splenic salvage** may be considered. In part, this is dependent on the relationship of the lesion to the splenic vessels, as well as the relationship of the splenic vessels to the pancreas.

N.T. Nguyen and C.E.H. Scott-Conner (eds.), *The SAGES Manual: Volume 2*   331
Advanced Laparoscopy and Endoscopy, DOI 10.1007/978-1-4614-2347-8_22,
© Springer Science+Business Media, LLC 2012

B. Patient Position and Room Setup

1. The insertion of an orogastric tube and Foley catheter is recommended.

2. A number of positions have been described, including supine, right lateral decubitus, and modified lithotomy or split leg. This chapter describes the operation as performed in modified lithotomy position with both arms tucked at the side. The surgeon stands between the patient's legs. As with other advanced upper abdominal procedures, this enhances access and facilitates a two-handed suturing and knot-tying technique.

3. The thighs must be parallel to the floor (rather than flexed at the hip and knee) so that movements of the instruments are not impeded.

4. If an arm needs to be out for anesthesia access, it should be the left one.

5. A bolster is placed beneath the left thoracic cage to elevate the left side 15–20°.

6. The camera operator stands to the right and the first assistant to the left side of the patient.

7. The video monitor is placed above the head of the patient in the midline. A suitable alternative position is near the patient's left shoulder.

8. A laparoscopic ultrasound should be readily available and used as needed to help locate the lesion and determine its relationship to the pancreatic duct and splenic vessels.

C. Trocar Position and Choice of Laparoscope (Fig. 22.1)

1. Place the first port just above and to the left of the umbilicus. This could be a 5- or 12-mm port depending on the diameter of the laparoscope used. Use an angled laparoscope (30 or 45°) to facilitate visualization of the left upper quadrant structures.

2. Place a 5-mm port in the epigastric midline.

3. Place a 12-mm port in the left midclavicular line at the level of the umbilicus or just below it. This port will be used for dissection and insertion of a laparoscopic linear stapler for transection of the splenic vessels and the pancreas. Thus, it must be low enough in the abdomen to allow the jaws of the stapler to open completely.

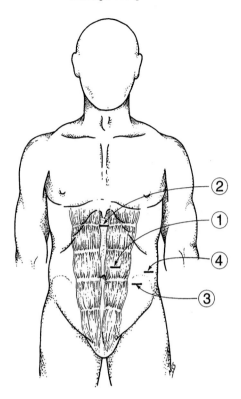

Fig. 22.1. Port placement. These sites are proper for distal pancreatectomy both with and without splenectomy. There should be at least a hand's breadth distance between ports 1, 3, and 4.

4. Place the fourth port (5-mm) in the left anterior axillary line. This site will be used for retraction and suction and irrigation.

5. All of the ports may need to be shifted cephalad in the obese patient.

D. Initial Dissection and Mobilization of the Pancreas

1. First explore the abdomen for other pathology or contraindications to proceeding with resection.

2. Position the angled laparoscope to look down on the abdominal structures.

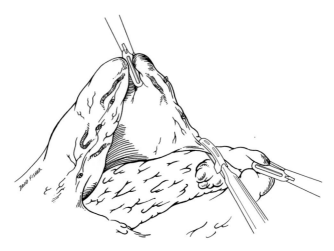

Fig. 22.2. Entering the lesser sac. The pancreas is exposed by dividing the gastrocolic omentum to enter the lesser sac. The tumor is seen in the tail of the pancreas.

3. **Enter the lesser sac** by dividing the gastrocolic omentum (Fig. 22.2).
   a. This is facilitated by superior retraction of the stomach (port 2) and lateral traction of the omentum (port 4). The operating port is 3.
   b. The dissection can be accomplished with ultrasonic shears or monopolar or bipolar energy.
   c. It is easier to stay outside of the gastroepiploic vessels.
   d. Wide mobilization of the gastrocolic omentum and posterior attachments of the stomach is required to fully visualize the pancreas.
   e. If distal pancreatectomy with splenectomy is being performed, the short gastric vessels may be divided using ultrasonic shears, bipolar energy, or clips.
   f. Retraction of the stomach can be accomplished using a Keith needle to pass a suture transabdominally and through the posterior wall of the stomach. It is then secured extracorporeally. Alternatively, a liver retractor may be used but this requires insertion of another 5-mm port in the epigastrium, just below the xiphoid process.
4. Incise the posterior peritoneum at the inferior border of the pancreas. Identify the inferior mesenteric vein and avoid it. With that exception, the plane is fairly avascular.

5. With the pancreas exposed, the laparoscopic ultrasound may be used to determine the location of the lesion and its relationship to the splenic vessels.

6. Proceed using a medial to lateral approach. Divide the spleno-colic ligament and visualize the splenorenal attachments.

7. Dissect the posterior aspect of the pancreas to ascertain involvement of the splenic vein and/or artery. If a benign lesion or a tumor of low malignant potential, the decision to remove or salvage the spleen is made. Each procedure is described separately in the sections that follow.

E. Distal Pancreatectomy with Splenectomy

1. Identify the splenic artery beneath the posterior peritoneum at the superior border of the pancreas.

2. Dissect the splenic artery by staying in the adventitial plane next to it (Fig. 22.3). The site of division should be at the planned line of pancreatic transection. The artery may be ligated using the laparoscopic linear stapler or clips. If clips are used,

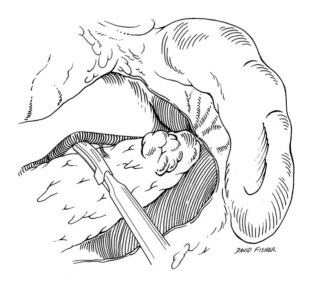

Fig. 22.3. Splenic artery. The splenic artery is identified along the superior border of the pancreas and dissected by staying in the adventitial plane next to it. The site of division should be at the planned line of pancreatic transection.

the artery is clipped doubly on the proximal and distal sides along with a pre-tied suture ligature on the proximal side for additional security.

3. Fully mobilize the posterior pancreas from the retroperitoneal tissues at the site of the previously divided artery. Elevate the gland medially (port 2) and laterally (port 4) with graspers to expose the area. The splenic vein should be on the posterior aspect of the gland. This is a delicate part of the operation and hemorrhage here must be avoided.

4. Once the posterior gland is fully mobilized, the dissector should be visible at the superior border of the pancreas at the previously divided splenic artery.

5. Pass the laparoscopic linear stapler through port 3 to divide the gland and splenic vein as a unit (Fig. 22.4). Two applications of the stapler are usually necessary to completely transect the pancreas. The staple height will depend on the thickness of the tissue but usually a closed staple height of 1.5–2 mm is

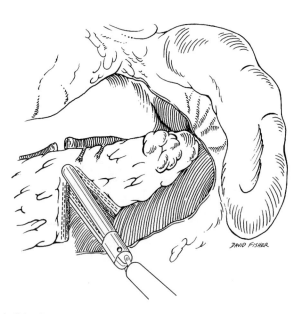

Fig. 22.4. Distal pancreatectomy with splenectomy. The pancreas and splenic vein are divided en bloc with a linear cutting stapler at the site of the previously divided splenic artery. The posterior aspect of the pancreas must be dissected completely to allow free passage of the stapler.

appropriate. A bioabsorbable reinforcement to the staple line may be used as well.

6. Adequate compression without fracturing the tissue is important.

   a. If the pancreas appears too thick or fibrotic for the stapler, the ultrasonic shears may be used to transect the pancreas. In this case, the pancreatic duct should be located and ligated using a nonabsorbable monofilament suture in figure-of-eight fashion. Additionally, the entire stump may be oversewn with a monofilament suture in running baseball fashion in two layers using gentle tissue handling technique.

   b. Alternatively, the stump may be secured using overlapping horizontal mattress sutures of a nonabsorbable suture. The pancreas may then be transected sharply and the pancreatic duct located and ligated as described above.

7. The remainder of the dissection of the pancreatic tail, splenorenal ligament, and splenodiaphragmatic attachments is facilitated by pancreatic division and occurs in avascular planes. The short gastric vessels can be ligated using an energy source or clip applier.

8. After the remaining attachments have been divided, remove port 3 and use a large specimen retrieval bag to remove the specimen from the abdomen. The pancreas can be divided from the spleen for separate extraction, allowing for a smaller extraction site.

9. Thoroughly check for hemostasis. Irrigate and place a closed suction drain via port 4. The operation is concluded in the usual fashion.

F. Pancreatectomy with Splenic Salvage

Splenic salvage is appropriate in the setting of benign disease or tumors with low malignant potential, and studies have demonstrated decreased morbidity when compared to distal pancreatectomy with splenectomy. It has been performed with and without (Warshaw technique) splenic vessel preservation. Preserving the splenic vessels requires advanced laparoscopic skills and meticulous dissection of small perforating branches to the pancreas. The Warshaw technique is easier to perform, but relies on the preservation of the short gastric and left gastroepiploic vessels. It should not be attempted if the spleen is enlarged. A laparoscopic distal pancreatectomy with splenic salvage using splenic vessel preservation is described below.

1. The short gastric vessels are preserved.
2. Laparoscopic ultrasound may again be helpful.
3. In general, there are multiple small branches from the splenic artery and vein to the pancreas that need to be dissected. Since the blood vessels are small, the ultrasonic shears or 5-mm titanium clips are good choices for hemostasis.
4. Vessel loops can be placed around the splenic vessels during dissection.
5. As in pancreatectomy with splenectomy, ports 2 and 3 are the operating ports with port 4 being the assisting port.
6. The spleen is inspected after dissection to determine whether it can indeed be salvaged.
7. The specimen is removed using a retrieval bag. Hemostasis, irrigation, aspiration, and optional placement of a closed suction drain complete the procedure.

G. Hand-Assisted Distal Pancreatectomy

The advantages of a hand-assisted operation include improved tactile feedback, it is technically easier, and manual compression can be used for bleeding. Further, even for a laparoscopic distal pancreatectomy, an incision typically needs to be enlarged for specimen extraction. If a hand port is utilized, it is usually placed at the beginning of the case in the upper midline or oriented along the left subcostal margin.

H. Robotic Distal Pancreatectomy

Robotic distal pancreatectomy has been reported, but the experience is still in its infancy and not widely performed. Although operative times are longer with the robotic procedure, initial reports do suggest there may be an improvement in maneuverability and the performance of complex tasks, such as dissection of the splenic vessels as well as postoperative outcomes.

I. Complications

1. Hemorrhage

a. **Cause and prevention**. The most common event leading to conversion to an open operation is the inability to control hemorrhage. Both of the splenic vessels are sources, but particularly the splenic vein. Dissection in the proper adventitial plane and gentle laparoscopic technique will limit this complication.

b. **Recognition and management**. Hemorrhage that cannot be controlled requires prompt conversion to a hand-assisted or open procedure. Temporary control may be obtained by exerting pressure with a grasper. Laparoscopic hemostatic techniques include vascular staples, titanium clips, monopolar or bipolar energy, ultrasonic energy, suturing and knot-tying capability.

2. Pancreatic Leak

a. **Cause and prevention**. Disruption of the pancreatic duct closure can lead to leakage of pancreatic juice. The enzymes in pancreatic fluid are caustic to surrounding tissue. Inspect the stump of the pancreatic remnant, and ligate the duct with a nonabsorbable suture if necessary.

b. **Recognition and management**. A closed suction drain is routinely placed at the cut end of the pancreas. The drainage fluid should be checked for amylase if there is any suspicion of pancreatic leak, such as high volume output or "dirty dishwater" quality of the fluid. Increased amylase is consistent with a pancreatic leak. Management is dependent on the clinical status of the patient. If there is no proximal obstruction of the pancreatic duct and no foreign body, the pancreatic leak should close. If the surgical drain has been removed, a percutaneous drain should be placed. Supportive measures, such as somatostatin analogues and total parental nutrition (TPN) may be started but have not been convincingly shown to impact outcome. A pancreatic stent or pancreatic duct sphincterotomy may also be performed if the patient is symptomatic or there is no improvement in the leak over time.

3. Infection

a. **Cause and prevention**. Pancreatic leak, hematoma, and seroma formation at the surgical site in the left upper quadrant can lead to abscess formation. Meticulous hemostasis, closure of the pancreatic duct, gentle handling of the pancreatic gland, and minimal use of electrocautery may decrease, but not eliminate, infection. There is no evidence that prophylactic antibiotics prevent infection in this setting. Most surgeons will place a closed suction drain at the time of surgery.

b. **Recognition and management**. Hiccoughs, fever, tachycardia, respiratory difficulty, sepsis, pleural effusion, and left upper quadrant pain are all signs of a left subphrenic abscess, best confirmed by CT scan. Antibiotics and percutaneous or operative drainage may be required.

Selected References

Knaebel HP, Diener MK, Wente MN, et al. Systematic review and meta-analysis of technique for closure of the pancreatic remnant after distal pancreatectomy. Br J Surg. 2005;92:539–46.

Nigri GR, Rosman AS, Petrucciani N, et al. Metaanalysis of trials comparing minimally invasive and open distal pancreatectomies. Surg Endosc. 2011;25:1642–51. http://www.springerlink.com/content/6370231125368j88/.

Vijan SS, Ahmed KA, Harmsen WS, et al. Laparoscopic vs open distal pancreatectomy: a single-institution comparative study. Arch Surg. 2010;145:616–21.

Warshaw AL. Distal pancreatectomy with preservation of the spleen. J Hepatobiliary Pancreat Sci. 2010;17:808–12.

Waters JA, Canal DF, Wiebke EA, et al. Robotic distal pancreatectomy: cost effective? Surgery. 2010;148:814–23.

Yamamoto M, Hayashi MS, Nguyen NT, et al. Use of seamguard to prevent pancreatic leak following distal pancreatectomy. Arch Surg. 2009;144:894–9.

23. Laparoscopic Whipple

Michel Gagner, M.D., F.R.C.S.C., F.A.C.S.,
F.A.S.M.B.S., F.I.C.S., A.F.C.(Hon.)

A. Introduction

Laparoscopic pancreatoduodenectomy, described in 1994, is increasingly performed for tumors in the periampullary area for pancreatic neoplasm and chronic pancreatitis. The last decade has seen an improvement in instrumentation, with better and more reliable staplers, new energy sources capable of dividing pancreatic tissue and surroundings with less blood loss, robotic-assisted technology, and improved surgical handsewn skills. Many academic institutions in the USA and worldwide have embarked on prospective and comparative studies of this operation, which may give a better quality of life after a debilitating gastrointestinal operation. It assumed that oncologic principles are respected, just as they are in laparoscopic colorectal resection, and laparoscopic gastrectomy for cancer just to mention a few.

B. Indications/Contraindications

1. Indications for this operation, performed laparoscopically, are essentially the same as for the open counterpart. These include malignant tumors of the periampullary region (distal bile duct carcinoma, ampullary carcinoma, and duodenal carcinoma), malignant islet cell tumors, pancreatic adenocarcirnoma, and chronic pancreatitis.
2. Relative contraindications include previous surgeries in the area with resulting severe adhesions, large pancreatic masses,

IPMN (intraductal papillary micinous neoplasm) (which may require an extensive pancreatectomy), and certain cases of chronic pancreatitis causing significant regional inflammation. Conditions that make it difficult to get a proper plane near large vessels, such as chronic inflammation or tumor encasement or invasion of the portal vein and/or superior mesenteric vein can be a challenge to manage laparoscopically. Peritoneal metastases may not necessarily contraindicate the procedure, if the surgeon believes that a "palliative Whipple" can be achieve with minimal morbidity. An example where this might be justified would be the presence of an ulcerated bleeding tumor in the duodenum.

3. The surgeon should have extensive experience in both pancreatic surgery and advanced laparoscopy, and be assisted by a competent team in this area, with accessible state of the art laparoscopic instrumentation, including laparoscopic ultrasonography.

C. Technique Description

1. Preoperative Considerations and Setup

a. Appropriate informed consent for this operation will include a possibility of conversion to an open operation, as this is quite high compared to other laparoscopic procedures (15–40%).

b. All radiological studies, including CT scan and /or 3-D imaging should be readily available to the surgeon intraoperatively. Detailed knowledge of the individual vascular anatomy (for example, the presence of an aberrant right hepatic artery originating from the superior mesenteric artery) should be obtained before surgery.

c. All equipment required should be working properly before the initiation of pneumoperitoneum.

d. Blood typing should have been done as blood transfusion intraoperatively may be necessary due to hemorrhage from the pancreatic transection, uncinate process transection or division of branches of the portal vein/mesenteric vein or splenic vein, but rarely from the inferior vena cava.

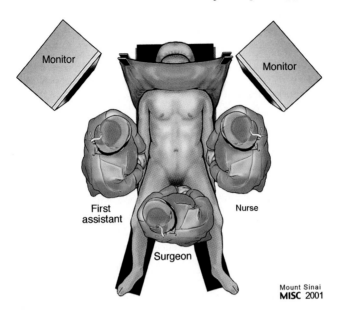

Fig. 23.1. Patient positioning, with operating room layout.

e. Prophylactic cephalosporin is administered intravenously at induction and DVT prophylaxis is used according to a standard protocol from the institution.

f. An operating table with a "split legs" function is preferable as the surgeon can dissect in a better position in the right upper quadrant of the abdomen, certain anastomosis are easier to be performed from the left side of the patient (Fig. 23.1). The table should provide excellent angulations, and should be able to lower sufficiently that the operating surgeon can perform hand-sewn without requiring a platform.

g. Fluoroscopy may be necessary as an adjunct to biliary cholangiography if biliary reconstruction dictates this part.

h. Monitors should be movable as they may be positioned at the head of the patient, or on the left or right side (Fig. 23.1).

i. Two insufflators permit a stable pneumoperitoneum, especially after specimen extraction. Due to the prolonged operative time, the patients should have a body warmer to prevent hypothermia.

2. Diagnostic Laparoscopy and Evaluation of Resectability

Assessment of resectability progresses in a manner similar to that employed during the initial phase of an open pancreatoduodenectomy. Here are the steps that I follow:

a. Use a 30-degree laparoscope to first seek peritoneal metastases, as these generally contraindicate performance of a laparoscopic Whipple operation. A laparoscopic palliative procedure can be performed at the same time, such as a gastroenterostomy for impending duodenal obstruction or a hepaticojejunostomy for biliary decompression (I do not do this if a biliary stent has been placed successfully) – see Chapter 25.

b. Next, enter the lesser sac to determine if there is regional invasion from the tumor bed. Do this by widely opening the gastro colic ligament. It may be necessary to sample nodes in the porta hepatis.

c. A diagnostic laparoscopic ultrasound with Doppler can also be used to evaluate the portal vein.

d. Dissect the inferior border of the pancreas, and bluntly displace the anterior walls of the superior mesenteric vein and portal vein.

e. Perform a wide Kocher maneuver, dissecting the retroperitoneal attachments of the duodenum, dissecting the pancreatic head from the vena cava and aorta to complete the assessment of resectability (Fig. 23.2). A laparoscopic Whipple can be performed if all of these planes are free of vascular invasion and free of peritoneal metastasis.

3. Resection

a. Trocar positions may be variable and will depend on body habitus, and precise location of the pancreatic head in relationship with the right costal margin. For the laparoscope a 10 mm trocar is minimum, as well as two trocars of 12 mm for the use of the laparoscopic staplers. Others can be 5 mm, usually for retraction and exposure in the right and left upper abdomen.

b. If the gallbladder is present, use it to retract the right lobe of the liver upward, and complete cholecystectomy at the end of the case.

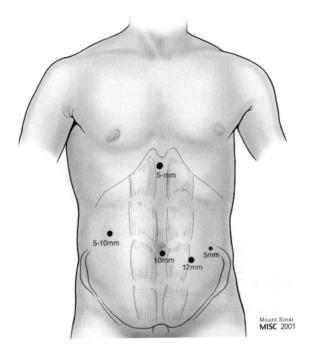

Fig. 23.2. Trocar positions.

c. First, isolate and transect the bile duct (after the biliary stent is removed). Use a stapler (60 mm long) with a white cartridge, (staple height of 2.5 mm) as this permit the avoidance of contaminated bile flowing in the peritoneal cavity.

d. Dissect the gastroduodenal artery from its origin and ligate it with a vascular stapler. I do not like to use clips in general as they may fall off and energy sources are unreliable in securing this relatively large artery.

e. Divide the proximal and distal duodenum with a blue cartridge (3.5 mm).

f. Divide the pancreas over the portal vein with the 5 mm ultrasonic shears. Some bleeders are suture ligated with absorbable 2–0 monofilament, with a hand-sewn technique.

g. Dissect the rest of the uncinate process from the vena cava and superior mesenteric artery with the harmonic scalpel.

h. Extract the specimen in a large plastic bag, and have the margins checked by microscopic examination by an experienced pathologist. Margins should be free of neoplasia before initiation of reconstruction.

4. Reconstruction

a. After a pylorus-preserving Whipple, the first anastomosis is the pancreaticojejunostomy. Pass the proximal jejunum through the ligament of Treitz in the natural tunnel. Hand sew the anastomosis laparoscopically in two layers, a first with 5–0 absorbable monofilament interrupted duct to a small jejunal opening on the antimesenteric side and a second layer on the capsule of the pancreas with the serosa of the jejunum.

b. Next, excise the distal staple line on the common bile duct. Create an end to side hepaticojejunostomy with a running 3–0 monofilament suture, posterior and anterior.

c. Finally, perform the pylorojejunostomy, either end-to-end or end-to-side, with a 3–0 absorbable monofilament. Alternatively, an EEA 21 can also be used.

d. The addition of closed suction drains of the Jackson Pratt type had been routine.

e. Close the mesenteric defect at the ligament of Treitz with 2–0 silk sutures to prevent an internal hernia.

5. Postoperative Considerations

An upper GI gastrografin swallow is done postoperatively to rule out any leaks, at which point a clear liquid diet is begun. Drains are removed by the 3rd or 4th day if amylase is not measures in the drain fluid. The diet is progressively advanced to five small feeds per day, CBC, biochemical profiles, amylasemia, and pancreasemia are measured. DVT prophylaxis is used until discharged, but antibiotics are not used postoperatively.

D. Results and Discussion

A majority of laparoscopic pancreatoduodenectomies are performed for malignancy (91.5%). Apart from a long operating time (448 min.), morbidity is acceptable at 28%, pancreatic fistula reasonable at 12% and mortality at 2.1%, with a hospital stay of 16 days. This is very similar to what I reported 15 years ago. Hospital stays can be reduced by half, approximately 8 days, for uncomplicated cases. I published a recent review of the literature, which included 146 laparoscopic Whipple procedures since 1994. The average patient was 59 years old, and laparoscopic Whipple procedures took a mean operating time of 439 min. The average blood loss was 143 mL; median hospital stay was 18 days; conversion rate was 46%; number of lymph nodes in the pathologic findings was 19; and mortalities related to the procedure was low at 1% and complication rate was 16%. Complications included 2 hemorrhages, 4 bowel obstructions, 1 stress ulcer, and 1 delayed gastric emptying, 4 cases of pneumonia, and 11 leaks.

Selected References

Gagner M, Pomp A. Laparoscopic pylorus preserving pancreatoduodenectomy. Surg Endosc. 1994;8(5):408–10.

Pugliese R, Scandroglio I, Sansonna F, Maggioni D, Costanzi A, Citterio D, et al. Laparoscopic pancreaticoduodenectomy: a retrospective review of 19 cases. Surg Laparosc Endosc Percutan Tech. 2008;18(1):13–8.

Dulucq JL, Wintringer P, Mahajna A. Laparoscopic pancreaticoduodenectomy for benign and malignant diseases. Surg Endosc. 2006;20(7):1045–50.

Palanivelu C, Jani K, Senthilnathan P, Parthasarathi R, Rajapandian S, Madhankumar MV. Laparoscopic pancreaticoduodenectomy: technique and outcomes. J Am Coll Surg. 2007;205(2):222–30.

Staudacher C, Orsenigo E, Baccari P, Di Palo S, Crippa S. Laparoscopic assisted duodenopancreatectomy. Surg Endosc. 2005;19(3):352–6.

Lu B, Cai X, Lu W, Huang Y, Jin X. Laparoscopic pancreaticoduodenectomy to treat cancer of the ampulla the Vater. JSLS. 2006;10(1):97–100.

Zheng MH, Feng B, Lu AG, Li JW, Hu WG, Wang ML, et al. Laparoscopic pancreaticoduodenectomy for ductal adenocarcinoma of common bile duct: a case report and literature review. Med Sci Monit. 2006;12(6):CS57–60.

Sa Cunha A, Rault A, Beau C, Laurent C, Collet D, Masson B. A single institution prospective study of laparoscopic pancreatic resection. Arch Surg. 2008;143(3):289–95 (discussion 295).

Gentileschi P, Gagner M. Laparoscopic pancreatic resection. Chir Ital. 2001; 53(3):279–89.

Ammori BJ. Laparoscopic hand assisted pancreaticoduodenectomy: initial UK experience. Surg Endosc. 2004;18(4):717–8.

Gagner M. Laparoscopic pancreatic surgery. In: Eubanks S, Swanstron L, Soper N, editors. Mastery of endoscopic and laparoscopic surgery, chap. 32. Lippincott Williams & Wilkins; Philadelphia 1999. p. 291–305.

Assalia A, Gagner M. Laparoscopic pancreatic surgery for islet cell tumors of the pancreas. World J Surg. 2004;28(12):1239–47.

Ammori BJ, Ayiomamitis GD. Laparoscopic pancreaticoduodenectomy and distal pancreatectomy: a UK experience and a systematic review of the literature. Surg Endosc. 2011;25(7):2084–99.

Palanivelu C, Rajan PS, Rangarajan M, Vaithiswaran V, Senthilnathan P, Parthasarathi R, Praveen Raj P. Evolution in techniques of laparoscopic pancreaticoduodenectomy: a decade long experience from a tertiary center. J Hepatobiliary Pancreat Surg. 2009;16(6):731–40.

Gagner M, Palermo M. Laparoscopic Whipple procedure: review of the literature. J Hepatobiliary Pancreat Surg. 2009;16(6):726–30.

Gagner M, Pomp A. Laparoscopic pancreatic resection: is it worthwhile? J Gastrointest Surg. 1997;1(1):20–5; discussion 25–6.

24. Laparoscopic Liver Resection

Paul D. Hansen, M.D.
Pippa Newell, M.D.

A. Introduction

The perioperative morbidity of hepatectomy has decreased significantly over the last two decades. This is largely due to improved perioperative monitoring and critical care medicine, and the development of new technologies and techniques within the fields of interventional radiology and surgery. In addition, patient selection has been refined with modern diagnostics and expanded surgeon experience. Finally, there has been a movement of higher risk cases toward hepatobiliary centers, where focused expertise and advanced supportive services are available to patient and surgeon.

Although general surgeons were swift to adapt laparoscopy for lower risk procedures, hepatobiliary surgeons have been more cautious in evolving their practices. There are several reasons for caution, the most important of which is the requirement for the hepatobiliary surgeon to acquire two separate high-level skill sets. In order to safely perform advanced laparoscopic liver resections, surgeons must first be experienced and knowledgeable in the anatomical and technical considerations of open hepatectomy. They must also have acquired a second skill set in advanced laparoscopic techniques; this includes the ability to translate the two dimensional visual field into a three dimensional understanding of pertinent anatomy, dexterity in vascular dissection and control, and laparoscopic suturing. In addition, laparoscopic liver resection requires proficiency and confidence in use of laparoscopic ultrasound.

To summarize, programs performing laparoscopic liver surgery should meet a number of criteria:

1. Their volume and experience in open liver resection should be substantial.
2. Surgeons should be trained in complex laparoscopy.

3. The operative nursing team should be dedicated and trained in both advanced laparoscopic techniques as well as advanced hepatobiliary techniques.

4. Supporting services, including intensive care units, postoperative nursing units, gastroenterology, and radiology should be comfortable and experienced with the care of hepatobiliary patients.

Laparoscopic liver surgery programs should focus on wedge resections and segmentectomies before advancing to more advanced liver resections.

B. Indications

In a consensus statement authored by 45 experts in hepatobiliary surgery (Buell et al.), it is reiterated that indications for liver resection should not be expanded because of the decreased morbidity related to laparoscopic approach. Therefore, indications for laparoscopic liver resection are the same as for open surgery. The laparoscopic approach was initially performed on patients with benign, small, and peripheral lesions, but as technologies and techniques improved and experience was gained, we have seen an increase in the complexity of resections, including the performance of lobectomies and trisegmentectomies.

1. Primary liver cancer
   a. The incidences of hepatocellular carcinoma (HCC) and intrahepatic cholangiocarcinoma (ICC) are increasing in the USA, the former mainly due to Hepatitis C viral infection and increasing incidence of nonalcoholic steatohepatitis.
   b. Liver resection is the best option for attempted curative treatment in selected patients with early stage HCC and no evidence of tumor thrombus in the inferior vena cava (IVC) or main portal vein, no extrahepatic disease, and minimal or no portal hypertension.
   c. Assessment of liver function reserve is paramount. The lower limit of liver remnant volume in patients with normal liver is 20–25%, but the volume necessary to prevent post resection liver failure in patients with cirrhosis has not been documented, and varies widely depending on the severity of cirrhosis. Several methods have been applied to estimate liver function, including computed tomography

(CT) volumetry, preoperative biopsy to grade fibrosis, and indocyanine green (ICG) clearance. In general, resection would not be considered in patients whose remnant liver volume is estimated to be less than 40%.

d. The risk of surgical resection in cirrhotic livers is higher than in normal liver due to reduced liver function reserve and limited capacity for liver regeneration. Candidates should have no evidence of portal hypertension (thrombocytopenia, varices). In large volume centers, the mortality of liver resections in patients with cirrhosis ranges from 1–8% compared with 1–5% in patients with normal liver. The extra morbidity and mortality is attributable to several factors including the following:

  i.   Increased risk of intraoperative bleeding, due to distorted anatomy, portal hypertension, and coagulopathy;

  ii. Postoperative liver failure, which occurs in 2–10% of patients undergoing major hepatectomy in high volume centers. This can occur because of inadequate liver remnant volume, but is often precipitated by bleeding or sepsis;

  iii. Ascites and malnutrition.

e. Overall outcomes following laparoscopic liver resection are similar to open liver resection in patients with a cirrhotic liver.

f. Because patients with primary liver cancer are now likely to live longer, reoperation for intrahepatic recurrence of HCC may become more common and has been reported as feasible and safe.

2. Metastatic disease

a. The majority of hepatectomies performed in the USA are for metastatic disease.

b. The treatment with best curative potential for patients with metastatic cancer is complete surgical extirpation. In patients with liver only metastases, curative liver resection requires complete removal of the tumor and a 1 cm margin of surrounding liver parenchyma.

c. In patients with an otherwise normal liver, the future liver remnant must include two contiguous liver segments with preserved vascular inflow and outflow, preserved biliary drainage, and a minimum of 20–25% of the original functional liver volume.

d. Indications for resection are expanding as case series have reported survival benefit to aggressive surgical treatment for metastatic colorectal cancer, as well as selected noncolorectal liver metastases.

e. The best results after laparoscopic liver resection are in patients with single lesions, 5 cm or less, located in peripheral liver segments 2–6.

f. Central and larger tumors necessitating major liver resections should be referred to centers performing high volumes of advanced laparoscopic liver surgery.

g. Advantage of laparoscopic approach: decreased recovery time and wound complications allowing for faster transition to adjuvant chemotherapy; because patients are surviving longer now, reoperation will become more frequent, and therefore efforts to minimize formation of adhesions are valuable; laparoscopic approach is useful for patients with bilobar disease who need staged resections to achieve an R0 resection.

h. 5-year survival following laparoscopic liver resection for selected patients with metastatic colon cancer is as high as 64% in some centers, and can be equivalent to outcomes following open resection.

i. Laparoscopic repeat hepatectomy seems to be safe, with comparable oncological outcomes to repeat open hepatectomy. Repeat laparoscopic liver resections following an initial laparoscopic approach are associated with lower blood loss and transfusion requirements.

C. Preoperative Planning

a. Anatomy of vascular inflow and outflow and the biliary system should be defined using preoperative imaging, such as multiphase contrast enhanced CT. Cholangiocarcinoma involving main bile ducts should be imaged with cholangiography for optimal planning.

b. Biliary obstruction caused by malignancy, most commonly cholangiocarcinoma, may call for preoperative drainage of the proposed liver remnant.

c. Similar to open surgery, central and large tumors may require trisegmentectomy or lobectomy, in which case portal venous embolization (PVE) may be indicated to increase the capacity of the future liver remnant. Standardized functional liver remnant volume (FLRV) is typically calculated using CT volumetry, taking into consideration patient's weight. In patients with liver disease, the volume increase of the proposed remnant following PVE is often less than in patients with normal livers, and lack of hypertrophy following PVE may portend postoperative liver failure. Patients who have undergone oxaliplatin-based and irinotecan-based chemotherapy are at relatively high risk for hepatic injury, such as steatohepatitis.

d. Indications for PVE are not formalized, but take into consideration preexisting liver disease, extent of planned resection, volume of liver replaced by tumor, patient comorbidities, such as diabetes, and patient size. For example, a patient with a large tumor replacing much of the right lobe is at lower risk for postoperative liver failure than a patient with multiple small tumors in the right lobe necessitating a comparable resection[25]. Proposed indications for PVE include an FLRV of ≤20% in patients with normal liver, ≤30% in patients who have undergone recent chemotherapy, and ≤40% in patients with cirrhosis.

D. Patient Position, Room Setup, Specialized Instruments

a. Patients are typically positioned supine or split leg. Arms should be extended because ports are often placed far laterally just below the costal margin or rarely through the intercostal space. The bed can be positioned in reverse Trendelenberg to drop the viscera away from the inferior edge of the liver during the dissection and mobilization phases.

b. A bump or wedge may be placed under the right posterior costal margin for large right-sided tumors, or the patient may be placed in a modified left lateral decubitus position for posterior right-sided tumors.

c. The ultrasound machine is typically placed adjacent to the arm opposite the operating surgeon.

d. Whether or not a purely laparoscopic procedure is planned, open and vascular instruments should be available in the room in case the need to convert to open arises; instruments for open liver surgery should be available and counted to allow for rapid conversion if necessary. Similarly, a backup electrocautery device, suction, and staple loads should be available in case of malfunction during parenchymal transection.

e. Instruments particularly helpful include: Two insufflators, liver retractors, and atraumatic graspers for exposure during transection.

f. Port placement and surgeon position are diagrammed in Fig. 24.1. In general, the surgeon faces the lesion, with an instrument in each hand, converging on the target at a 90-degree angle. A 30° to 45° angled scope is used and centered between the surgeon's two instrument ports. Assistant ports are positioned laterally to allow optimal retraction and suction and minimal obstruction of view.

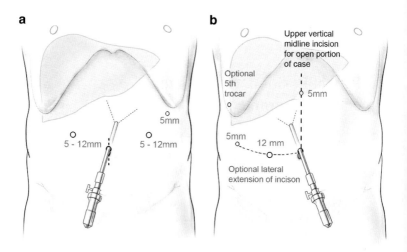

Fig. 24.1. (**a**) Port placement for left lateral sectionectomy. Ultrasound probes typically pass through 10-mm trocars while staplers require 12-mm trocars. (**b**) Port placement for hybrid right hepatectomy. © Corinne Sandone, printed with permission.

E. Techniques for Parenchymal Division

There is neither a consensus nor any validated randomized data demonstrating the superiority of one method of parenchymal transection over another. The patient's central venous pressure should be kept low to minimize blood loss during transection.

a. A number of new technologies have been developed for hepatic parenchymal transection.
    i.   Electrocautery devices include both monopolar and bipolar coagulating/cutting devices, and saline-linked cautery (TissueLink).
    ii. Ultrasonic tissue division technologies include ultrasonic scalpel/shears (Harmonic, AutoSonix), and continuous ultrasound aspirator (CUSA).
    iii. Hydro-jet technologies (as well as the CUSA) disrupt cells, leaving behind the vascular and biliary structures, which may then be cauterized, clipped, tied, or stapled.
b. Stapler hepatectomy
    i.   Stapled transection of isolated vasculature provides clean and reliable ligation. It is critical to assure that there are no clips or loose staples in the jaws prior to firing the stapling device, as these will tear the new staple line as the cutting blade is advanced.
    ii. 1–1.5 cm thick bites of parenchyma can also be transected with the stapler, although this has been associated with slightly higher incidence of postoperative bile leak.
    iii. The stapler technique has the advantage of allowing for rapid division of parenchyma and control of large structures encountered therein.
c. Clips and ties for short hepatic veins along the IVC
    i.   During anatomic resections, many of the short hepatic veins are small enough that they can be controlled with electrocautery or ultrasonic shears. Rarely, these veins can be greater than 5 mm in diameter, necessitating ties. Clips can be rapidly deployed but are more likely to be dislodged.
d. The Pringle maneuver or portal triad clamping is typically reserved for bleeding and is not generally performed during laparoscopic liver resections.
    i.   Preparation for vascular control with a vessel loop may be advisable during anatomical resections or large segmentectomies.

  ii. Bleeding is typically controlled laparoscopically if it is minor. A dry field is of paramount importance and for this reason, it cannot be stressed enough that surgeons undertaking laparoscopic liver resection have a thorough understanding of the vascular anatomy and be facile with laparoscopic suturing and other techniques of hemorrhage control.

  iii. The need for conversion to open for major or uncontrolled hemorrhage should be a rare occurrence, but must be anticipated. Preparation includes development of a pre-orchestrated process that can be rapidly implemented.

 e. Portal structures are most commonly dissected, individually identified, and divided in their extrahepatic location.

 f. The intrahepatic approach in which the portal structures are divided within the parenchyma of the liver has been described in several case series as safe and feasible. The portal pedicle is approached by making a small incision in front of the hilar plate, the right side of the gallbladder bed, and/or the round ligament perpendicular to the hepatic hilum where it connects to the caudate lobe. The right anterior, right posterior, and left medial sheaths can be reached by combining these incisions. A vascular clamp is passed across the pedicle and the parenchyma is allowed to demarcate. The endovascular stapler is then positioned in the same location and the structures are divided as long as the line of demarcation remains the same.

F. Choice of Operative Technique

 a. Pure laparoscopy
  i. Technique introduced and practiced by French surgeons.
  ii. Becoming standard of care for left lateral sectectomy (resection of segments II and III).

 b. Hand-assist
  i. Allows for palpation of margins during transection and for gentle retraction during mobilization.
  ii. Considerations when choosing location of port include location of tumor and surgeon handedness.
  iii. Posterior wedge resections and right hepatectomies in particular can be facilitated with hand ports.
  iv. The hand-port site may be used for specimen extraction.

c. Hybrid technique
  i. Americans have expanded use of hybrid technique, which is defined as laparoscopic mobilization of the liver followed by open ligation of portal structures and parenchymal transection.
  ii. The advantage over a straight open technique is that it allows the transection to be performed through a vertical midline incision, typically a less painful incision than the bilateral subcostal or Chevron incision.

G. Ultrasound

Whether performing open or laparoscopic liver resections, ultrasound is a vital technique for the surgeon to master. Understanding the size, shape, and location of the target tumors relative to vital internal hepatic structures is critical to performing a safe and successful resection. With this information, the surgeon can ensure a tumor free remnant, they can plan a transection line with an appropriate margin, and they can anticipate the intersection of major structures which need to be divided in a controlled fashion.

a. Technology
  i. Laparoscopic probes are all currently available as a 10-mm wand. They may have a flexible or rigid tip with a linear or curvilinear array.
  ii. The typical frequency used for contact liver sonography is between 5 MHz and 10 MHz. Lower frequencies (5–7 MHz) provide a slightly lower resolution, but allow deeper penetration into the liver. This may be helpful with cirrhotic or fatty livers. Higher frequencies (7.5–10 MHz) penetrate less deeply, but provide higher resolution. The surgeon should be facile with selecting a frequency that provides the optimal image for a given clinical scenario.
b. Technique
  i. Staging laparoscopy is performed prior to laparoscopic liver resection. A thorough evaluation of the liver will determine how many tumors are present, whether the presumed liver remnant is free of tumor, and will confirm the target tumor's relationship to vital hepatic structures and the planned line of transection.

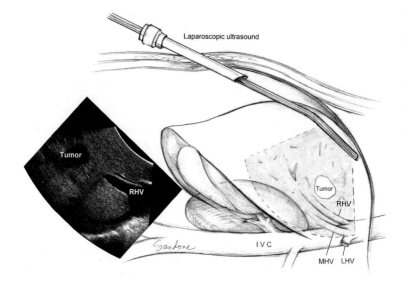

Fig. 24.2. Ultrasound traces the dimensions of the tumor and defines its proximity to vital structures. In addition, it can be used to map out portal and hepatic venous structures which cross the line of transection. © Corinne Sandone, printed with permission.

    ii.   The liver should be scanned in a preplanned and thorough fashion, identifying the individual segmental portal pedicles and hepatic venous drainage. See Fig. 24.2.

    iii.   After selecting a transection plane, the surgeon can make note of the position and depth of each vascular structure they anticipate dividing during the transection. Preplanning the transection will prevent surprises and minimize blood loss.

H. Hepatectomy

For any type of liver resection, location of ports is planned such that the camera is centered between the surgeon's primary working instruments during the principle portions of the case. Subxiphoid and far lateral ports can be useful for mobilization and retraction of both lobes.

    a.   Wedge resection

        i.   Ultrasound is initially used to define size of tumor and to identify adjacent vascular and biliary structures to be avoided or incorporated, allowing for approximately 1 cm margin of normal tissue surrounding the target tumor. Ultrasound should be repeated during resection to ensure margins are adequate.

    ii.   Ultrasonic scalpel can provide adequate hemostasis for most superficial wedge resections.

b.   Left lateral sectectomy (resection of segments II and III)

    i.   The laparoscopic approach is becoming the standard of care due to its demonstrated safety and minimization of morbidity.

    ii.   Ports are typically placed in a subcostal array. See Fig. 24.1a.

    iii.   Ultrasound is used to visualize proximity of tumor to segment 2 and 3 branches of main left portal structures.

    iv.   Divide the falciform ligament from the round ligament to the vena cava.

    v.   Divide the left triangular ligament from the left of the vena cava continuing along the diaphragm to the left lateral border. Be aware of possible phrenic veins crossing near this ligament.

    vi.   The gastrohepatic ligament is divided from the hepatoduodenal ligament to the right crus.

    vii.   Divide the tissue bridge between segments 3 and 4b.

    viii.   Dissect out the left hepatic vein by taking the peritoneum overlying the middle and left veins at the level of the IVC from the superior approach. The bifurcation between the middle and left veins may be slightly intraparenchymal.

    ix.   If the anterior/superior approach proves difficult, the left vein can be dissected from an inferior approach by retracting the left lateral lobe upward (see Fig. 24.3a). The vein should be divided with an endovascular stapler after the portal inflow is divided (See Fig. 24.3c).

    x.   The parenchymal transection line follows the falciform ligament along the ligamentum teres toward the medial border of the left hepatic vein (See Fig. 24.3b). Care is taken to transect the liver just lateral to the main left portal structures.

    xi.   Place the specimen inside a nonpermeable specimen bag and remove through an expanded incision. Margins can be inked if they are in question. For benign disease, the specimen can be morcellated and removed through a smaller incision.

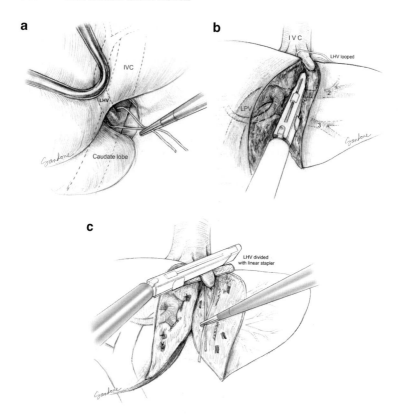

Fig. 24.3. (**a**) The left hepatic vein can be exposed and controlled by retracting the left lateral lobe anteriorly. (**b**) The segment II and III portal structures are typically transected close to the main left portal vein with a 2.5 mm (*white*) cartridge loaded on the endovascular stapler. (**c**) The left hepatic vein is transected with a 2.0 mm (*gray*) load. Care should be taken to avoid narrowing the middle hepatic vein and IVC. © Corinne Sandone, printed with permission.

    c.   Anterior segmentectomy
         i.   Ports are placed according to preoperative studies and intraoperative ultrasound visualization of tumors.
        ii.   Inflow and outflow vessels and bile ducts are divided intraparenchymally, using endoscopic staplers.
       iii.   Proximity of the mass to vital structures is assessed real-time with ultrasound, and line of transection is reassessed

during parenchymal division to ensure clear margins and to anticipate larger vascular or biliary structures which could need stapler or suture control.

d. Right lobectomy, hybrid technique

    i. Purely laparoscopic major liver resections are typically reserved for specialized centers performing high volumes of laparoscopic hepatobiliary surgery. Key steps in the purely laparoscopic approach described by Gayet include isolation and division of hepatic inflow, control of hepatic outflow, division of hepatic parenchyma, division of hepatic outflow, and specimen retrieval.

    ii. For a planned hybrid right hepatectomy, ports are placed as shown in Fig. 24.1b.

    iii. The falciform is divided followed by both right and left triangular ligaments, exposing the confluence of the right hepatic vein and the IVC.

    iv. The attachments to the hepatic flexure of the colon, the retroperitoneum and the right diaphragm are released with the ultrasonic scalpel. This is facilitated by either a triangle liver retractor or hand-assisted port.

    v. The IVC is exposed and the short hepatic veins are serially dissected and divided with ultrasonic scalpel. Medium-sized vessels are ligated with ties or clips before being divided. Large or accessory right hepatic veins may require division with a stapler. The caudate ligament which wraps around the vena cava may also require stapler transection.

    vi. The right hepatic vein is identified and a vessel loop is passed around the base of the vein.

    vii. A midline laparotomy is made from the xiphoid to above the umbilicus and the right portal structures are dissected free and divided in an open fashion. The right hepatic vein is divided and the parenchymal division is performed, using ultrasound to verify the location of the tumor relative to major portal and hepatic vein branches as often as necessary to guarantee a safe and adequate resection.

    viii. The midline incision can be extended laterally through the right abdominal ports if necessary for exposure.

I. Ultrasound-guided Biopsy and Ablation

a. Laparoscopic ultrasound-guided biopsy is a useful technique for obtaining tissue biopsy.

b. The key to successful biopsy is identifying the target tissue and approaching the target with the biopsy needle in the same plane as the linear array of the ultrasound. This allows the surgeon to track the needle though the liver parenchyma on its approach to the target.

c. Firing the biopsy mechanism typically leaves a small air track within the target allowing confirmation of an accurate biopsy.

d. A number of different thermal ablation technologies are currently available to the surgeon. While resection of tumors is still largely considered the gold standard, experience with thermal ablation is growing and results suggest that in selected scenarios, ablation may be the treatment of choice.

   i. Cryoablation is no longer widely used as it is an expensive technology and has been associated with high local recurrence rates following percutaneous application.

   ii. Radiofrequency ablation (RFA) uses a rapidly alternating electrical current to excite ions within the target tissue, causing frictional heating and tissue destruction.

   iii. Microwave energy excites water molecules generating heat and again causing tissue destruction.

e. Thermal energy is an effective method of ablating tumors and a margin of surrounding tissue.

   i. If the heat is applied thoroughly, ablation can be as effective as resection in extirpating target tumors.

   ii. Ablation, however, is heavily reliant on exact, ultrasound-guided placements of the ablation probe within the tumor, and overcoming any local cooling effect of nearby vasculature.

   iii. RFA and microwave ablation must be used with great caution within 2 cm of central biliary structures as these can be damaged, resulting in severe complications.

J. Cyst Fenestration

a. Indicated for large, symptomatic simple liver cysts.

b. Ultrasonic scalpel is useful for transecting thin portions of liver parenchyma at the base of the cysts.

c. The surgeon should consider use of a stapler when dividing two cysts immediately adjacent because biliary and vascular structures can be trapped between two separately enlarging cysts.

d. If adequately mobile, omentum can be placed inside the fenestrated cyst bed to minimize reaccumulation of cyst fluid, particularly in cysts in which <50% of the wall has been removed.

K. Outcomes and Complications

In spite of the initial reticence of liver surgeons, laparoscopic liver resections have now become more commonplace. This transition occurred concomitantly with improved outcomes. Nguyen et al. reviewed all laparoscopic liver resections reported in the literature prior to 2009, with an overall morbidity and mortality of 10.5% and 0.3% in the 2,804 patients included. While the authors openly admit there is selection bias in that only 25% of the surgeries involved major resections, these numbers indicate that laparoscopic liver resections have safety profiles comparable to open surgeries when performed by surgeons with expertise in both complex laparoscopy and hepatobiliary surgery.

Selected References

Abdalla EK. Portal vein embolization (prior to major hepatectomy) effects on regeneration, resectability, and outcome. J Surg Oncol. 2010;102(8):960–7.

Asiyanbola B, Chang D, Gleisner A, et al. Operative mortality after hepatic resection: are literature-based rates broadly applicable? J Gastrointest Surg. 2007;12:842–51.

Belghiti J, Hiramatsu K, Benoist S, Massault PP, Sauvanet A, Farges O. Seven hundred forty-seven hepatectomies in the 1990s: an update to evaluate the actual risk of liver resection. J Am Coll Surg. 2000;191(1):38–46.

Buell JF, Cherqui D, Geller DA, et al. The international position on laparoscopic liver surgery: the Louisville statement, 2008. Ann Surg. 2009;250(5):825–30.

Castaing D, Vibert E, Ricca L, Azoulay D, Adam R, Gayet B. Oncologic results of laparoscopic versus open hepatectomy for colorectal liver metastases in two specialized centers. Ann Surg. 2009;250(5):849–55.

Hirohashi K, Tanaka H, Tsukamoto T, et al. Limitation of portal vein embolization for extension of hepatectomy indication in patients with hepatocellular carcinoma. Hepatogastroenterology. 2004;51(58):1084–7.

Imamura H, Seyama Y, Kokudo N, et al. One thousand fifty-six hepatectomies without mortality in 8 years. Arch Surg. 2003;138(11):1198–206.

Kennedy TJ, Yopp A, Qin Y, et al. Role of preoperative biliary drainage of liver remnant prior to extended liver resection for hilar cholangiocarcinoma. HPB (Oxford). 2009;11(5):445–51.

Kneuertz PJ, Maithel SK, Staley CA, Kooby DA. Chemotherapy-associated liver injury: impact on surgical management of colorectal cancer liver metastases. Ann Surg Oncol. 2011;18(1):181–90. Epub 2010 Jul 20.

Kooby DA, Fong Y, Suriawinata A, et al. Impact of steatosis on perioperative outcome following hepatic resection. J Gastrointest Surg. 2003;7(8):1034–44.

Machado MA, Makdissi FF, Galvao FH, Machado MC. Intrahepatic Glissonian approach for laparoscopic right segmental liver resections. Am J Surg. 2008;196(4):e38–42. Epub 2008 Jul 2009.

Manizate F, Hiotis SP, Labow D, Roayaie S, Schwartz M. Liver functional reserve estimation: state of the art and relevance for local treatments: the western perspective. J Hepatobiliary Pancreat Sci. 2009;17(4):385–8.

Nguyen KT, Gamblin TC, Geller DA. World review of laparoscopic liver resection-2,804 patients. Ann Surg. 2009;250(5):831–41.

Poon RT, Fan ST. Liver resection in cirrhosis of the liver. In: Blumgart LH, editor. Surgery of the liver, biliary tract, and pancreas, vol. 2. 4th ed. Philadelphia, PA: Saunders Elsevier; 2007.

Roayaie S, Bassi D, Tarchi P, Labow D, Schwartz M. Second hepatic resection for recurrent hepatocellular cancer: a western experience. J Hepatol. 2010;2010:10.

Sarpel U, Hefti MM, Wisnievsky JP, Roayaie S, Schwartz ME, Labow DM. Outcome for patients treated with laparoscopic versus open resection of hepatocellular carcinoma: case-matched analysis. Ann Surg Oncol. 2009;16(6):1572–7. Epub 2009 Mar 1574.

Vauthey J-N, Chaoui A, Do K-A, et al. Standardized measurement of the future liver remnant prior to extended liver resection: methodology and clinical associations. Surgery. 2000;127(5):512–9.

25. Laparoscopic Palliation for Pancreatic Cancer

Chan W. Park, M.D.
James A. Dickerson II, M.D.
Aurora D. Pryor, M.D.

A. Introduction

The role of laparoscopy in the management of pancreatic cancer continues to evolve. With advancements in minimally invasive surgery (MIS) techniques, laparoscopy has become an accepted approach to initial surgical inspection of the peritoneal cavity and can play a key role in determining resectability of pancreatic cancer. Contemporary surgical management of pancreatic cancer now incorporates innovative MIS techniques beyond just the "first-look," and even in cases of unresectable cancer, laparoscopy offers the patient viable therapeutic options to palliate underlying disease symptoms and maintain the quality of life while significantly minimizing associated surgical morbidity. These patient derived benefits of an MIS approach can be significant since nearly 80% of pancreatic cancer patients are deemed unresectable and require palliative surgical options. This chapter outlines techniques for laparoscopic palliation of pancreatic cancer and discusses key surgical considerations for patient management.

B. Defining Resectability and the Need for Palliative Treatment

1. **Laparoscopic Inspection of the Peritoneal Cavity**
   Laparoscopy has become an accepted approach to initial surgical inspection of the peritoneal cavity and can play a key role in

determining resectability of pancreatic cancer. Studies report variable outcomes due to variability in the extent of the peritoneal exploration (superficial survey versus more thorough exploration of retrogastric area, lymph node evaluation, laparoscopic ultrasound, and peritoneal washings/cytology); however, laparoscopic peritoneoscopy does appear to increase diagnostic sensitivity and specificity. A more detailed discussion of this procedure as applied to pancreatic cancer is presented elsewhere in this manual (see Chapter 23).

2. **Laparoscopic Cholangiography**

Biliary obstruction (often resulting in jaundice) is commonly associated with pancreatic cancer, and the specific anatomic location(s) of the biliary obstruction will determine the best palliative surgical option. Thus, once curative surgical resection has been contraindicated, the patency of the biliary tree must be defined. While preoperative imaging studies (CT, radionuclide study, etc.) may preclude the need for invasive evaluation of the biliary tree, laparoscopic transcystic cholangiography is recommended if any uncertainty exists.

C. Palliative Procedures for Pancreatic Cancer

Weight loss, jaundice, and abdominal pain are common symptoms of pancreatic cancer, and laparoscopic palliative procedures can be undertaken to alleviate these symptoms. Outcomes and complication rates are quite favorable, with minimal mortality and morbidity rates reported in the literature. The biggest benefit of laparoscopic palliative procedures appears to be in patient reported "quality of life"; one of the primary goals of palliative therapy.

1. **Bypass Procedures**

Obstructive symptoms (both enteric and biliary) are commonly associated with pancreatic cancer. However, if the patient does not have any evidence of biliary obstruction, an enteric bypass (gastrojejunostomy) procedure may be all that is indicated. If the patient exhibits biliary obstruction a biliary bypass procedure must be chosen based on the anatomic level of the obstruction. A cholecystojejunostomy procedure requires patency of the cystic duct to allow decompression of the biliary tree, but a higher level biliary-enteric bypass procedure, such as a choledochojejunostomy is required when the cystic duct is obstructed. Alternatives to these laparoscopic approaches include endoscopic, combined laparoendoscopic, and percutaneous biliary decompression procedures, but in-depth discussion of these procedures are beyond the scope of this chapter.

a. **Enteric Bypass Procedure: Gastrojejunostomy**

    i. **Laparoscopic gastrojejunostomy** is indicated for bypass of distal gastric, pyloric, or duodenal obstruction, generally when the patient is not considered to be a candidate for a more definitive procedure. This procedure can be used alone or in conjunction with biliary-enteric bypass procedures.

b. **Biliary Bypass Procedures: Cholecystojejunostomy and Choledochojejunostomy**

Endoscopic biliary stenting has equivalent short-term outcomes and is generally preferred over surgery. However, if endoscopic procedures prove unsuccessful or if the expected length of survival exceeds 6 months (the need for re-intervention increases over time), laparoscopic biliary bypass procedures are indicated.

    i. **Laparoscopic cholecystojejunostomy** is indicated when bypass of the biliary tract is needed and the cystic duct is known to be patent. The procedure is most commonly used to palliate unresectable malignancies of the region of the ampulla of Vater. It may also be used in chronic pancreatitis. Endoscopic/internal stenting is an alternative procedure.

    ii. **Laparoscopic choledochojejunostomy** is indicated when bypass of the biliary tract is needed, but the cystic duct is not patent. However, due to the anatomic and physiologic characteristics of the common bile duct, this procedure may be more technically challenging. Newer techniques of choledochojejunostomy creation, including sutureless anastomoses, utilization of surgical stents, and combination approaches incorporating endoscopy, ultrasound, and/or fluoroscopy, have been presented in the literature.

c. **Combined Biliary and Enteric Bypass Procedures:**

    i. **Laparoscopic cholecystojejunostomy (or choledochojejunostomy) and gastrojejunostomy** can be combined into a double-bypass procedure when both biliary and gastric diversion are indicated. There are some minor modifications in the surgical approach that must be incorporated when combining these bypass procedures.

2. **Other Palliative Procedures**
   a. **Laparoscopic celiac plexus block** has been shown to effectively reduce pain and improve overall quality of life with minimal risk. Since pain is a common presenting symptom and nearly all patients with pancreatic cancer will experience pain during the course of their disease, multiple medical and minimally invasive therapeutic options exist. While image-guided percutaneous techniques have been traditionally utilized, these procedures are not without complications and failures. The laparoscopic celiac plexus block procedure is a relatively simple procedure which can be performed exclusively, but it is best when performed during the initial cancer screening operation or in combination with a bypass procedure; avoiding the need for a second trip to the operating room.

D. The Surgical Approach

Initial patient positioning and operating room setup are similar for all of the aforementioned procedures, with minor differences specific to each procedure.

1. **Initial Patient Positioning and Room Setup**
   a. Position the patient supine on the operating table with both arms extended.
   b. The table position will change significantly throughout the operation, and extra care in safely securing the patient on the operating table is mandatory.
   c. The surgeon stands at the right side of the patient. Some surgeons prefer to stand between the patient's legs, particularly if a sutured anastomosis is planned.
   d. Place the monitors at the head, in positions similar to those used for laparoscopic cholecystectomy.

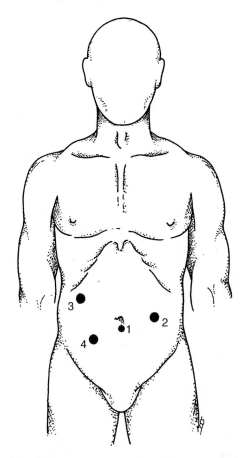

Fig. 25.1. **Trocar Placement for Gastrojejunostomy.** A standard umbilical or subumbilical location for trocar 1 places the laparoscope in good position. If you plan to perform a biliary bypass procedure, it is recommended that trocar 3 be upsized to 10- or 12-mm in order to achieve a favorable angle for stapler insertion. This will also enable passage of a 10-mm laparoscope through trocar 3 for "internal" visualization of the anastomoses. Trocar 4 must be placed low enough to allow sufficient working distance to open the jaws. As with all advanced laparoscopic procedures, trocar placement is crucial, and careful consideration to assure good alignment and positioning are recommended.

2.   **Trocar Position and Choice of Laparoscope (Fig. 25.1)**
   a.   Place the first trocar at or just below the umbilicus. An angled laparoscope (30°) is recommended to facilitate visualization.

b. Place a 5-mm trocar to the left of the midline, lateral to the rectus, at a position slightly higher than the level of the umbilicus. Place another trocar (5 mm for gastrojejunostomy or 12 mm for cholecystojejunostomy) in the right subcostal region. These two trocars will be used for manipulation and suturing.

c. The fourth trocar will be used for the endoscopic stapling device, and an appropriately sized (12 mm) trocar is recommended. This trocar is placed to the right of the midline, lateral to the rectus, at a position at about the level of the umbilicus. Placement of this trocar must be low enough to allow sufficient working space within the abdomen. If the trocar is placed too close to the gallbladder, it will be difficult to manipulate the stapling device (remember that to properly open the device, the jaws must be completely out of the trocar). Take care to ensure that you are satisfied with the alignment and spatial relationships before placing this trocar.

3. **Performing the Gastrojejunostomy**

a. Trocar placements are similar (Fig. 25.1) except that trocar 2 may be placed lower on the left side (to create sufficient working distance from the stomach).

b. Identify the ligament of Treitz and run the bowel to a point at least 50 cm distal to the ligament of Treitz. Verify that the loop selected passes comfortably up to the stomach in an antecolic fashion; if the loop does not pass easily, try selecting a more distal small bowel site (and hence farther from the ligament of Treitz). Alternatively, a retrocolic window may be created in the transverse mesocolon to allow passage of the selected loop of bowel; however, this requires additional dissection and eventual suture closure of the created mesenteric defect.

c. Choose a dependent site, low on the greater curvature of the stomach. Instillation of air via a nasogastric (NG) tube or use of the endoscope can help elevate the stomach and make it easier to identify a favorable site.

d. Place two stay sutures to approximate the stomach and the jejunum.

e. Make two enterotomies; pass and fire the stapling device with a 3.5-mm cartridge (Fig. 25.2). The 60-mm stapler provides an adequate lumen. If this is not available, perform

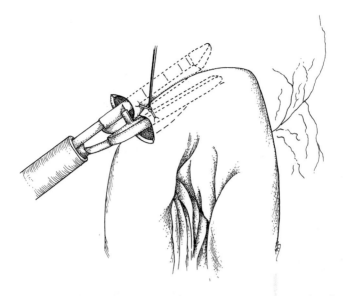

Fig. 25.2. **Gastroejunostomy-Stapled Anastomosis.** A stay suture placed prior to creation of the enterotomy opening helps align the stomach and jejunum for stapler insertion. (An alternative technique, without the use of a stay suture, has also been described). Use of a 60-mm stapler with a 3.5-mm cartridge is recommended. A stay suture placed prior to creation of the enterotomy opening helps align the stomach and jejunum for stapler insertion. (An alternative technique, without the use of a stay suture, has also been described). Use of a 60-mm stapler with a 3.5-mm cartridge is recommended. Some advocate keeping the stapler closed for 1–1.5 min; gentle compression may facilitate hemostasis.

a second firing of the 30-mm device, taking care to extend the staple line directly back from the apex.

i.   **Alternate technique (no stay sutures)**: After verifying appropriate reach and selecting the anastomotic site, enterotomies are created in both the stomach and jejunum. First, insert the narrow end of the linear stapler and gently close, but do not fire the stapler. This will serve to hold the jejunal loop in position. Next, deliver the stapler and jejunal loop, up toward the stomach and open the jaws, taking care not to drop the jejunal loop. Pass the wide end of the stapler into the stomach. Use atraumatic graspers to position the jejunum and stomach in proper alignment. Close and fire the stapler.

f.   Close the enterotomies with suture or with the endoscopic stapler. We prefer to utilize a continuous/running suture closure. First, an anchoring suture is placed at one end of the opening, but after the knot is secured, the suture tail is left long (Fig. 25.3). The enterotomy opening is then closed by running a continuous suture beginning at the opposite end of the opening and working toward the anchoring suture. Upon completion of the closure, one of the long tails of the anchoring suture is used to tie the final knot.

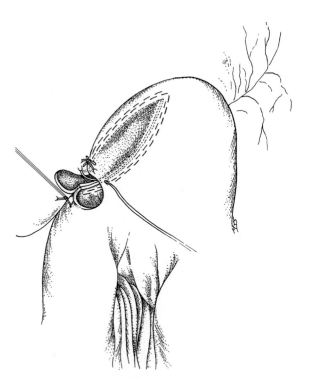

Fig. 25.3. Gastrojejunostomy Enterotomy Closure. After creation of the stapled anastomosis, the common enterotomy opening is closed with running suture. An interrupted anchoring suture is first placed at one end of the opening (through both stomach and jejunum), and a running suture is then started from the opposite end (working toward the anchoring suture) to close the opening. The two sutures are then tied together at the conclusion of the closure.

g. Inspect the staple line. Endoscopic visual inspection of the anastomosis (for hemostasis) and testing of the anastomosis with air under saline (for leaks) are recommended. Alternatively, instillation of air/methylene blue into the NG tube may be used to test the anastomosis for leaks.

4. **Performing the Cholecystojejunostomy**

a. Identify the ligament of Treitz and select a loop of jejunum as previously described. Again, verify that the loop passes comfortably up into the right upper quadrant.

b. Place two stay sutures (1 cm apart) to approximate the jejunum to the gall bladder.

    i. An alternative technique, without the use of stay sutures, may be used as previously described.

c. Use electrocautery or endoscopic scissors to make two stab incisions, each large enough to accommodate one jaw of the endoscopic linear stapling device (approximately 8 mm long). Suction the bile from the gallbladder, note its color, and send a sample for culture. The gallbladder bile should be golden. If the gallbladder bile is white (hydrops) the cystic duct is not patent, and the procedure should not be performed (see Complications, Section E).

d. Pass the endoscopic linear stapling device, with a 3.5-mm cartridge, from trocar 4. Place one jaw within each stab wound (Fig. 25.4). Take care to ensure that the jaws pass into the lumen of the two viscera rather than into a submucosal plane. When you are satisfied, close the stapler and fire it. Open the stapler and remove it from the region of the anastomosis. Some advocate keeping the stapler closed for 1–1.5 min, feeling that this period of gentle compression facilitates hemostasis.

e. Inspect the staple line for bleeding. Irrigate the staple line and check the color of the effluent (see Complications, Section E).

f. Close the stab wounds with suture (Fig. 25.5). An alternative method is to close the opening with an endoscopic linear stapling device.

g. Inspect the completed anastomosis and place a closed suction drain in proximity. If there is omentum, place it in the right upper quadrant as well. Irrigate the abdomen and close in the usual fashion.

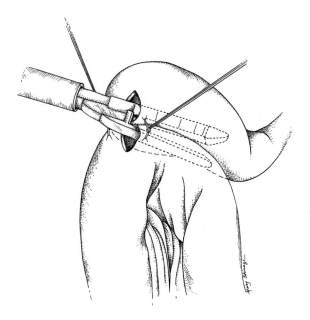

Fig. 25.4. **Cholecystojejunostomy-Stapled Anastomosis.** Stay sutures placed prior to creation of the enterotomy/opening helps align the gallbladder and jejunum for stapler insertion. (An alternative technique, without the use of a stay suture, has also been described). Use of a 60-mm stapler with a 3.5-mm cartridge is recommended (adapted from Bogen GL, Mancino AT, Scott-Connor CE. Laparoscopy for staging and palliation of gastrointestinal malignancy. Surg Clin North Am 1996;76:557–569).

5. **Performing the Choledochojejunostomy**

This procedure is technically challenging, and MIS technical proficiency is required. The use of linear staplers for this procedure is limited by the anatomic location and size of the common bile duct. The utilization of laparoscopic suturing devices and highly skilled surgical assistants are recommended.

a. Identify the ligament of Treitz and select a loop of jejunum as previously described.

   i. The loop of jejunum is delivered to the common bile duct in antecolic fashion.

   ii. Alternatively, a Roux-en-Y reconstruction with an end-to-side anastomosis to the common bile duct may be easier to perform. However, this will necessitate a distal small bowel anastomosis.

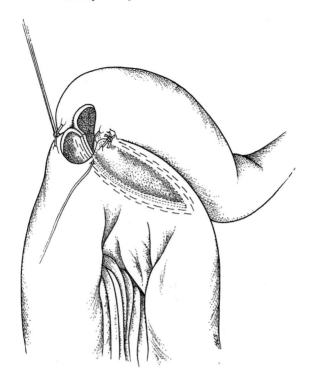

Fig. 25.5. **Cholecystojejunostomy Enterotomy Closure.** After creation of the stapled anastomosis, the common enterotomy opening is closed with running suture. An interrupted anchoring suture is first placed at one end of the opening (through both gallbladder and jejunum), and a running suture is then started from the opposite end (working toward the anchoring suture) to close the opening. The two sutures are then tied together at the conclusion of the closure (adapted from Bogen GL, Mancino AT, Scott-Connor CE. Laparoscopy for staging and palliation of gastrointestinal malignancy. Surg Clin North Am 1996;76:557–569).

b. Isolate the common bile duct and create a vertical (parallel to the axis of the duct) ~2 cm choledochotomy incision on the anterior surface of common bile duct; away from the blood supply at the 3 and 9 o'clock positions (Fig. 25.6).

   i. Do not use electrocautery or energy devices

   ii. Proper retraction of the liver with dedicated retraction devices is recommended:

   – Nathanson-type liver retractor may be placed through a separate stab incision placed in the sub-xiphoid space.

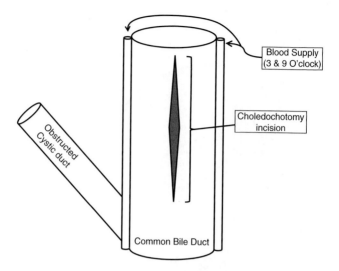

Blood Supply
(3 & 9 O'clock)

Choledochotomy
incision

Obstructed
Cystic duct

Common Bile Duct

Fig. 25.6. Choledochotomy for Choledochojejunostomy. After isolating the common bile duct a vertical (parallel to the axis of the duct) choledochotomy incision is created with sharp dissection (~2 cm in length). The choledochotomy incision must be placed carefully on the anterior surface of common bile duct; away from the blood supply at the 3 and 9 o'clock positions. No electrocautery or energy devices are used, and proper retraction of the liver with dedicated retraction devices is recommended.

      –   Articulating or "fan" type of liver retractor may be placed through a separate trocar placed along the right subcostal margin.

c. Suction the bile from the biliary tree, and prepare for creation of the anastomosis.

    i. If needed, an additional trocar placed on the assistant's side will greatly improve dexterity.

d. Create a jejunal enterotomy utilizing electrocautery or endoscopic scissors.

e. Absorbable suture is utilized to create the anastomosis in single-layer fashion.

    i. The first suture line is created between the farthest edges (from the surgeon) of the choledochotomy and enterotomy incisions. This suture line may be created

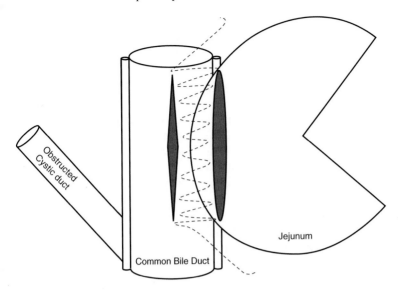

Fig. 25.7. **Choledochojejunostomy Anastomosis.** After performing both cho-ledochotomy and jejunal enterotomy, absorbable suture is utilized to create the anastomosis in single-layer fashion. The first suture line is created between the farthest edges (from the surgeon) of the choledochotomy and enterotomy inci-sions. This suture line may be created in a continuous, running fashion; utilizing full-thickness needle passes through both the common bile duct and jejunum. (The final suture line is completed with interrupted sutures placed strategically along the remaining edges of the choledochotomy and enterotomy incisions to create a water-tight seal).

       in a continuous, running fashion; utilizing full-thickness needle passes through both the common bile duct and jejunum (Fig. 25.7).

ii.   The final suture line is completed with interrupted sutures placed strategically along the remaining edges of the choledochotomy and enterotomy incisions to create a water-tight seal.

iii.   Alternatively, two long absorbable sutures may be placed ~1 mm apart at the apex of the choledochot-omy incision. Each suture is then utilized to create one "side" of the anastomosis in continuous, running fashion. As one suture line is created, the needle moves farther and farther away from the originating apex and travels toward the destination apex. Upon completion of one half of the anastomosis, the remaining long suture is utilized to finish the second half.

f. Inspect the anastomosis for bleeding. Irrigate the suture line and check the color of the effluent (see Complications, Section E).

g. Inspect the completed anastomosis and place a closed suction drain in proximity. If there is omentum, place it in the right upper quadrant as well. Irrigate the abdomen and close in the usual fashion.

6. **Performing the Laparoscopic Celiac Plexus Block**

a. Trocar placement and initial setup are similar (Fig. 25.1), and this facilitates execution of the celiac plexus block concurrent with other palliative procedures.

   i. If laparoscopic celiac plexus block is the only procedure being performed, 5-mm trocars are usually all that is required.

   ii. Steep reverse Trendeleberg patient positioning allows bowel and intra-abdominal contents to "drop" away from the surgical field.

b. ~50 mL of a 50% ethanol solution should be prepared for injection.

   i. 20 mL will be injected on each side of the aorta; into the periaortic fat.

c. With the liver retracted anteriorly, the stomach is retracted laterally; exposing the gastrohepatic ligament.

d. Electrocautery can be utilized to dissect through the gastrohepatic ligament and enter the lesser sac.

   i. The left gastric artery, celiac trunk, and peri-aortic fat are visualized.

e. Utilizing a 23-gauge needle the peri-aortic fat pad is injected with the prepared ethanol solution. (20 mL on each side)

   i. Prior to injection, gentle aspiration is recommended to prevent direct injection into a vascular structure.

   ii. If laparoscopic injection needle/equipment is unavailable, a percutaneous approach may be employed. (Needle may be introduced through a small stab incision at the level of the celiac trunk).

E. Complications

1. **Leakage of the gastrojejunostomy**
   a. **Cause and prevention**: To minimize the possibility of leakage, test the gastrojejunostomy by air under saline irrigation using an endoscope, or by instillation of methylene blue through an NG tube. Reinforce any areas that appear weak or are leaking.
   b. **Recognition and management**: A localized collection or generalized peritonitis may result. Fever, ileus, abdominal tenderness, and distention are symptoms. A Gastrografin upper gastrointestinal series may demonstrate the site of leakage.
      i. Revision of the anastomosis will likely be required.
      ii. Successful temporary management with endoscopic placement of an expanding, covered stent has been reported.
2. **Leakage of the biliary bypass (cholecystojejunostomy and choledochojejunostomy)**
   a. **Cause and prevention**: Bile is a detergent and will go through a pinhole; hence, small leaks at biliary-enteric anastomotic sites are common. Many surgeons routinely place a closed suction drain in close proximity to a biliary-enteric anastomosis so that any such leakage is easily recognized and controlled. The resulting bile leak usually subsides spontaneously in the absence of distal obstruction.
   b. **Recognition and management**: Bilious output from the closed suction drain should be monitored and outputs recorded. Excessive (more than 100–200 mL/day) or prolonged (>1 week) output may be a sign of distal obstruction. A radionuclide biliary scan is an easy, noninvasive way to confirm that the jejunal loop is patent. The scan will show passage of radionuclide into the distal small intestine if the loop is patent. Sequential scans over time will confirm rapid transit of bile through the gut. If the loop is obstructed or the leak is very large, the radionuclide will pass out through the drain or puddle in the right gutter. Distal obstruction is generally mechanical in nature and requires operative correction.

If no drain has been placed, a subphrenic collection or generalized peritonitis may result. Generally, this is signaled by fever or ileus, and diagnosed by computed tomography or ultrasound. A localized collection may be amenable to percutaneous drainage. Generalized peritonitis will usually require exploration, with repair of the leak and establishment of adequate external drainage. Similar concerns about distal obstruction of the jejunal loop exist and should be kept in mind.

3. **Bleeding from the staple line**

    a. **Cause and prevention**: All gastrointestinal stapling devices are designed to approximate tissues without strangulating or devascularizing them. The potential for bleeding always exists. The rich submucosal blood supply of the stomach makes it particularly prone to staple line bleeding. To avoid this complication, inspect the staple line carefully before closing the stab wounds. Use of the suction irrigator to irrigate the staple line and to carefully inspect the color and quantity of the effluent is helpful. The effluent should be clear or bilious. Finally, endoscopic visualization of the finished anastomosis is highly recommended.

    b. **Recognition and management**: If the effluent is persistently bloody, suspect a staple line bleed and place the laparoscope into the lateral port. You can then advance the laparoscope through the stab wounds to look inside. Cauterize or suture-ligate any bleeding points under direct vision. Use cautery with caution to avoid thermal damage and delayed perforation.

4. **Failure of the cholecystojejunostomy to produce biliary diversion**

    a. **Cause and prevention**: Obstruction of the anastomosis by blood clot can cause recurrent jaundice. This can be avoided if hemostasis is carefully checked as noted earlier. An unrecognized blocked cystic duct will also cause the anastomosis to fail. Avoid this complication by defining the individual anatomy with preoperative imaging and/or intraoperative cholangiogram. A cholecystojejunostomy requires a patent cystic duct to allow decompression of the proximal biliary tree. If the cystic duct is blocked by tumor, this conduit will not function. At laparoscopy, the gallbladder should appear grossly distended (Courvoisier's sign). The cystic duct should be dilated and the gallbladder should contain bilious material. White bile (hydrops) indicates the presence of cystic duct obstruction and is a contraindication to performing a cholecystojejunostomy.

i. Cholangiography is the best way to delineate biliary anatomy. If you are uncertain about the anatomy, perform a transcystic cholangiogram by placing a needle in the gallbladder and injecting contrast. The cholangiogram should visualize the common duct.

b. **Recognition and management**: If the cystic duct is not patent, if a cholecystojejunostomy does not produce biliary diversion, or if the conduit fails as the tumor grows, stenting, transhepatic drainage, or a choledochojejunostomy should be considered. Decision to employ one of these procedures should be based upon careful consideration of the anatomy and the patient's overall medical condition.

5. **Failure of the choledochojejunostomy to produce biliary diversion**

a. **Cause and prevention**: Again, obstruction of the anastomosis by blood clot can cause recurrent jaundice. Meticulous inspection is mandatory to ensure hemostasis and to prevent this complication. In addition, creating a wide diameter (minimum 1 cm) anastomosis is recommended.

b. **Recognition and management**: If the choledochojejunostomy does not produce biliary diversion, stenting, and transhepatic drainage should be considered. Decision to employ one of these procedures should be based upon careful consideration of the anatomy and the patient's overall medical condition.

6. **Obstruction of the jejunum at the anastomotic site**

a. **Cause and prevention**: Problems during the construction of the anastomosis, particularly during closure of the enterotomies, can narrow the lumen of the jejunal loop or even totally obstruct it. This causes a high small bowel obstruction. Avoid this complication by taking care not to narrow the jejunal lumen, particularly if you use the stapler to close the enterotomies. Visually inspect the anastomosis after you construct it, and if it does not look right, consider revising it.

b. **Recognition and management**: Signs of high small bowel obstruction (vomiting, inability to tolerate feeds) suggest the diagnosis, which may be confirmed by Gastrografin upper gastrointestinal series. The anastomosis must be revised or a jejunojejunostomy (to bypass the obstruction) constructed.

7. **Distal mechanical obstruction of the jejunal loop**

a. **Cause and prevention**: Avoid kinking by visually verifying that the chosen site allows the jejunum to lie in a comfortable and loose position as it passes over the transverse colon. Rarely, a trocar site hernia may present as small bowel obstruction.

b. **Recognition and management**: Distal obstruction may cause the anastomosis to leak. If the anastomosis does not leak, obstructive symptoms of distention, inability to tolerate feedings, and vomiting suggest the diagnosis. The diagnosis may be confirmed by flat and upright abdominal films, hepatoiminodiacetic acid scan (cholecystojejunostomy), or Gastrografin upper gastrointestinal series (gastrojejunostomy). Generally, revision of the anastomosis will be required.

Selected References

Allen PJ, Chou J, Janakos M, Strong VE, Coit DG, Brennan MF. Prospective evaluation of laparoscopic celiac plexus block in patients with unresectable pancreatic adenocarcinoma. Ann Surg Oncol. 2011;18(3):636–41.

Amori BJ. Pancreatic surgery in the laparoscopic era. JOP. 2003;4(6):187–92.

Artifon ELA, Rodrigues AZ, Marques S, Halwan B, Sakai P, Bresciani C, Kumar A. Laparoscopic deployment of biliary self-expandable metal stent (SEMS) for one-step palliation in 23 patients with advanced pancreatico-biliary tumors – a pilot trial. J Gastrointest Surg. 2007;11:1686–91.

Bogen GL, Mancino AT, Scott-Conner CEH. Laparoscopy for staging and palliation of gastrointestinal malignancy. Surg Clin North Am. 1996;76:557–69.

Chang L, Stefanidis D, Richardson WS, Earle DB, Fanelli RD. The role of staging laparoscopy for intraabdominal cancers: an evidence-based review. Surg Endosc. 2009; 23:231–41.

Chekan EG, Clark L, Wu J, Pappas TN, Eubanks S. Laparoscopic biliary and enteric bypass. Semin Surg Oncol. 1999;16:313–20.

Cogliandolo A, Scarmozzino G, Pidoto RR, Pollicino A, Florio MA. Laparoscopic palliative gastrojejunostomy for advanced recurrent gastric cancer after Billroth I resection. J Laparoendosc Adv Surg Tech A. 2004;14:43–6.

Gentileschi P, Kini S, Gagner M. Palliative laparoscopic hepatico- and gastrojejunostomy for advanced pancreatic cancer. JSLS. 2002;6:331–8.

House MG, Choti MA. Palliative therapy for pancreatic/biliary cancer. Surg Clin North Am. 2005;85:359–71.

Kooby DA, Chu CK. Laparoscopic management of pancreatic malignancies. Surg Clin North Am. 2010;90:427–46.

Mayo SC, Austin DF, Sheppard BC, Mori M, Shipley DK, Billingsley KG. Evolving preoperative evaluation of patients with pancreatic cancer: does laparoscopy have a role in the current era? J Am Coll Surg. 2008;208:87–95.

Mittal A, Windsor J, Woodfield J, Casey P, Lane M. Matched study of three methods for palliation of malignant pyloroduodenal obstruction. Br J Surg. 2004;91:205–9.

Stefanidis CM, Stanelle EJ, Mansour J, Hinshaw JL, Rikkers LF, Rettammel R, Mahvi DM, Cho CS, Weber SM. Staging laparoscopy enhances the detection of occult metastases in patients with pancreatic adenocarcinoma. J Surg Oncol. 2009;100:663–9.

Strong VE, Dalal KM, Malhotta VT, Cubert KH, Coit D, Fong Y, Allen PJ. Initial report of laparoscopic celiac plexus block for pain relief in patients with unresectable pancreatic cancer. J Am Coll Surg. 2006;203:129–31.

26. Laparoscopic Splenectomy[*]

Namir Katkhouda, M.D., F.A.C.S.

A. Laparoscopic Splenectomy

1. Preoperative Requirements and Workup

Laparoscopic splenectomy is a difficult procedure that should only be performed by an experienced laparoscopic surgeon or under the direct supervision of such a surgeon. As always, the entire team should be adequately prepared.

a. Arrange for the patient to be vaccinated against pneumococcus, H. influenza, and meningococcus at least two weeks prior to surgery.

b. It is essential that patients presenting with idiopathic thrombocytopenic purpura (ITP) are worked up appropriately by the referring hematologists. The anesthesiologist must make sure that there is a suitable blood and platelet supply in the operating room prior to the start of the procedure.

c. Check the instrument set personally to ensure everything is available, specifically clip appliers, atraumatic graspers, liver fan retractors, and an irrigation suction machine with the capacity for hydrodissection. Always have an open tray with a number 10 or 20 blade immediately available in case there is a need for conversion. Harmonic shears (Ethicon Endosurgery Inc.) are especially useful because they can reduce the number of clips used during division of the short gastric vessels, and can also function as a grasper.

d. Place an orogastric tube to decompress the stomach.

---

[*] This chapter was contributed by Robert V. Rege, MD in the previous edition.

N.T. Nguyen and C.E.H. Scott-Conner (eds.), *The SAGES Manual: Volume 2* *Advanced Laparoscopy and Endoscopy*, DOI 10.1007/978-1-4614-2347-8_26, © Springer Science+Business Media, LLC 2012

2. Patient Positioning

a. Proper patient positioning is critical. Safely secure the patient on a beanbag with the left side up at a 60° angle in reverse Trendelenburg and the left arm positioned as for a left lateral thoracotomy (Fig. 26.1). This allows gravity to retract the abdominal organs and maximize the working space. This is the "hanging spleen" technique described by Delaitre and Gagner. The surgeon stands on the patient's right side facing the *left*

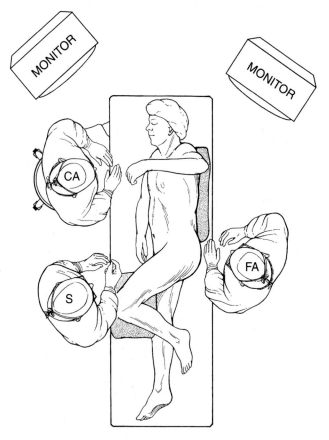

Fig. 26.1. Operating room set up for laparoscopic splenectomy. *S* surgeon, *FA* first assistant, *CA* camera assistant sitting on a chair. (From Katkhouda N. Advanced laparoscopic surgery: techniques and tips, 2nd ed. New York, NY: Springer; 2011. Reprinted with kind permission of Springer Science+Business Media).

monitor, with the camera assistant on the same side sitting on a stool to the surgeon's left. The first assistant is on the opposite side, but the three members of the team all look at the left monitor to avoid mirror imaging and discoordination with the critical first assistant.

b.   When inserting the trocars, ensure that the patient is positioned in reverse Trendelenburg. Combined with a 60° tilt, this position has two important effects. First, gravity pulls the stomach and small bowel in a rostral direction out of the operative field. Second, the spleen is kept hanging from the diaphragm by its phrenic attachments, thus placing the gastrosplenic vessels under tension, simplifying dissection and division of the vessels later in the operation. In the anterior approach, the hilar vessels are controlled first, and the phrenic attachments are divided at the end of the operation. In contrast, with a posterior approach, the lateral attachments are divided first, the spleen is mobilized laterally and the hilar vessels are controlled later, as done in open surgery.

3. Port Placement

a.   Four to five 12 mm ports are needed for this operation (Fig. 26.2). After insufflation using a Veress needle, insert the first trocar in the left upper quadrant approximately five finger breadths below the costal margin, moving the camera closer to the spleen. This will permit full exploration of the abdominal cavity to check for the presence of accessory spleens and other intra-abdominal lesions that might require laparoscopic management.

b.   Insert a port on each side of the umbilical port in a triangulated manner, for the right and left hands of the surgeon. Place another trocar laterally under the left costal margin for the first assistant. An optional subxiphoid trocar can be inserted for an irrigation/suction device or for a fan retractor used by the camera assistant if needed.

4. Surgical Anatomy

Splenic vascularization may be distributed or nonbranching (Fig. 26.3). Knowledge of the patient's vascular anatomy will help decide on the most appropriate dissection technique. The terminal branches of the splenic artery are depicted. Knowledge of the anatomy of the spleen is critical,

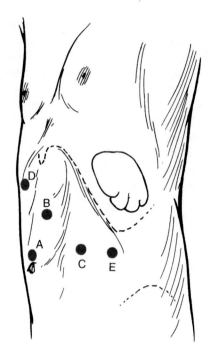

Fig. 26.2. Port positions for laparoscopic splenectomy: (**a**) umbilical telescope, (**b**) surgeon's left hand, (**c**) surgeon's right hand, (**d**) subxiphoid port for irrigation/suction or an assistant's grasper, (**e**) first assistant's grasper. (From Katkhouda N. Advanced laparoscopic surgery: techniques and tips, 2nd ed. New York, NY: Springer; 2011. Reprinted with kind permission of Springer Science+Business Media).

and two special features are of interest. First, as a rule, notched spleens and those with prominences have more entering arteries than those with smooth borders. Second, the tail of the pancreas lies close to the hilum of the spleen and is in direct contact with the spleen in about 30% of cases, and within 1 cm of the spleen in 40%. Caution is therefore recommended before firing a linear cutter across the hilar vessels.

5. Technique

a. Anterior Approach

The procedure follows these key steps:

- Division of the short gastric vessels and opening the lesser sac (Fig. 26.4).

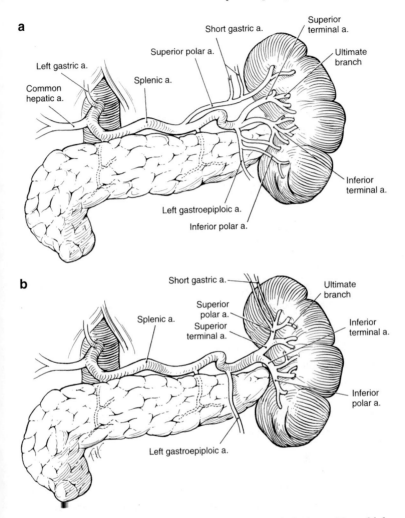

Fig. 26.3. Vascularization of the spleen: (**a**) **Distributed** type with multiple splenic notches, and (**b**) **Magistral** type with few splenic notches. (From Katkhouda N. Advanced laparoscopic surgery: techniques and tips, 2nd ed. New York, NY: Springer; 2011. Reprinted with kind permission of Springer Science + Business Media).

- Exposure of the tail of the pancreas.
- Division of the splenocolic ligament.
- Lateral and superior retraction of the inferior pole of the spleen and division of the inferior pole vessels.

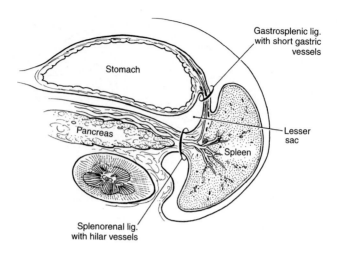

Fig. 26.4. Access to the hilar vessels through the lesser sac. Figure depicts ligaments of the posterior mesogastrum. (From Katkhouda N. Advanced laparoscopic surgery: techniques and tips, 2nd ed. New York, NY: Springer; 2011. Reprinted with kind permission of Springer Science+Business Media).

- Division of the hilar vessels.
- Division of the phrenic attachments.
- Extraction of the spleen in a bag.

i. Division of the Short Gastric Vessels and Exposure of the Tail of the Pancreas

The first step is to divide the short gastric vessels and enter the lesser sac along the greater curvature of the stomach. This proceeds as for a Nissen fundoplication with the exception that the dissection is carried out much closer to the spleen than to the stomach. The first assistant gently grasps the fatty tissue surrounding the short gastric vessels and retracts it superiorly while the surgeon gently retracts the stomach to the right. This will expose the short gastric vessels, which are subsequently controlled with the harmonic shears. Use additional clips for larger vessels if needed. Continue the division superiorly and then inferiorly until the tail of the pancreas is completely exposed

ii. Exposure of the Inferior Pole of the Spleen and Division of the Inferior Pole Vessels

The next step is exposure of the inferior pole of the spleen. The first assistant retracts the spleen superiorly and laterally with a closed Babcock clamp to expose the splenic flexure of the colon. With your left hand, retract the transverse colon inferiorly, exposing the splenocolic ligament. Divide it with the harmonic shears to allow safe dissection of the inferior pole of the spleen. Once the splenocolic ligament has been divided, lateral and superior retraction will expose the inferior pole vessels that branch from the main splenic vessels. Next, divide the inferior pole vessels, permitting full mobilization of the inferior pole of the spleen. These vessels are usually large in size and should be clipped or divided using an endo-GIA with a white load. We do not recommend the use of the harmonic shears on these vessels, as it will not achieve efficient hemostasis. Uncontrollable bleeding from these vessels can result in an early conversion to open surgery.

iii. Division of the Hilar Vessels and Phrenic Attachments

In order to expose the hilar vessels, opposing retraction by the first assistant and the surgeon is required. The first assistant retracts the mobilized inferior pole of the spleen superiorly and laterally. The surgeon gently pushes the exposed tail of the pancreas down, creating access to the hilum and the main splenic vessels. Division of the hilar artery and vein is a critical step that should be performed meticulously and carefully to avoid any bleeding. Use of a blunt right-angled dissector is safe.

There are two choices for ligation of the splenic vessels at the hilum of the spleen: transection of the vessels in the case of a bundled vasculature with one firing of a 30 mm endolinear cutter using vascular staples (or a more formal division of the artery and vein separately between clips in the case of a distributed or branching vasculature (Fig. 26.5). Using a combination of clips and staplers should also be done very cautiously, as clips can result in misfiring of the stapler and subsequent bleeding from a partially divided vessel.

Finally, divide the attachments of the spleen to the diaphragm, allowing full mobilization of the spleen.

iv. Extraction of the Spleen in a Bag

The next step is introduction of the retrieval bag. A good trick is to push the bag to the diaphragm with the opening of the bag facing the surgeon. This will allow introduction of the spleen into the bag using a "surfing" technique. Grab the spleen by its attachments and rolled it onto its back, using hilar and fatty attachments as a handle. Then, shove it into the bag with a gentle sliding motion (Fig. 26.6).

Close the bag and remove it and the umbilical port. The fascia of the umbilical port can be slightly enlarged to allow extraction of the bag.

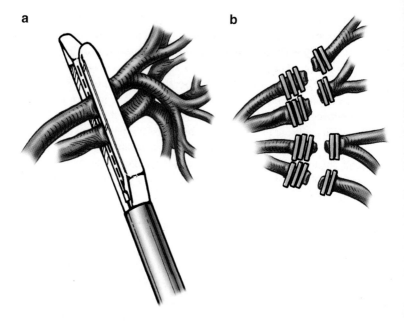

Fig. 26.5. Division of the splenic vessels: (**a**) firing of the cutter and simultaneous control of both vessels; or (**b**) separate control of the artery and vein using large clips. (From Katkhouda N. Advanced laparoscopic surgery: techniques and tips, 2nd ed. New York, NY: Springer; 2011. Reprinted with kind permission of Springer Science + Business Media).

The introduction of two fingers (or a Kelly clamp) to squeeze the spleen between the fingers and the anterior abdominal wall will enable morcellation of the spleen and extraction of both the bag and the splenic fragments. Take care not to drop any fragments in the abdomen, as this can lead to splenosis and recurrent disease.

v. Final Steps of the Procedure

Replace the ports. Carefully check the area of the spleen for hemostasis. A drain is very rarely needed. This depends on the surgeon's experience and in particular on the degree of trauma to the tail of the pancreas during the dissection. If a drain is used, bring it out through a separate incision to avoid herniation of small bowel while removing the drain through a large port site.

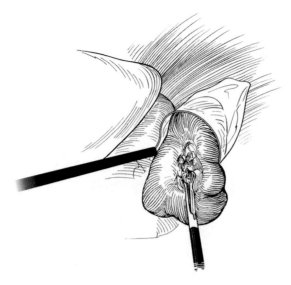

Fig. 26.6. Placement of the spleen into a retrieval bag. (From Katkhouda N. Advanced laparoscopic surgery: techniques and tips, 2nd ed. New York, NY: Springer; 2011. Reprinted with kind permission of Springer Science + Business Media).

b. Posterior Approach

Laparoscopic splenectomy can also be performed via a posterior approach. The benefit of this approach is improved exposure of the hilar vessels compared to the anterior approach; however, in the anterior approach, the hilar vessels are controlled earlier in the procedure, which reduces the risk of uncontrollable bleeding later in the procedure.

The procedure follows these key steps:

- Division of the splenocolic ligament.
- Division of the inferior pole vessels.
- Division of the phrenic attachments.
- Exposure and division of the hilar vessels.
- Division of the short gastric vessels.
- Extraction of the spleen in a bag.

The surgeon begins the procedure by taking down the inferior pole vessels, as described for the anterior approach. After division of these vessels, the spleen is gently retracted medially and the splenophrenic ligament is divided using the harmonic shears (Fig. 26.7). This dissection

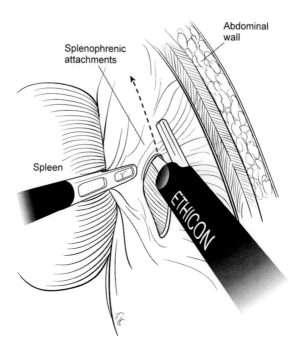

Fig. 26.7. Posterior approach for laparoscopic splenectomy; initial division of the splenophrenic ligament. (From Katkhouda N. Advanced laparoscopic surgery: techniques and tips, 2nd ed. New York, NY: Springer; 2011. Reprinted with kind permission of Springer Science+Business Media).

continues superiorly until the short gastric vessels are encountered. Careful dissection of the splenorenal ligament is done at this point, with extreme attention given to avoid injury to the left adrenal gland. Next, the short gastric vessels are divided using the harmonic shears and clips as needed. The hilar vessels will now be in view, and can be dissected with a right angle dissector before being divided separately or together with a vascular endo-GIA (Fig. 26.8). Next, the short gastric vessels are divided using the harmonic shears. The rest of the operation is performed as described in anterior approach.

c. Postoperative Course

The postoperative course following laparoscopic splenectomy is straightforward. Amylase and lipase levels should be checked on the first postoperative day to ensure there has been no pancreatic injury during the operation. A clear liquid diet is initiated if the levels are normal, and the patient can be discharged home once the diet has been tolerated.

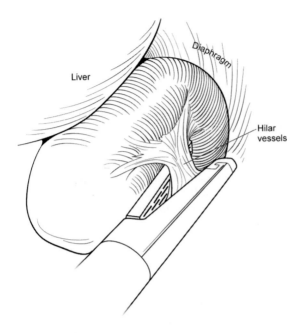

Fig. 26.8. Posterior approach; division of the pedicle with a stapler using the white vascular load. (From Katkhouda N. Advanced laparoscopic surgery: techniques and tips, 2nd ed. New York, NY: Springer; 2011. Reprinted with kind permission of Springer Science + Business Media).

6. Management of Complications

Bleeding constitutes a major problem. Two etiologies are possible:

- Bleeding from an unnamed vessel, such as a short gastric vessel or a branch of the inferior or superior pole vessels.
- Bleeding from a major vessel, such as the splenic artery or vein.
- Bleeding from a splenic injury.

a. Control of an Unnamed Vessel

Laparoscopic control of an unnamed vessel should always be attempted and is usually successful. The first step is to pull back on the scope to protect the lens from blood. The vessel is then clamped using an atraumatic grasper. The grasper should be long and flat without teeth. Irrigation and aspiration of the surgical site should follow to evaluate the rate of bleeding. If the bleeding has been controlled, clips are placed appropriately. Sometimes, electrocautery will control the situation and allow safe placement of the clips. Compression using a laparoscopic 2 cm×2 cm gauze can control the bleeding, allowing the operative site to be cleaned in preparation for hemostasis.

b. Control of a Major Vessel

The situation is different when a major vessel is injured. Examples are the splenic vein or artery, or the direct terminal branches of the main trunk. Flow is usually very high in these vessels, and blood reaching the left upper quadrant of the abdomen will obscure the view. In these circumstances, one can try to control the bleeding using the steps described previously, using a larger atraumatic instrument, such as a bowel clamp to grasp the whole hilum. If this is not successful, it is usually wise to convert the patient rapidly through an open left subcostal incision.

c. Splenic Injury

Another possibility is an injury to the spleen itself during the dissection. A forceful retraction, for example, can tear the capsule. Although resultant bleeding may obscure the dissection, simple compression with a 2 cm×2 cm surgical gauze together with appropriate electrocautery should control bleeding. If a combination of bleeding from the spleen and a minor vessel occurs, it is not possible to control both at the same time. It is recommended to either grab the bleeding vessel with a grasper while cauterizing the capsule, or control the capsular bleeding with a 2×2 gauze and compression while the bleeding vessel is clipped.

d. Maneuver of Last Resort During Bleeding of the Hilar Vessels

In the event of a splenic injury in traditional open surgery, the surgeon rapidly mobilizes the splenic attachments after inserting a large piece of gauze to compress the hilum. The surgeon's left hand retracts the splenic handle and the right hand clamps the vessels "en bloc" using large and long Kelly clamps. The same maneuvers can be realized laparoscopically if the surgeon and assistant have very good laparoscopic skills.

The hilum is compressed using a large 4×4 gauze and the bleeding controlled. As the short gastric vessels and the inferior attachments are already divided, the surgeon should promptly divide the phrenic attachments to mobilize the spleen. Once the spleen is mobilized, the assistant can retract the whole spleen superiorly with an open fan retractor, and the surgeon fires one or two shots of a linear cutter with vascular staples. This should be done quickly and staying as close as possible to the spleen to avoid pancreatic injury.

If this maneuver is not successful, conversion to an open procedure should be initiated.

B. Laparoscopic Partial Splenectomy

It is also possible to perform a partial laparoscopic splenectomy. In order to accomplish this, it is important to identify the inferior pole vessels, or any vessel per se, that is supplying the territory that has to be removed. Once the vessel is isolated using a right angle dissector, clips are placed and the vessel is divided, immediately producing a zone of ischemia in the spleen (Fig. 26.9). Once this has been achieved, harmonic shears are used to perform a partial splenectomy. Our preference is to use harmonic shears as they allow permanent hemostasis. It is important to leave 2 or 3 mm of zonal ischemia tissue on the remaining

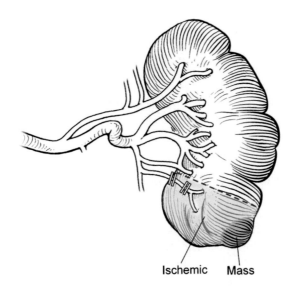

Ischemic   Mass

Fig. 26.9. Partial splenectomy. Ligation of the inferior polar vessels in this example that delineates a segmental zone of ischemia. (From Katkhouda N. Advanced laparoscopic surgery: techniques and tips, 2nd ed. New York, NY: Springer; 2011. Reprinted with kind permission of Springer Science + Business Media).

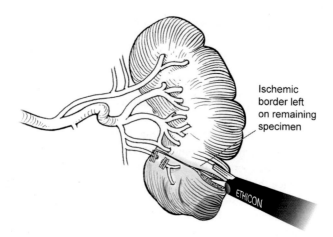

Fig. 26.10. Partial splenectomy. Division of the splenic parenchyma using the Harmonic shears, just beneath the line of ischemic demarcation. (From Katkhouda N. Advanced laparoscopic surgery: techniques and tips, 2nd ed. New York, NY: Springer; 2011. Reprinted with kind permission of Springer Science+Business Media).

healthy spleen, and divide the spleen in the ischemic territory to avoid massive bleeding (Fig. 26.10). Once the partial splenectomy is performed, fibrin sealant is sprayed on the remaining tissue to further enhance hemostasis. The specimen will be removed as described previously.

C. Hand-Assisted Splenectomy

In the case of splenomegaly, as defined by a spleen over 20 cm in size, it is possible to use a hand-assisted technique (HALS). An incision is made for the nondominant hand the same size as the surgeon's glove size (7.5 → 7.5 cm, 8 → 8 cm, etc.), and a gelport is inserted to allow comfortable manipulation of the spleen. It is important to place this incision rather away from the camera on the right side of the patient to avoid interaction between the hand and the scope. The procedure is then performed as described above.

Selected References

Brunt LM, Langer JC, Quasebarth MA, Whitman ED. Comparative analysis of laparoscopic versus open splenectomy. Am J Surg. 1996;172(5):596–9.

Cadiere GB, Verroken R, Himpens J, Bruyns J, Efira M, De Wit S. Operative strategy in laparoscopic splenectomy. J Am Coll Surg. 1994;179(6):668–72.

Delaitre B. Laparoscopic splenectomy: the 'hanged spleen' technique. Surg Endosc. 1995;9:528–9.

Katkhouda N, Umbach T, Kaiser A. Splenectomy: anterior laparoscopic approach. Probl Gen Surg. 2002;19:24–8.

Katkhouda N, Manhas S, Umbach TW, Kaiser A. Laparoscopic splenectomy. J Laparoendosc Surg. 2001;11:383–90.

Katkhouda N, Mavor E. Laparoscopic splenectomy. Surg Clin N Am. 2000;80:1285–97.

Katkhouda N, Hurwitz M. Laparoscopic splenectomy for hematologic disease. Adv Surg. 1999;33:141–61.

Katkhouda N, Hurwitz MB, Rivera RT, et al. Laparoscopic splenectomy: outcome and efficacy in 103 consecutive patients. Ann Surg. 1998 Oct;228(4):568–78.

Katkhouda N, Waldrep D, Feinstein D, et al. Unresolved issues in laparoscopic splenectomy. Am J Surg. 1996;172:585–90.

Phillips EH, Carroll BJ, Fallas MJ. Laparoscopic splenectomy. Surg Endosc. 1994; 8(8):931–3.

Poulin EC, Thibault C. Laparoscopic splenectomy for massive splenomegaly: operative technique and case report. Can J Surg. 1995;38(1):69–72.

Poulin BC, Thibault C, Mamazza J. Laparoscopic splenectomy. Surg Endosc. 1995;9(2): 172–6.

Trias M, Targarona EM, Balague C. Laparoscopic splenectomy: an evolving technique. A comparison between anterior and lateral approaches. Surg Endosc. 1996;10(4): 389–92.

Uranus S, Pfeifer J, Schauer C, et al. Laparoscopic partial splenic resection. Surg Laparosc Endosc. 1995;5(2):133–6.

27. Laparoscopic Adrenalectomy[*]

Catherine A. Madorin, M.D.
William B. Inabnet, M.D.

A. Anatomy

The adrenal glands are retroperitoneal organs located anteromedial to the superior pole of the kidneys. The adrenal glands are encased in Gerota's fascia and surrounded by fat. A layer of loose connective tissue separates the adrenal gland from the kidney.

1. The right adrenal is bordered anteriorly by the liver, anteromedially by the inferior vena cava (IVC), and posteriorly by the liver and diaphragmatic reflection. The right adrenal vein is short and wide and typically enters the IVC posteriorly.
2. The left adrenal is bordered by the peritoneum anteriorly, the stomach superiorly and the tail of the pancreas inferiorly. The left adrenal vein exits inferiorly and merges with the inferior phrenic vein to empty into the left renal vein.
3. Blood supply is abundant and is provided by the aorta, inferior phrenic, and renal arteries. Each of these supplies arteries that branch freely before entering the adrenal gland, with upward of 50 small arteries penetrating the capsule.

B. Indications

The presence of a unilateral functioning (hormone-secreting) adrenal adenoma is a common indication for laparoscopic adrenalectomy. Incidentally discovered adrenal masses, or incidentalomas, should first

---

[*]This chapter was contributed by Ahmad Assalia MD and Michel Gagner MD in the previous edition.

N.T. Nguyen and C.E.H. Scott-Conner (eds.), *The SAGES Manual: Volume 2*   401
Advanced Laparoscopy and Endoscopy, DOI 10.1007/978-1-4614-2347-8_27,
© Springer Science+Business Media, LLC 2012

be evaluated for functionality or malignancy, even in the absence of symptoms. Adenomas >4 cm should be resected due to the increased risk of malignancy. Small, nonfunctioning incidentalomas may be followed by observation.

1. Pheochromocytoma. The presence of pheochromocytoma is a strong indication for surgery. Preoperative blood pressure control is achieved by alpha-blockade; this will also help reverse the relative hypovolemia associated with pheochromocytoma. Surgical principles include early ligation of the adrenal vein and minimal manipulation of tissue so as not to disrupt the capsule.

2. Cushing syndrome. Adrenalectomy for ACTH-independent Cushing syndrome is curative, and is recommended for all patients with unilateral adenomas. Adrenalectomy for subclinical Cushing syndrome is recommended for young patients (<50 years) and those with suppressed ACTH, hypertension, or diabetes mellitus. Asymptomatic patients with normal ACTH levels or high-risk surgical patients may be observed. Cushing syndrome due to nodular hyperplasia often involves both glands and may require bilateral adrenalectomy. Patients who undergo adrenalectomy for Cushing syndrome must receive steroid replacement therapy to prevent adrenal insufficiency.

3. Aldosteronoma. Resection of aldosterone-secreting adenomas is curative in up to 70% of patients. A preoperative response to aldosterone receptor antagonists is predictive of successful postoperative outcome. Age >50 years, male sex, and the presence of multiple nodules are associated with poor response. Idiopathic adrenal hyperplasia is best treated medically as the response to adrenalectomy is variable. Adrenal venous sampling-guided unilateral adrenalectomy can be considered in select cases of hyperplasia and can also be helpful in select cases of micro aldosterone-producing adenomas.

4. Cancer. Adrenocortical carcinomas are rare and aggressive tumors. Adrenal masses >6 cm are highly suspicious for cancer. Common features of carcinoma include invasion of surrounding structures, lymphadenopathy, necrosis, and hemorrhage. Open adrenalectomy is indicated for all stages of cancer. Metastases to the adrenal glands are common, most often from melanoma, lung, and breast cancer. Biopsy of lesions should only be performed after exclusion of pheochromocytoma. Indications for adrenalectomy are dependent on the type of cancer and the absence of extraadrenal metastases.

C. Operative Approach

Multiple laparoscopic approaches have been described. No one technique has been shown to be clearly superior to another. The most common approaches are:

1. Anterior transabdominal with the patient supine.
2. Lateral transabdominal with the patient in lateral decubitus.
3. Retroperitoneal with the patient prone or lateral. A retroperitoneal approach may be ideal for nonobese patients with previous abdominal surgery and for those undergoing bilateral adrenalectomy.

The two most popular approaches, lateral transabdominal and retroperitoneal, are described here. References at the end include descriptions of the anterior transabdominal (supine) approach.

D. Transabdominal Lateral Adrenalectomy

1.   Patient position and setup

a. Position the patient in lateral decubitus with knees bent. Breaking the OR table will distract and enlarge the distance from the costal margin to the iliac crest and maximize space for trocar placement. This position allows other tissue and organs overlying adrenal glands to fall away from the retroperitoneum (Fig. 27.1).

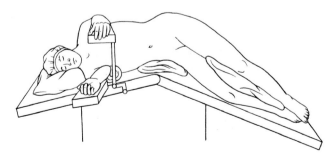

Fig. 27.1. Patient positioning for lateral transabdominal adrenalectomy.

b.   Prep widely from the nipple to the anterior superior iliac spine, the midline anteriorly, and the spine posteriorly.

c.   Both open and closed techniques may be used to initiate pneumoperitoneum. This is done at the level of the anterior axillary line, 2 cm below the costal margin. A 5 or 10 mm trocar is placed at this location and will serve as the camera port. A 30° laparoscope is preferred.

2.   Left Adrenalectomy

a.   Initiate pneumoperitoneum by an open or closed technique. Place the camera trocar (5 or 10 mm) is placed in the mid-clavicular line 2 cm below the costal margin. A 30° laparoscope is preferred (Fig. 27.2).

b.   Place two additional 5 mm trocars 2 cm below the costal margin in the epigastrium and anterior axillary line. Occasionally, a fourth trocar is placed at the posterior axillary line.

c.   Establish a plane along the anterior surface of the left kidney lateral and dorsal to the spleen and tail of pancreas. Incise splenorenal ligament and mobilize laterally until the left crus of the diaphragm is reached. Gravity will allow the spleen and tail of pancreas to fall medially away from the kidney, permitting visualization of the adrenal gland.

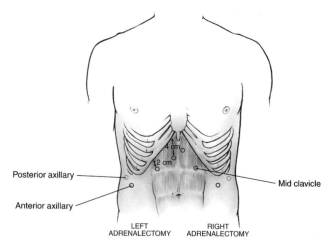

Fig. 27.2. Trocar placement for left and right adrenalectomy.

d. The correct plane of dissection is avascular. Mobilize supe-
    riorly to the diaphragm and the greater curve of stomach.
    Dissect along anterior surface of the kidney and adrenal
    gland until the inferior and medial border of the adrenal are
    exposed. If fat prevents visualization, the medial and infe-
    rior borders may be identified by ballottement of the retro-
    peritoneal tissue along the anterior surface of the kidney.

e. Isolate the left adrenal vein at the inferior pole of the adre-
    nal gland. Divide it between clips or with a vessel sealing
    device (Fig. 27.3).

f. Dissect in a superior and lateral direction. Take small blood
    with electrocautery, ultrasonic energy or a vessel sealing
    device.

g. Identify and ligate the inferior phrenic artery.

h. Retrieve the specimen in an endoscopic bag through the
    medial 10 mm cannula. Alternatively, the gland can be
    morcellated to avoid the need to extend the incision for
    retrieval.

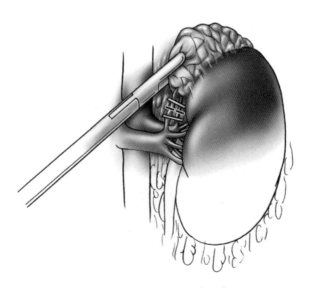

Fig. 27.3. Sequential steps in laparoscopic left adrenalectomy.

3. **Right Adrenalectomy**

   a.   Place a liver retractor in the epigastric port and retract the liver superiorly.

   b.   Mobilize the liver by incising the retroperitoneal attachments of the right lobe of the liver, including the triangular ligament, thus revealing the anterior surface of the adrenal gland. Mobilization of the hepatic flexure of the colon and/or the duodenum is rarely necessary.

   c.   Expose the medial border of the IVC to identify the adrenal vein. The right vein is typically short and broad, entering the IVC posteriorly at a right angle. The right adrenal vein can be ligated with clips, or secured with a vessel sealing device or endoscopic stapler with a vascular load. Rarely, the adrenal vein may drain into the right hepatic or renal vein (Fig. 27.4).

   d.   An arterial branch of the inferior phrenic artery is often located at the superomedial aspect of the gland, superior to the adrenal vein, and requires careful control. As with left adrenalectomy, dissect in a medial to lateral, and inferior to superior direction, dividing small vessels and attachments until completely mobilized.

   e.   Remove the adrenal gland with an endoscopic bag.

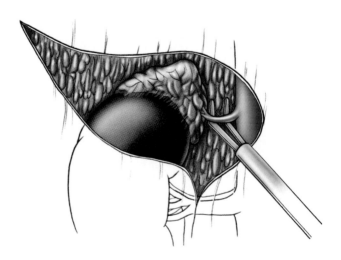

Fig. 27.4. Sequential steps in laparoscopic right adrenalectomy.

E. Retroperitoneal Endoscopic Adrenalectomy: Posterior Approach

1.   Patient position and setup
   a.   Place the patient in a prone jackknife position with the table flexed at the waist to maximize the space between the twelfth rib and iliac crest.
   b.   Prep the patient from the scapula to the mid-buttocks.

2.   Trocar placement (Fig. 27.5)
   a.   Make a 1.0–1.5 cm transverse incision below and lateral to the twelfth rib and sharply enter the retroperitoneal space with scissors. Use the index finger to develop the retroperitoneal space medial and lateral to the incision.
   b.   Insert a 10 mm trocar with a small balloon to help prevent the leakage of CO_2. Insufflate the retroperitoneum to

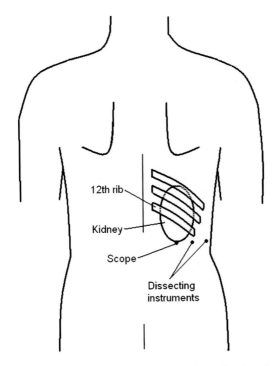

Fig. 27.5. Trocar placement for retroperitoneal endoscopic adrenalectomy.

20 mm Hg and use a zero-degree endoscope to develop the retroperitoneal space. Change to a 30° endoscope.

c.   Place a second trocar (5 or 10 mm) 5 cm medial to the initial port, but lateral to the rectus spinae muscles.

d.   Place a third trocar (5 or 10 mm) 5 cm lateral to the initial port, at the posterior axillary line. The placement of a fourth trocar is rarely necessary.

3.   Left adrenalectomy

a.   Mobilize the upper pole of the kidney and gently retract downward. Here, the insertion of a fourth trocar may aid in retraction.

b.   Begin dissection of the adrenal gland bluntly at the medial and caudal aspects of the gland.

c.   Identify the left adrenal vein in the space between the gland and the upper pole of the kidney. Vascular clips or an energy sealing device can be used to ligate the vein.

d.   Continue dissection laterally and cranially. Remove the gland with an endoscopic retrieval bag.

4.   Right adrenalectomy

a.   Mobilize the upper pole of the kidney and gently retract downward. Here, the insertion of a fourth trocar may aid in retraction.

b.   Using a two handed technique, mobilize the lateral and inferior borders of the gland.

c.   Identify the vena cava. Dissect the gland from the vena cave to permit identification of the short right adrenal vein running posterolaterally into the IVC. Vascular clips or an energy sealing device can be used to ligate the vein. In the case of a very broad vein, an endoscopic stapler with vascular load may be used.

d.   Continue dissection medially, laterally, and cranially.

e.   Remove the gland with an endoscopic retrieval bag.

F. Complications

Both laparoscopic transperitoneal and endoscopic retroperitoneal adrenalectomy may be performed with minimal morbidity and mortality. The overall 30-day morbidity is approximately 7%, with mortality rates of less than 1%. Recent studies suggest that the two approaches have comparable complication rates. Complications, however, may be severe when they occur, with hemorrhage being the most common intraoperative complication. Nearby organs, including the spleen, pancreas, liver, and colon are also vulnerable to damage during adrenal dissection.

1. **Intimate knowledge of the anatomy**, delicate handling of tissues, and meticulous attention to hemostasis are necessary to avoid hemorrhagic complications.
   a. Superior renal pole arteries are present in 15% of people and may be vulnerable to injury.
   b. Occasionally, the left adrenal gland may extend medially to the hilum of the kidney and bleeding may indicate injury to the renal vessels.
   c. Excessive traction on the spleen may cause tearing of the capsule and subsequent hemorrhage.
   d. Pancreatic parenchyma may be damaged with blunt dissection in the retroperitoneum, leading to hemorrhage or pancreatitis.

2. **Postoperative adrenal insufficiency** and **postoperative hemorrhage** will both manifest as hypotension. Adequate preparation with steroid replacement for select patients and high clinical suspicion for hemorrhage are essential to avoid potentially catastrophic results.

Selected References

Berber E, Tellioglu G, Harvey A, Mitchell J, Milas M, Siperstein A. Comparison of laparoscopic transabdominal lateral versus posterior retroperitoneal adrenalectomy. Surgery. 2009;146:621–6.

Gagner M. Laparoscopic adrenalectomy. Surg Clin North Am. 1996;76:523–37.

Gagner M, Lacroix A, Bolte E. Laparoscopic adrenalectomy in Cushing's syndrome and pheochromocytoma. N Engl J Med. 1992;327:1003–6.

Gagner M, Pomp A, Heniford BT, Pharand D, Lacroix A. Laparoscopic adrenalectomy: lessons learned from 100 consecutive procedures. Ann Surg. 1997;226:238–47.

Gupta PK, Natarajan B, Pallati PK, Gupta H, Sainath J, Fitzgibbons Jr RJ. Outcomes after laparoscopic adrenalectomy. Surg Endosc. 2011;25:784–94.

Kebebew E, Siperstein AE, Duh QY. Laparoscopic adrenalectomy: the optimal surgical approach. J Laparoendosc Adv Surg Tech. 2001;11:409–13.

Lee J, El-Tamer M, Schifftner T, et al. Open and laparoscopic adrenalectomy: analysis of the national surgical quality improvement program. J Am Coll Surg. 2008;206: 953–61.

Lombardi CP, Raffaelli M, De Crea C, et al. Endoscopic adrenalectomy: is there an optimal operative approach? Results of a single-center case–control study. Surgery. 2008; 144:1008–15.

Morris L, Ituarte P, Zarnegar R, et al. Laparoscopic adrenalectomy after prior abdominal surgery. World J Surg. 2008;32:897–903.

Schreinemakers JM, Kiela GJ, Valk GD, Vriens MR, Rinkes IH. Retroperitoneal endoscopic adrenalectomy is safe and effective. Br J Surg. 2010;97:1667–72.

Siperstein AE, Berber E, Engle KL, Duh QY, Clark OH. Laparoscopic posterior adrenalectomy: technical considerations. Arch Surg. 2000;135:967–71.

28. Endoscopic Retrograde Cholangiopancreatography: General Principles*

Melissa S. Phillips, M.D.
Jeffrey M. Marks, M.D.

A. Indications

Prior to the development of endoscopic retrograde cholangiopancreatography (ERCP), examination of the extrahepatic biliary tree and pancreatic duct was possible only during laparotomy. In 1968 William McCune, a surgeon, and his colleagues first reported the endoscopic visualization of the pancreatic duct. Initially developed as a diagnostic procedure, ERCP has become an indispensable tool in the therapeutic management of pancreaticobiliary disease, replacing what had routinely required surgical intervention. The developments of computed tomographic scans, endoscopic ultrasonography, percutaneous transhepatic cholangiography, and magnetic resonance imaging have not diminished the importance of ERCP, but have replaced many of the diagnostic indications for ERCP. These imaging modalities have far less associated morbidity and complications as compared to ERCP. ERCP continues to offer the advantage over these imaging modalities, including direct visualization of the ampullary region and direct access to the distal common bile duct. Because the situation where these benefits outweigh the risk reduction offered by the above mentioned less-invasive imaging modalities, ERCP has become predominantly a therapeutic tool, with the development of numerous endoscopic adjuncts for intraluminal imaging, stricture dilation, stone removal, and pancreaticobiliary stenting. Therapeutic ERCP is discussed in Chap. 29. The diagnostic role for

---

*This chapter was contributed by Harry S. Himal, M.D. in the previous edition.

N.T. Nguyen and C.E.H. Scott-Conner (eds.), *The SAGES Manual: Volume 2*
Advanced Laparoscopy and Endoscopy, DOI 10.1007/978-1-4614-2347-8_28,
© Springer Science+Business Media, LLC 2012

Table 28.1. Indications for ERCP.

Visualization of ampulla of Vater
Adenomas
Carcinoma
Surveillance in patients with polyposis syndromes
Cholangiography (Figs. 28.1–28.4)
Cholestatic jaundice of unknown cause
Choledocholithiasis
Cholangitis
Carcinoma of the bile duct
Bile duct stricture
Bile duct injury
Pancreatography (Figs. 28.5 and 28.6)
Chronic pancreatitis
Pancreatic carcinoma
Pancreatic ascites
Pancreatic pseudocyst
Pancreatic trauma
Gallstone pancreatitis

ERCP remains situations where a concomitant therapeutic intervention may be performed and cases where sphincter of Oddi manometry is needed to evaluate patients with suspected sphincter of Oddi dysfunction. ERCP also allows introduction of a choledochoscope into the bile duct without need for operative choledochotomy. This allows for direct visualization of lesions and may facilitate tissue diagnosis through brushings or biopsies. Advances in intraductal imaging, such as optical coherence tomography, may lead to an increased list of diagnostic indications in the future. Specific indications for ERCP are listed in Table 28.1, and representative radiographs are shown in Figs. 28.1 through 28.6.

B. Facilities and Equipment

ERCP requires the following facilities:
1. An X-ray room capable of both fluoroscopy and endoscopy. A room dedicated to ERCP is most convenient. This may include either a fixed fluoroscopy table or a mobile fluoroscopic C-arm and fluorocompatible table.
2. Equipment for performance of general anesthesia. Due to the complexity of ERCP, as well as the fact that many patients

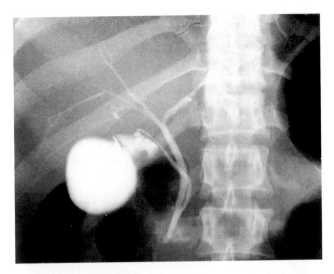

Fig. 28.1. Normal cholangiogram with visualization of the gallbladder.

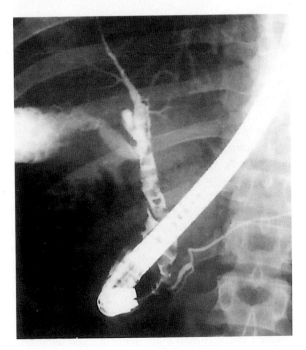

Fig. 28.2. ERCP performed in patient with cholestatic jaundice. The cholangio-gram demonstrates multiple stones within the common bile duct and gallbladder.

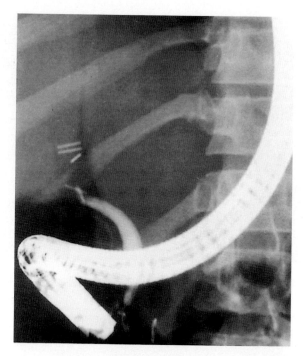

Fig. 28.3. Common bile duct transection during laparoscopic cholecystectomy. Note the clips across the proximal common bile duct with lack of filling of the duct above this level.

requiring this procedure can have extensive comorbidities, general endotracheal anesthesia rather than conscious sedation may be necessary. This can be provided in an operating room setting or an endoscopy suite with dedicated equipment and personnel for delivery of general anesthesia.

3. The ERCP endoscope, referred to as a duodenoscope (Fig. 28.7), is a side-viewing videoendoscope with a single working channel and an adjustable elevator adjunct at the distal end of the scope which allows for upward manipulation of endoscopic tools passed through the biopsy channel. The biopsy channel diameter and outer diameter of the endoscope come in varied sizes. The therapeutic endoscope has a 3.7 mm channel and 14 mm outer diameter. The diagnostic endoscope has a 2.8 mm channel and a 10 mm outer diameter. The duodenoscope has standard suction, irrigation, and both upward and left right maneuverability similar to a gastroscope.

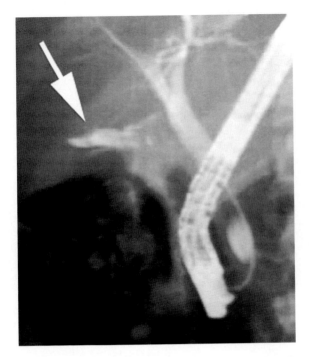

Fig. 28.4. ERCP following laparoscopic cholecystectomy. Note the contrast extravasation consistent with a Duct of Lushka leak.

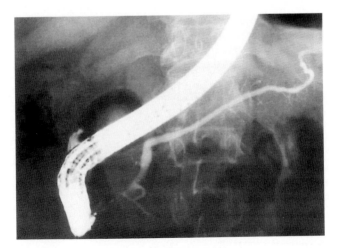

Fig. 28.5. Normal pancreatogram obtained during ERCP.

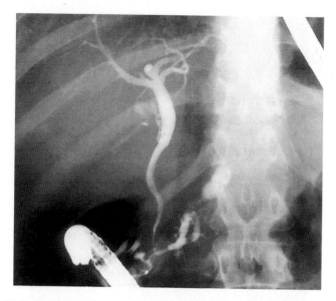

Fig. 28.6. Pancreatic duct in a patient with chronic pancreatitis demonstrating dilatation and strictures. The common duct is also visualized and demonstrates extrinsic compression by the pancreatic mass.

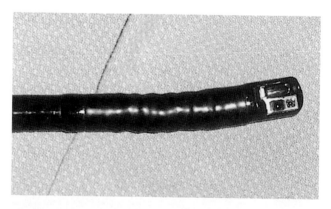

Fig. 28.7. The side-viewing duodenoscope used for ERCP allows direct visualization, biopsy, and cannulation of the ampulla of Vater.

C. Patient Preparation

1. The technique and possible complications should be explained to the patient and informed consent should be obtained. A knowledgeable, informed patient will cooperate with the endoscopist so that the procedure can be done quickly and safely. The complications associated with ERCP are discussed in Chap. 30.

2. The patient is made NPO for 8 h prior to the procedure. The coagulation status of the patient should be considered if a therapeutic ERCP (sphincterotomy, biopsy, or stone extraction) is planned or if the patient has evidence of liver dysfunction.

3. Intravenous access should be obtained in all patients for the administration of conscious sedation. Patients with possible biliary obstruction, cholangitis, or choledocholithiasis should receive antibiotics directed at common biliary flora. Patients should be monitored with telemetry, blood pressure, and pulse oximetry. We also encourage the use of dedicated capnography if available. A dedicated nurse should monitor for adverse events throughout the procedure.

4. The patient should then be placed in the prone position with the head turned to the right (Fig. 28.8). In patients with cervical

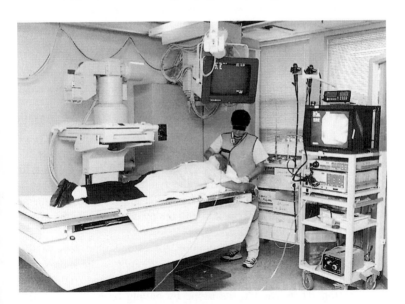

Fig. 28.8. X-ray facilities to carry out ERCP include fluoroscopy. Note the position of the patient, endoscopic cart, and fluoroscopic monitor.

arthritis or obesity, a roll may be placed in the cranial–caudal direction under the right shoulder, converting the patient to a mix between the prone and lateral position. This will facilitate the endoscopist's access to the mouth.

5. Analgesia and conscious sedation are then administered. Chapter 39 detailed sedation administration and monitoring. The author's prefer a step-wise titration of intravenous fentanyl and midazolam. Topical anesthesia may also be applied to the oropharynx if desired. A bite block is placed the patient's mouth to prevent damage to the duodenoscope.

6. Other medications should be available, including glucagon (used to decrease duodenal peristalsis), atropine (used to treat increased vagal activity), and kinevac (a CCK analog used to help identify biliary secretion from the major papilla in difficult cases).

D. Passing the ERCP Scope: Normal Anatomy

1. Test the duodenoscope for all functions (suction, irrigation, and maneuverability) before use. Apply water-soluble lubricant. Then, gently insert the duodenoscope through the bite block into oropharynx. As the duodenoscope is a side-viewing instrument, passage of the scope is essentially a blind procedure. Difficult passage can be facilitated by having the patient swallow or repositioning the patient. Never force the advancement of the duodenoscope as this can lead to perforation.

2. Then, introduce the scope through the esophagus and into the stomach. Commonly, the scope will follow the greater curve of the stomach and head directly toward the pylorus (Fig. 28.9). Because of the side-viewing orientation, the endoscopist will not be able to view and enter the pylorus simultaneously.

3. Using a combination of gentle rotation and scope advancement, advance the endoscope through the pylorus and into the proximal duodenum (Fig. 28.10).

4. To facilitate better positioning for cannulation, remove the redundancy from the scope by transitioning to the short scope position. To do this, turn the dials to the "up" and "right" position. Then, shorten the scope by pulling back slowly on the

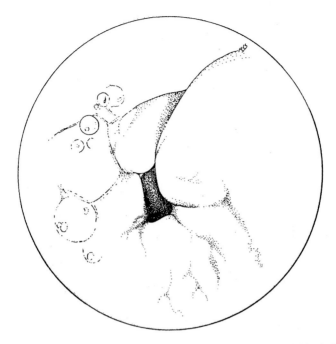

Fig. 28.9. View of pylorus from a side viewing duodenoscope. Bubbles indicating bile provide a clue to the location of the distal stomach when orientation of the side-viewing endoscope is difficult.

endoscope until the ampulla of Vater is visualized (Fig. 28.11). Once the papilla is seen, make small adjustments using the dials to center it in the working space. Then, lock the dials to maintain positioning.

5. Examine the papilla with an attempt to identify the orifice and the likely orientation of the common bile duct and pancreatic duct. Usually, the two ducts share a common channel with a single orifice. The pancreatic duct often heads in the direction of the 02:00 h position and the common bile duct in the direction of the 10:00 h position (Fig. 28.12). In the situation where there are two orifices, the more superior of the two is the bile duct.

6. Advance the cannula toward the papilla using a combination of catheter advancement with the right hand, changing the angle of the catheter using the elevator with the left thumb, and manipulation of the position of the endoscope. It is best to

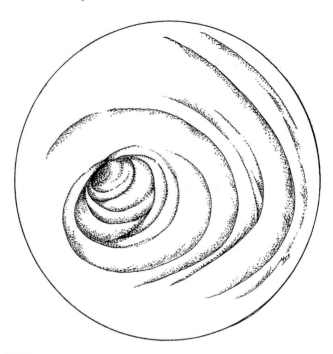

Fig. 28.10.   View of the proximal duodenum.

cannulate the duct of interest first (Fig. 28.13). For pancreatic cannulation, the endoscopist should position the cannula at a right angle to the duodenal wall and the papilla should be approached in a left to right direction. For cannulation of the common bile duct, the cannula should be directed cephalad and should approach the papilla in a right to left approach (Fig. 28.14). Once access has been obtained to a duct, the authors prefer to advance a 0.035 in. guidewire under fluoroscopic guidance.

7.   Tips for difficult cannulation include:

   a.   Bile duct cannulation can be improved by deflecting the tip of the cannula upward, using the curve of the cannula in combination with the elevator function of the scope (Fig. 28.15). This allows the cannula to follow the roof of the common channel into the common bile duct selectively.

   b.   If unsuccessful, consider changing to a different catheter (Fig. 28.16) with different tips and angles to aid in selective cannulation. Consider using a sphincterotome with a

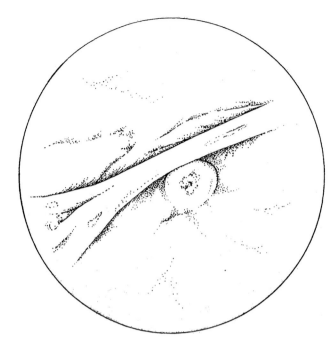

Fig. 28.11. Endoscopic visualization of the ampulla of Vater. A transverse fold of mucosa overlying the ampulla is frequently seen, as shown here.

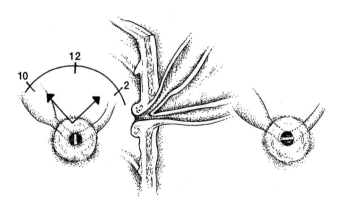

Fig. 28.12. Orientation of the pancreatic and bile ducts. When the papilla is viewed en face, the bile duct is directed in the 10:00 h position and the pancreatic duct in the 02:00 h direction. The septum separating the orifices may be oriented in any direction.

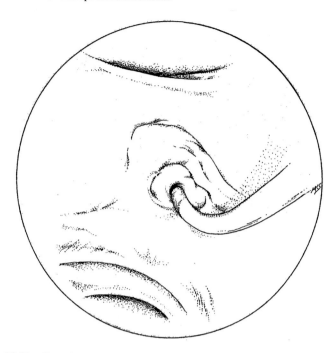

Fig. 28.13. Cannulation of ampulla of Vater.

cutting wire that can bow the tip of the cannula, as this can allow a greater cephalad orientation of the catheter for selective bile duct cannulation.

c. If neither duct can be entered, try impacting the catheter against the papilla and gently injecting a small amount of contrast. This may allow for filling of the desired duct and give a radiographic road map to allow for cannulation.

d. The double wire technique may also offer a treatment option. If the undesired duct is repeatedly cannulated, advance the guidewire into that duct and leave it in place while completely removing the cannula. Then, using the direction of the wire as a guide for the undesired duct, introduce the cannula with new guidewire into the desired duct.

8. Water-soluble contrast injection under fluoroscopic guidance will then help to delineate anatomy and reveal multiple patholo-gies. In patients with an obstructed system, such as those with

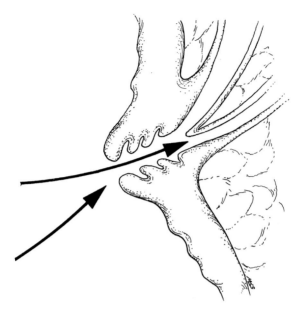

Fig. 28.14. Cephalad directionality during cannulation helps direct the catheter into the common bile duct preferentially while cannulation directed perpendicular to the duodenal wall selects for the pancreatic duct.

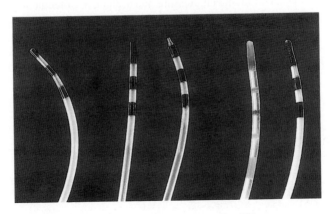

Fig 28.15. Catheters used for cannulation of ampulla of Vater.

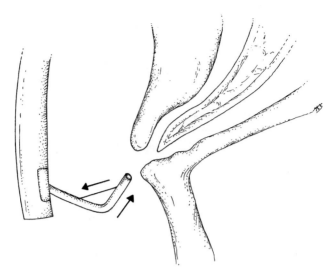

Fig. 28.16. The use of a sphincterotome can help guide the catheter entry in the cephalad direction, allowing selective entry of the bile duct. This can be further facilitated by tightening the cutting wire which results in a bowing of the catheter.

jaundice or cholangitis, excessive contrast injection may lead to elevated intraductal pressure and seeding of potential infection. It is also crucial to avoid acinarization, which may be caused by overinjection of the pancreatic duct, as this may lead to an increased risk of postprocedural pancreatitis.

9. Once access to the desired duct has been obtained, multiple therapeutic options are available and are discussed in Chap. 29.

Selected References

Baron TH, Fleischer DE. Past, present and future of endoscopic retrograde cholangiopancreatography. Perspective on the national institutes of health consensus conference. Mayo Clin Proc. 2002;77:407–12.

Calleti G, Brocchi E, Agostini D. Sensitivity of endoscopic retrograde pancreatography in chronic pancreatitis. Br J Surg. 1982;69:507–9.

Cameron JL. Chronic pancreatic ascites and pancreatic pleural effusions. Gastroenterology. 1978;74:134–40.

Frick MP, Feinberg SB, Goodale RL. The value of endoscopic retrograde cholangiopancreatography in suspected carcinoma of the pancreas and indeterminate computer tomography results. Surg Gynecol Obstet. 1982;155:177–82.

Gaisford WS. Endoscopic retrograde cholangiopancreatography in the diagnosis of jaundice. Am J Surg. 1976;132:699–704.

Ghazi A, Washington M. Endoscopic diagnosis and management of diseases of the pancreas and hepatobiliary tract. Probl Gen Surg. 1990;7:1610–74.

Himal HS. Common duct stones: the role of preoperative, intraoperative, and postoperative ERCP. Semin Laparosc Surg. 2000;7:237–45.

Kozarek R, Gannan R, Baerg R, Wagonfeld J, Ball T. Bile leak after laparoscopic cholecystectomy: diagnostic and therapeutic application of endoscopic retrograde cholangiopancreatography. Arch Intern Med. 1992;152:1040–3.

Laraja RD, Lobbato VJ, Cassaro S, Reddy S. Intraoperative endoscopic retrograde cholangiopancreatography (E.R.C.P.) in penetrating trauma of the pancreas. J Trauma. 1986;6:1146–7.

McCune WS, Shorb PE, Moscowitz H. Endoscopic cannulation of the ampulla of Vater: a preliminary report. Ann Surg. 1968;167:752–6.

Neoptolemos JP, Carr-Locke DC, London NJ, Bailey IA, James D, Fossard DP. Controlled trial of urgent endoscopic retrograde cholangiopancreatography and endoscopic sphincterotomy versus conservative treatment for acute pancreatitis due to gallstones. Lancet. 1988;2:979–83.

O'Connor M, Kolars J, Ansel H, Silvis S, Vennes J. Preoperative endoscopic retrograde cholangiopancreatography in the surgical management of pancreatic pseudocysts. Am J Surg. 1986;151:18–24.

Oi L. Fiberduodenoscopy and endoscopic pancreatocholangiography. Gastrointest Endosc. 1970;17:59–62.

Sherman S, Lehman GA. E.R.C.P. and endoscopic sphincterotomy induced pancreatitis. Pancreas. 1991;6:350–67.

Vennew JA, Bond JH. Approach to the jaundiced patient. Gastroenterology. 1983;84:1615–9.

29. Therapeutic Endoscopic Retrograde Cholangiopancreatography

Brian J. Dunkin, M.D., F.A.C.S.

A. Introduction

This chapter focuses on four categories of diseases that may be treated with therapeutic endoscopic retrograde cholangiopancreatography (ERCP): (1) common bile duct (CBD) stones, (2) malignancy of pancreatic or biliary origin, (3) pancreatitis, and (4) abdominal pain of possible pancreaticobiliary origin.

B. Access to the Bile and Pancreatic Ducts

To perform therapeutic procedures in the bile or pancreatic ducts, the opening to the papilla of Vater must often be enlarged. This is done through the creation of a sphincterotomy. Figure 29.1 illustrates the most common relationship of the CBD and pancreatic duct (PD) to the papilla of Vater. The muscular sphincter of Oddi surrounds the intramural portions of the CBD and PD and must be divided to enlarge the papillary opening.

1) **Pull sphincterotomy**: The most common device used to perform a sphincterotomy is a "pull" sphincterotome (Fig. 29.2). This is a plastic cannula with a monofilament wire mounted on the tip and connected to electrocautery. The tip of the sphincterotome is placed within the ampulla and directed toward the CBD. The wire is then "bowed" across the roof of the papilla and energy applied. The roof of the papilla and intramural portion of the CBD are divided along with the sphincter of Oddi. Care is taken to ensure that the length of the cut remains within

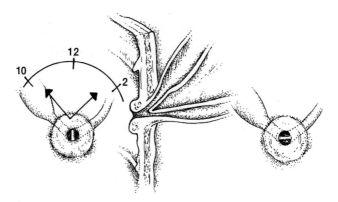

Fig. 29.1. The septum separating orifices to the pancreatic and bile ducts can be oriented in any direction from horizontal to vertical. When papilla is viewed en face, the course of the bile duct is usually toward the 10:00 h position and the pancreatic duct toward the 02:00 h position, although some variation exists.

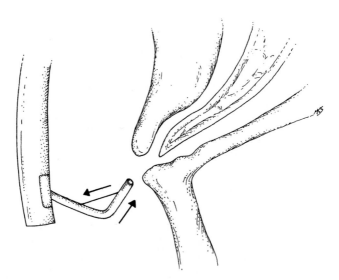

Fig. 29.2. Illustration of a pull sphincterotome. Electrocautery wire is bowed across the "roof" of the papilla and used to cut superiorly.

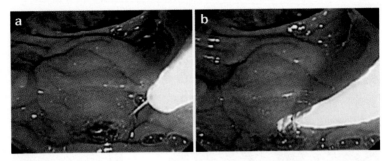

Fig. 29.3.   Needle-knife sphincterotome cutting on top of an impacted gallstone. (a) Impacted stone at papilla. (b) Initiating needle knife sphincterotomy.

the intramural portion of the CBD and avoids the retroduodenal artery—a branch of the gastroduodenal artery. The pull sphincterotomy technique can be used to widen the opening into the CBD, PD, or minor papilla (papilla of Santorini).

2) **Needle knife (precut) sphincterotomy**: On occasion, the endoscopist cannot gain access to the CBD or PD to perform a pull sphincterotomy. In these instances, a needle-knife sphincterotome may be used to perform a free-hand cut of the sphincter (Fig. 29.3). This catheter has a fine wire that can be extended beyond the tip to deliver electrocautery. The endoscopist engages the tissue at the papillary orifice and then cuts superiorly with short bursts of energy. This free-hand needle-knife or "precut" sphincterotomy can provide access to the intramural portion of the CBD when traditional cannulation techniques are unsuccessful.

C. Common Bile Duct Stones

ERCP is most commonly performed to remove stones from the CBD. The procedure begins with gaining access to the CBD and performing a biliary sphincterotomy. Two devices are then available to use for extraction.

1) **Balloon extraction**: The simplest method of stone extraction is to pass a balloon catheter above the CBD stone, inflate it, and then pull the balloon down the CBD and deliver the stone out of

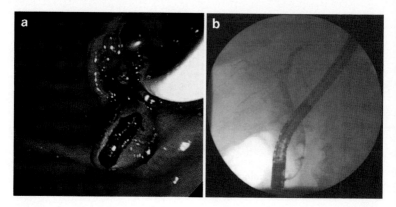

Fig. 29.4. (**a**) Balloon extraction of a common bile duct stone. (**b**) Radiograph showing balloon extraction of a CBD stone.

the sphincterotomized papilla (Fig. 29.4). The balloon can be passed in this manner multiple times to deliver more than one stone. After all stones have been removed, the balloon can then be inflated in the distal CBD while contrast is injected above it to perform an "occlusion cholangiogram" and confirm that no residual stone material has been left behind. ERCP extraction balloons come in various sizes to accommodate different sized CBDs and stones.

2) **Basket extraction**: Stone baskets can be used as an alternative to balloons. The basket is passed into the CBD alongside or above the targeted stone. It is then opened, trapping the stone within the basket (Fig. 29.5). The basket and stone are withdrawn out of the sphincterotomized papilla. As with the balloon, the basket can be passed multiple times into the CBD to remove more than one stone. Retrieved stones are simply dropped into the duodenum and the basket reintroduced into the CBD.

3) **Lithotripsy**: Some stones are too large to remove with simple balloon or basket extraction. In these situations, lithotripsy can be used to break the stone(s) into pieces. Three methods of lithotripsy are commonly available. Choosing among them depends on the availability of technology, familiarity of the endoscopist with each modality, and the size/configuration of the stone(s).

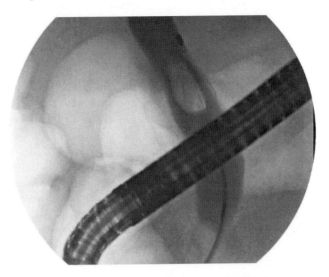

Fig. 29.5. Radiograph showing basket extraction of a CBD stone.

a) **Mechanical lithotripsy**: One advantage of basket stone extraction is that the device can be used to mechanically crush stones if necessary. The handle of the basket device is connected to a specialized pistol grip that is used to forcefully close the basket over the stone until it fractures. The fragments are then removed with the basket or a balloon.

b) **Electrohydraulic lithotripsy (EHL)**: Stones may be fractured using a shock wave applied directly to the surface. An electrohydraulic probe consists of two coaxially isolated electrodes at the tip of a flexible catheter capable of delivering electric sparks in short rapid pulses that generate pressure waves to fracture the stone. Because of the danger of applying this energy to the wall of the CBD, the procedure is most commonly done under direct endoscopic visualization using choledochoscopy (described later in this chapter).

c) **Laser lithotripsy**: This device creates a shock wave via a flexible quartz fiber delivering light from a laser. The 504-nm pulsed-dye laser produces a pulse that is absorbed on the stone surface creating a plasma cloud that rapidly expands and contracts creating the shock wave that fractures the stone. As in EHL, the energy is applied under direct vision using choledochoscopy to avoid damage to the surrounding CBD wall.

4) **Decompression**: On occasion, the CBD cannot be cleared of all stones or debris during one procedure. This may be because there is too much material to clear or that circumstances prevent performing a complex procedure, such as a critically ill patient with cholangitis or a pregnant woman in whom radiation exposure must be minimized. In these circumstances, decompression of the CBD provides effective drainage and allows for scheduling an elective completion procedure at a more optimal time. There are two methods of providing temporary decompression of the CBD.

a) **Plastic stent**: Small plastic tubes can be passed through the working channel of the endoscope and pushed into position in the CBD. These stents range in size from 7 to 11.5 French and come in various lengths. They also have either fixation flaps or a pigtail configuration to prevent migration (Fig. 29.6). The stent is typically positioned with the proximal end in the common hepatic duct and the distal end in the duodenum. To improve drainage, multiple stents are sometimes placed next to each other. Plastic stents remain patent for about 2–3 months after which they must be exchanged or removed.

b) **Nasobiliary drain (NBD)**: It is possible to decompress the biliary system by placing a drain via the nose down the

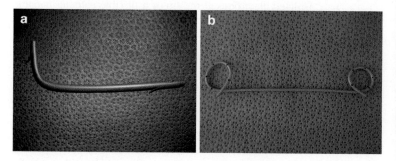

Fig. 29.6. Plastic biliary stents with flap (**a**) and pigtail configuration (**b**).

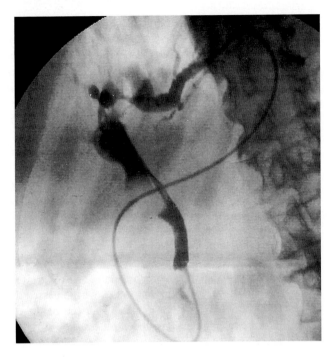

Fig. 29.7.   Radiograph of a nasobiliary tube in place.

esophagus, across the stomach and duodenum, and into the CBD (Fig. 29.7). The side holes in the NBD allow for bile to drain from the CBD into the duodenum, and the transnasal placement enables removal without repeat endoscopy. NBDs are used more commonly outside of the USA for temporary decompression of the biliary tree or instillation of solutions into it.

D. Pancreaticobiliary Malignancy

Over 50,000 new cases of pancreas, gallbladder, or extrahepatic biliary tract malignancy are diagnosed each year and ERCP is often used for sampling or decompression in these cases.

1) **Sampling**: Pancreas cancer often presents with painless jaundice from obstruction of the CBD at the intrapancreatic portion. While endoscopic ultrasound (EUS)-guided biopsy has become the gold standard for gaining a tissue diagnosis when necessary, ERCP can be used to confirm the diagnosis while also providing decompression of the obstructed biliary tree. Tissue sampling during ERCP is done with a cytology brush or biopsy forceps.

   a) **Cytology brush**: A cytology brush can be passed via the endoscope into the biliary or pancreatic duct. Most commonly in pancreas cancer, it is used to brush the area of CBD narrowing at the intrapancreatic portion. When cytology brush biopsies confirm a diagnosis of pancreas cancer, they can be helpful, but often the yield is low with a sensitivity as low as 8%. Balloon dilation of the strictured CBD prior to brush cytology does not seem to improve the diagnostic yield, but repeat brushing may.

   b) **Biopsy**: Biopsy forceps can sometimes be passed into the CBD to acquire tissue samples. This can be done under fluoroscopic guidance or under direct vision using per oral choledochoscopy (technique described later in this chapter). Studies show that using a biopsy forceps under direct vision improves the sensitivity of detecting malignancy to about 64%.

2) **Decompression**: CBD obstruction from pancreas malignancy may be treated with decompression in patients deemed surgically unresectable or in those undergoing neoadjuvant chemo/radiation therapy. Decompression is accomplished by placing plastic or metal stents.

   a) **Plastic stents**: As described above, plastic stents can be used effectively for decompressing biliary obstruction. Given their limited patency, plastic stents should be used only in those cases expected to require decompression for less than 90 days. If longer periods of decompression are required, a metal stent should be considered.

   b) **Self-expanding metal stent (SEMS)**: These metal stents are constrained on a 7–10 French delivery system passed down the working channel of the endoscope. When deployed, they open to their full diameter and have a wire mesh consistency (Fig. 29.8). They can be coated with an impermeable covering and come in a variety of lengths

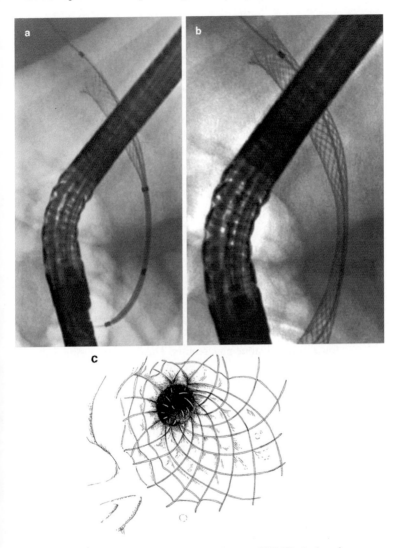

Fig. 29.8. Radiograph self-expanding metal stent (SEMS) deployed across a CBD stricture. (**a**) Initial deployment of SEMS. (**b**) SEMS deployed. (**c**) Endoscopic view of deployed SEMS.

with a maximum diameter of 10 mm. SEMSs have traditionally been designed with a partial impermeable cover that leaves the open cell weave of the ends of the stent exposed. Tissue ingrowth occurs at these open cells and fixes the stent into position to prevent migration. Removal after tissue ingrowth is difficult, so SEMSs have been used most often as palliation for malignant CBD obstruction when surgery is not an option. More recently, fully covered SEMSs have become available which are easy to remove from the CBD. This has fostered the use of SEMS for temporary decompression of the biliary tree because of improved patency and less need for reintervention compared to plastic stents. Biliary SEMSs have an average patency rate of over 300 days if covered compared to less than 150 days for plastic stents.

E. Pancreatitis

ERCP is used to lessen the severity of acute pancreatitis and manage the complications of chronic pancreatitis.

1) **Acute pancreatitis**: Multiple randomized, controlled, prospective studies have investigated the utility of early ERCP and endoscopic sphincterotomy (ES) to lessen the severity of symptoms from gallstone pancreatitis. The data demonstrates that in severe attacks of biliary pancreatitis (>3 Ranson's criteria) early ERCP with sphincterotomy and stone extraction can lessen the severity of the course of pancreatitis. It is also beneficial in those cases of pancreatitis with signs and symptoms suggestive of biliary obstruction. ERCP with placement of a biliary stent may be used to temporarily prevent future attacks of gallstone pancreatitis. It may also be used in pregnant patients to get them through delivery before they undergo definitive management of their biliary tract disease.

2) **Pancreatic pseudocyst**: Simple pancreatic pseudocysts which are enlarging or causing symptoms can be endoscopically decompressed. This is done either transmurally through the wall of the stomach or duodenum or transpapillary via the pancreatic duct.

   a) **Transmural drainage**: Endoscopy can be used to create a fistula between a pseudocyst and the intestinal tract to affect drainage. This is most commonly done across the wall of the stomach or duodenum. The procedure begins by localizing the optimal place for drainage. This can be done by observing where there is prominent compression into the lumen of the stomach or duodenum or by using EUS. Once the drainage site is chosen, an aspiration needle is advanced across the intestinal wall into the cyst cavity. Fluid is aspirated and contrast injected to confirm proper location. A needle knife is then used to cut an opening across the intestinal wall into the cyst. A guide wire is advanced under fluoroscopic guidance into the cyst cavity and a dilation balloon used to dilate the opening into the cyst. Through this opening, multiple side-by-side plastic stents or a covered SEMS are placed for drainage. The stents are usually left in place for 4–12 weeks and then removed after imaging has confirmed resolution of the cyst.

b) **Transpapillary**: Pancreatic pseudocysts that communicate with the pancreatic duct may be drained transpapillary. After the pancreatogram confirms communication, a pancreatic stent is placed across the papilla, through the pancreatic duct, and out into the cyst. This route of drainage is least commonly available, but is as effective as transmural drainage with less risk of bleeding.

F. Abdominal Pain of Possible Pancreaticobiliary Origin

Chronic pancreatitis and sphincter of Oddi dysfunction (SOD) are two conditions that cause abdominal pain and may be amenable to therapeutic ERCP.

1) **Chronic pancreatitis**: Chronic irritation of the pancreas can lead to fibrosis and stricture of the PD. This in turn can cause pancreatic duct stone formation. ERCP can be used to relieve both conditions.

a) **Stricture**: PD strictures may be dilated and PD stents placed to improve drainage.

b) **Stones**: PD stones may be amenable to the same stone extraction techniques described for CBD stones. However, PD stones are often impacted tightly and cannot be removed by the usual means. In these instances, a PD stent can be placed proximal to the stone to effect drainage and then extracorporeal shock wave lithotripsy (ESWL) used to break the stone into smaller fragments. The stent and fragments are subsequently extracted.

c) **Pancreas divisum**: During normal embryologic development, the dorsal and ventral pancreatic ducts join and the pancreas drains through the papilla of Vater. However, in some instances, the ducts do not fuse and a small portion of the head of the pancreas drains via the ventral PD through the papilla of Vater (major papilla) while the majority of the pancreas drains via the dorsal PD via the papilla of Santorini (minor papilla). Frequent drainage via the minor papilla is not adequate causing PD hypertension with recurrent attacks of pancreatitis. These patients may benefit from a minor papilla sphincterotomy and/or placement of a PD stent.

2) **SOD**: Chronic abdominal pain may be caused by SOD—a condition of abnormal resting hypertension or intermittent spasm of the sphincter of Oddi resulting in pancreatitis. There are three types of SOD: Type 1—pain, abnormal laboratory tests, dilated biliary, or pancreatic ducts, Type 2—pain plus either abnormal laboratory tests or dilated duct(s), and Type 3—pain only. Types 1 and 2 are amenable to ERCP and ES. It is important to confirm the diagnosis with sphincter of Oddi manometry. High sphincter of Oddi pressures (>40-mmHg), coupled with a dilated CBD/PD and/or delayed drainage of contrast, may benefit most from ES.

G. Determinants of Complications from Therapeutic ERCP

Multiple factors can predispose to the development of complications following ERCP. They are categorized into patient, procedure, and operator factors.

1) **Patient factors**: Younger age (<60 years old) and SOD are associated with higher rates of ERCP-induced pancreatitis. Some studies have shown as high as a 30% incidence of pancreatitis in young women with SOD undergoing an ES. Coagulopathy increases the risk of hemorrhage following sphincterotomy.

2) **Procedure factors**: Difficulty in cannulating the papilla is associated with a higher rate of complications following ERCP. Associated factors that suggest difficult cannulation include multiple pancreatic injections of contrast and performance of a precut sphincterotomy.

3) **Operator factors**: The experience of the endoscopist seems to be a factor in predicting complications from ERCP. One or fewer procedures per endoscopist per week, fewer than 40 endoscopic sphincterotomies per year, and fewer than 150 ERCPs per year are all associated with increased risk of complications.

H. Other Indications for ERCP

In addition to those described above, there are a few other disease processes that can be treated with ERCP.

1) **Postcholecystectomy bile leak**: Bile leakage after cholecystectomy usually manifests with increased abdominal pain and possibly associated sepsis. Radiologic imaging of the abdomen confirms the leak and associated biloma and percutaneous drainage is a mainstay of therapy. Once the leak is controlled, ERCP is useful in diagnosing the etiology of the leak and possibly treating it. Bile duct injury after cholecystectomy can be classified into categories. Figure 29.9 illustrates the Strasberg–Soper modification of the Bismuth classification of bile duct injuries. Injuries A and D can be successfully managed with ERCP and placement of a plastic biliary stent. The stent allows the bile to drain preferentially into the duodenum causing the leak to seal. It is not necessary for the stent to be placed across the area of leak for successful management. Cystic duct stump leaks (type A) treated in this manner often seal within hours and reoperative surgery is not usually required.

2) **Traumatic pancreatic duct leak**: Blunt abdominal trauma can sometimes lead to traumatic disruption of the pancreatic duct which leads to peripancreatic inflammation. As in bile duct leaks, pancreatic duct leaks may be successfully treated with PD stenting. It is preferred to place the stent across the area of leak, but even if this cannot be accomplished a stent distal to the leak may provide preferential drainage of pancreatic enzymes into the duodenum and allow the leak to heal.

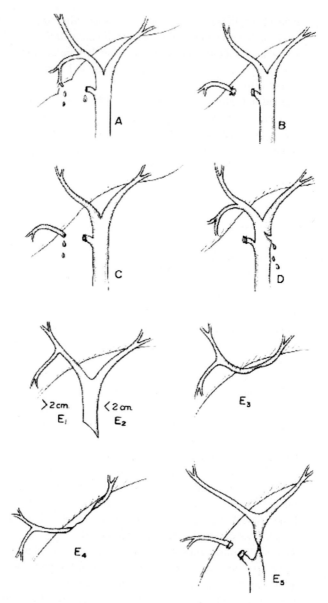

Fig. 29.9. Strasberg–Soper classification of bile duct injuries following cholecystectomy.

3) **Benign biliary stricture**: Strictures of the CBD can frequently occur from benign pathology, such as chronic pancreatitis, ischemic injury after biliary surgery, or anastomotic stricture after bile duct reconstruction. These benign strictures can frequently be managed with endoscopic dilation and stenting. Balloon dilators for the biliary tract are available in a variety of diameters and lengths and can be used to dilate an anastomotic or ischemic stricture. Dilation alone, however, usually does not result in successful management and is often accompanied by placement of one or more biliary stents. In strictures from chronic pancreatitis, for instance, multiple plastic stents are placed side by side across the sphincterotomized papilla into the strictured area of the bile duct. This allows for scar remodeling around the stents as well as biliary drainage both through and around the stents. Successful management often requires keeping the stents in place for up to a year with periodic changes. More recently, fully covered SEMSs have been used for benign strictures of the CBD with good success and less need for reintervention when compared to plastic.

4) **Periampullary adenoma**: Ampullary adenomas are premalignant neoplasms arising from the mucosal epithelium of the papilla of Vater. They may occur sporadically or as part of familial adenomatous polyposis (FAP). While the treatment of benign ampullary neoplasm is controversial, one method of excision is endoscopic ampullectomy. A standard monopolar diathermic snare like that used in colonic polypectomy is used to remove the ampulla—preferably en bloc. The procedure is associated with a high rate of pancreatitis (up to 80% in some series) and a pancreatic stent is usually placed to reduce this incidence. Surveillance endoscopy is based on the pathologic findings and usually done at 6- or 12-month intervals.

I. Per Oral Choledochoscopy/Pancreatoscopy

It is possible to perform choledochoscopy or pancreatoscopy at the time of ERCP. The choledochoscope is passed down the working channel of the duodenoscope and up into the desired duct. This is called a "mother–daughter scope" configuration with the duodenoscope serving as the "mother" scope and the choledochoscope as the "daughter" scope

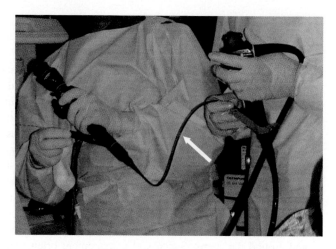

Fig. 29.10.   Image of a mother–daughter (*arrow*) scope configuration.

(Fig. 29.10). Traditionally, this configuration required two endoscopists, although recent advances in technology have provided a single operator system. Direct visualization into the CBD and PD can be useful in defining strictures of unclear etiology, gaining better tissue samples, managing large or impacted stones with laser or electrohydraulic lithotripsy, or assuring that a duct is completely clear of stones and debris. Choledochoscopy and pancreatoscopy require a sphincterotomy and dilated ducts to allow passage of the choledochoscope.

Selected References

Kozarek R, Kodama T, Tatsumi Y. Direct cholangioscopy and pancreatoscopy. Gastrointest Endosc Clin N Am. 2003;13(4):593–608.

Martin JA, Haber GB. Ampullary adenoma: clinical manifestations, diagnosis, and treatment. Gastrointest Endosc Clin N Am. 2003;13(4):649–70.

Silverstein FE, Tytgat G. Endoscopic retrograde cholangiopancreatography and sphincterotomy. In: Wolfe MM, editor. Gastrointestinal endoscopy, Thieme New York, NY. 3rd ed. 1997. p. 238–60.

Sherman S, Lehman GA. Endoscopic retrograde cholangiopancreatography, endoscopic sphincterotomy and stone removal, and endoscopic biliary and pancreatic drainage. In: Yamada T, Alpers DH, Laine L, Owyang C, Powell DW, editors. Textbook of gastroenterology, vol. 2. Philadelphia, PA: Lippincott Williams & Wilkins; 1999. p. 2718–46.

Mark D, Lefevre F, Bohn RL, Finkelstein B. Endoscopic retrograde cholangiopancreatography. Evid Rep Technol Assess. Rockville, MD: AHRQ Publication; 2002;50:02-E017.

30. Complications of Endoscopic Retrograde Cholangiopancreatography*

Melissa S. Phillips, M.D.
Jeffrey M. Marks, M.D., F.A.C.S.

Endoscopic retrograde cholangiopancreatography (ERCP) is a commonly performed procedure that is not without risks. It allows a less invasive way to treat biliopancreatic lesions, but is associated with a 7% complication rate and a 0.3% mortality rate. Risks associated with ERCP include those similar to other endoscopic procedure, such as those related to conscious sedation, drug reaction, and cardiopulmonary complication. There are also risks specifically related to the diagnostic and therapeutic aspects of ERCP which are discussed here in more detail.

A. Pancreatitis

1. **Cause and prevention**: Pancreatitis is the most common complication following ERCP. When searching the literature, it is clear that a set value for the definition of postprocedural pancreatitis has not been consistently established. As many as 60% of patients may develop transient hyperamylasemia after ERCP. Clinical pancreatitis, defined as abdominal pain in combination with an amylase level above three times the upper limit of normal, occurs in approximately 5% of patients. Most cases of post-ERCP pancreatitis (>90%) are mild to moderate and self-limited. Unfortunately, there have been rare cases of fatal necrotizing post-ERCP pancreatitis reported. Post-ERCP pancreatitis

---

*This chapter was contributed by Morris Washington, M.D., and Ali Ghazi, M.D., in the previous edition.

has an increased incidence in therapeutic ERCP when compared to diagnostic ERCP. It is more common in younger patients, females, and those with previous or recurrent pancreatitis. Patients undergoing ERCP for suspected sphincter of Oddi dysfunction also have an increased risk for post-ERCP pancreatitis.

a.   **The exact mechanism** that initiates post-ERCP pancreatitis is still unproven, but it is believed by many to have a mechanical component. It has been proposed that an increase in pancreatic intraductal pressure with release of pancreatic enzyme from acini into the pancreatic parenchyma is the underlying pathology, supporting the idea that pancreatic duct stenting may decrease the risk. This increased intraductal pressure may be further exacerbated by hydrostatic pressure from contrast injection. Proposed mechanisms for increasing intraductal pressure and thus pancreatitis include the following:

   i.   Difficulty with cannulation leading to overmanipulation of the papilla of Vater, causing trauma and spasm of the sphincter of Oddi.

   ii. Repeated injection into the pancreatic ductal system in an attempt to access the bile duct.

   iii. Overzealous injection of contrast media into the pancreatic ductal system, resulting in a complete outline of the pancreas on X-ray known as acinarization.

   iv. Thermal injury to the papilla of Vater from the electrocautery used during endoscopic sphincterotomy leading to increased edema and impaired emptying.

   v.   Placement of large endobiliary stents without a sphincterotomy, causing obstruction of the pancreatic duct orifice.

   Other considerations have been given to the ideas that post-ERCP pancreatitis is related to a chemical or allergic reaction to contrast injection, enzymatic injury from intraluminal activation of intestinal contents, and infectious causes. More research is needed to understand the role of these factors on the pathogenesis of post-ERCP pancreatitis.

b.   **Prevention of ERCP-induced pancreatitis**: Intuitively, better technique during cannulation and sphincterotomy should lower the incidence of post-ERCP pancreatitis;

however, this has been difficult to study and document. Nevertheless, the following technical considerations may be helpful in the prevention of post-ERCP pancreatitis.

i. Avoid unnecessary diagnostic ERCPs if a less invasive alternative (such as MRCP or US) is available.

ii. Good positioning of the duodenoscope facilitates immediate cannulation to avoid trauma to the papilla that can occur with repeated attempts.

iii. Selective cannulation of the common bile duct avoids injection into the pancreatic ductal system if a pancreatogram is not required.

iv. Minimize the use of contrast injection with the goal of filling only the main pancreatic duct and avoid acinarization. A larger syringe delivers less hydrostatic pressure during contrast injection and thus may avoid inadvertent overfilling of the pancreatic ductal system. Consider guide wire use rather than injection to confirm location.

v. If repeated access to a cannulated duct is needed, such as would be the case in therapeutic ERCP, or if the initial cannulation has been difficult, access should be maintained with the use of a guide wire.

vi. During sphincterotomy, avoid excess use of energy. If possible, use the "cut" function rather than the "coagulation" function to decrease the amount of edema and tissue injury. Another option includes use of the Erbe, which auto adjusts the blend based on tissue resistance. Precut sphincterotomy should be used only by those comfortable with this technique because of the higher risk for pancreatitis and bleeding.

There have been many attempts at pharmacologic prevention of post-ERCP pancreatitis using atropine, glucagon, calcitonin, and steroids, all of which have shown limited efficacy in experimental and clinical trials. Other agents, including somatostatin (which suppresses pancreatic secretion), nonsteroidal anti-inflammatory drugs and IL-10 (which promote the anti-inflammatory process), allopurinol (which works to inhibit free radical production), and gabexate (which works as a protease inhibitor), have shown initial promise, but further trials have failed to support the use of these medications. Additional clinical investigations in the form of randomized controlled trials are needed to document the efficacy of pharmacologic prevention of pancreatitis prior to generalized use.

2. **Treatment**: Most cases of post-ERCP pancreatitis are mild to moderate in severity and resolve with conservative treatment, including bowel rest, pain control, and intravenous hydration. In a small number of patients, pancreatitis may be more severe, requiring treatment in the intensive care unit. Treatment of pancreatitis as a result of ERCP is no different than the treatment from other causes. Oral intake should be restricted in these patients and parenteral nutrition instituted. Ranson's criteria can be used to risk stratify patients, and imaging studies may be needed to monitor for complications of the disease process. Inflammatory phlegmons or pseudocysts may develop in the acute phase, take several weeks to resolve, and require drainage. Large pseudocysts that persist with conservative therapy longer than 8 weeks require internal drainage either surgically or endoscopically through a cystogastrostomy. Repeat endoscopic intervention or percutaneous transhepatic drainage may be required if adequate biliary decompression was not established during the initial procedure. In patients who develop pancreatic necrosis with subsequent infection, exploration with pancreatic debridement and necrosectomy is required as a lifesaving measure.

B. Hemorrhage

1. **Cause and prevention**: As is true with any other invasive procedure, hemorrhage following ERCP is related to many factors, including technical approach and preoperative optimization. Patients with obstructive jaundice or other signs of liver dysfunction must be evaluated before the procedure is undertaken by checking coagulation parameters, specifically a prothrombin time (PT), as they may have impaired vitamin K absorption. This is particularly important for patients undergoing therapeutic ERCP as the patient may require an endoscopic biliary or pancreatic sphincterotomy to allow access to the duct for further therapeutic treatments. If the ERCP can be delayed, treatment with vitamin K to correct the PT should be undertaken. For those who

require an urgent intervention, fresh frozen plasma must be administered. It is recommended that patients who are taking antiplatelet medications discontinue these medications for 7–10 days before an endoscopic sphincterotomy if the patient's other medical conditions allow. Again, if the intervention cannot be delayed, consideration should be given to a platelet transfusion. Most cases of bleeding encountered during ERCP are mild and self-limited, presuming that the patient has a normal coagulation profile. However, endoscopic biliary or pancreatic sphincterotomy is a predisposing factor to clinically significant bleeding, which is reported in 2% of cases. Half of patients with clinically significant bleeding are diagnosed at the time of sphincterotomy while the other half present later, up to 1 week after the original procedure which can be induced by sloughing of the eschar at a previous sphincterotomy site. Patient factors, such as coagulopathy, renal or hepatic failure, and cholangitis before the procedure, have been shown to increase the bleeding risk. Anatomic factors, such as the presence of periampullary diverticula or papillary stenosis, and technical factors, such as sphincterotomy length or low case volume, have also been associated with increased risk.

Prevention of bleeding can be accomplished by identifying patients at risk, treating coagulopathies, and following careful technique. While it is difficult to document the exact role of technique in preventing clinically significant bleeding following sphincterotomy, the following guidelines may help reduce bleeding.

a. Maintain proper orientation of the wire at the 11:00 h position. Perform the sphincterotomy in sequential steps rather than a long, less-controlled cut.

b. Use a blended cutting/coagulation current, such as the Erbe, which adjusts the blend of current based on tissue resistance.

c. Tailor the size of the sphincterotomy to the task at hand. Avoid unnecessary extension of the sphincterotomy above the transverse fold.

d. Avoid forceful extraction of large stones by using a mechanical lithotripter.

e. Consider endoscopic balloon dilation to reduce bleeding in high-risk patients, but be aware that there may be a higher pancreatitis rate from this intervention.

2. **Treatment**: As mentioned earlier, most cases of ERCP-related bleeding are self-limited and often stop spontaneously. Patients with clinically relevant bleeding are most commonly managed with medical or endoscopic therapies. In patients with refractory cases, angiography and surgery offer additional therapies. Standard care for a patient with clinically significant hemorrhage should be undertaken in all patients, including large-bore IV access, close hemodynamic monitoring, serial hematocrit values, and, if needed, blood transfusion.

Medical treatment modalities for ERCP-related bleeding are discussed in the prevention section and include correction of coagulation and/or platelet abnormalities. Endoscopic therapies are the mainstay for treating ampullary bleeding. If bleeding is discovered at the time of sphincterotomy, simple approaches, such as applying mechanical compression to the bleeding area using an endoscopic balloon for tamponade, may suffice. Injection of epinephrine is the most commonly used endoscopic treatment for post-ERCP hemorrhage. Using a sclerotherapy or variceal injection needle, a few milliliters of 1:10,000 epinephrine solution can be delivered to the localized area of bleeding with good results. A small chance for rebleeding following treatment remains, but the overall efficacy of this treatment is high. The use of electrocautery may also assist in the control of hemorrhage if a visible vessel or single point of bleeding is encountered; however, care must be taken to avoid inadvertent thermal injury to surrounding areas. Endoscopic clips may also be applied. Care must be taken to prevent occlusion of the biliary or pancreatic orifice during placement, increasing the risk for pancreatitis or obstruction.

In situations where endoscopic and medical management fail to control the hemorrhage, consideration must be given to more aggressive treatment modalities. If there are experienced interventional radiology capabilities available, selective embolization of the bleeding branch of the gastroduodenal artery can be performed in an attempt to avoid a surgical intervention. If successful, the patient must be monitored after the procedure for the rare complication of end-organ ischemia. If angiography is unsuccessful in obtaining control of the hemorrhage, operative treatment must be performed. Exploration of the abdomen through a midline incision, including a Kocher maneuver for mobilization of the duodenum, should be performed. Through an anterior duodenotomy, ampulla of Vater can be accessed and suture ligation can be used to control the site of hemorrhage. As is true with endoscopic clip application, care must be taken to avoid narrowing of the biliary or pancreatic orifice, leading to an increased rate of pancreatitis. If the patient is hemodynamically stable and the ERCP treatment was aborted for bleeding, surgical treatment of the original pathology can be performed. In a hemodynamically challenged patient, bleeding should be controlled but other elective treatments should be deferred.

C. Cholangitis

1. **Cause and prevention**: The overall incidence of cholangitis following ERCP is low, around 1% in many large studies, but is one of the most potentially morbid complications. In patients who do not have evidence of biliary obstruction, cholangitis following ERCP is exceedingly rare. Because of the low incidence of cholangitis in these patients, there has been no established role for prophylactic antibiotics when undergoing ERCP. In patients with a biliary obstructions and jaundice, however, there are impaired host defenses that make the patient more susceptible to the development of cholangitis. Jaundiced patients undergoing stenting of malignant biliary strictures, those having combined percutaneous endoscopic procedures, those with hilar strictures of both benign and malignant etiologies, and those who have had failed or incomplete biliary drainage after ERCP are at the highest risk. Antibiotic prophylaxis in these high-risk patients has been shown to decrease the risk of subsequent cholangitis. Antibiotics should be tailored to cover enteric flora, with the author's preference being piperacillin/tazobactam or ciprofloxacin.

   Postprocedural cholangitis can be decreased by proper ERCP technique. When working in a setting concerning for biliary obstruction, care should be taken to inject as little contrast as possible to avoid increasing intraductal pressure. Place a wire across any recognized stricture before injecting contrast to assure a patent lumen and avoid overfilling of the proximal biliary tree. Every attempt should be made to obtain adequate biliary decompression when obstruction is demonstrated. This can be accomplished using ERCP therapeutics, radiographic, or surgical intervention. No matter the path chosen, prompt treatment of the biliary obstruction is important.

2. **Treatment**: Patients presenting with a septic presentation must have other infectious complications, such as acute cholecystitis or liver abscess, ruled out, but treatment for cholangitis cannot be delayed. As mentioned above, incomplete biliary drainage is the most important risk factor for the development of cholangitis. If the patient develops classic signs of Charcot's triad, including fever, right upper quadrant pain, and jaundice, systemic antibiotics should be initiated and immediate drainage is indicated. In patients with a previously placed biliary stent, consideration must be given to occlusion of the stent as a cause for cholangitis. If endoscopic drainage options fail to decompress the biliary obstruction, urgent percutaneous or surgical decompression procedures must be performed. If the patient is allowed to progress to hypotension, mental status changes, or septic shock, risk of mortality is high.

D. Perforation

1. **Cause and prevention**: All endoscopic procedures carry an associated risk for perforation, often related to traumatic passage or manipulation of the endoscope/endoscopic instruments. ERCP is unique in that in addition to the standard perforation risks there are additional risks for retroperitoneal duodenal or biliary perforation. When combined, the risk for any type of perforation is rare, occurring in less than 0.6% of cases, but each requires prompt diagnosis and treatment to avoid associated morbidity. Retroperitoneal duodenal perforations are the most common location and can be misdiagnosed as pancreatitis on presentation. These perforations are often a result of an extensive endoscopic sphincterotomy that continues beyond the portion of the bile duct contained by the duodenum. Bile duct perforations may result from forceful cannulation or as a complication of therapies for biliary strictures.

    As compared to patients with free perforation, patients with retroperitoneal duodenal perforations present in a more indolent fashion, often complaining of abdominal or back pain. As mentioned, this can lead to an initial misdiagnosis of pancreatitis unless further complications are appropriately investigated. Patients presenting with a retroperitoneal perforation may also have associated fever or leukocytosis. CT scans are more sensitive than plain films for demonstrating retroperitoneal air or contrast. The presence of retroperitoneal air on imagining must be interpreted within the context of the clinical appearance as cases of benign retroperitoneal air without perforation have been described. The presence of fluid in the retroperitoneum may be, however, a more concerning finding when concerned for perforation as this fluid may represent bile or enteric contents. The following technical considerations may help to avoid this complication.

a. Maintain proper orientation during the endoscopic sphincterotomy.

b. Avoid using a "precut" technique unless absolutely necessary.

c. Perform the sphincterotomy in a stepwise fashion, limiting the extent of the sphincterotomy to only that needed for the specific therapy.

d. Do not extend the sphincterotomy beyond the transverse duodenal fold.

2. **Treatment**: Treatment for perforation must be considered in the context of patient conditions and predisposing factors. Treatment for a patient with a large ampullary carcinoma may be different from a patient with a benign common duct stricture based on the impact of perforation-related changes on figure interventions. Patients with free abdominal perforation often require urgent laparotomy; however, patients with retroperitoneal perforations can often be managed conservatively with good outcomes. Conservative management includes bowel rest with nasogastric tube decompression and broad-spectrum antibiotic coverage. Serial abdominal examinations should be performed. If the patient clinically worsens (or fails to improve) with this treatment, surgical intervention should be performed. A midline laparotomy with Kockerization of the duodenum should be performed to reveal the posterior wall which is the most likely site of perforation. This site may then be treated either by primary closure or an omental patch based on the induration of the surrounding tissues. A pyloric exclusion procedure with gastrojejunostomy and distal feeding jejunostomy should be considered. A drain should also be left in place for anastomotic monitoring.

E. Rare Complications

There are rare complications of ERCP that can occur; some are unique to ERCP and others can occur with any endoscopic procedure targeting the upper gastrointestinal tract. They are listed here so that one may have a general knowledge of them:

1. Cardiopulmonary dysfunction.
2. Oversedation or adverse medication reactions.
3. Esophageal or gastric perforations.
4. Mallory–Weiss tears.
5. Hepatic and splenic hematomas.
6. Stone extraction basket entrapment or impaction.
7. Proximal stent migration.
8. Hepatic abscess or biloma formation.
9. Papillary stenosis.
10. Recurrent choledocholithiasis.

Selected References

Andriulli A, Loperfido S, Napolitano G, Niro G, Valvano MR, et al. Incidence rates of post-ERCP complications: a systematic survey of prospective studies. Am J Gastroenterol. 2007;102(8):1781–8.

Aronson N, Flamm CR, Bohn RL, Mark DH, Speroff T. Evidence-based assessment: patient, procedure, or operator factors associated with ERCP complications. Gastrointest Endosc. 2002;56(6 Suppl):S294–302.

Baillie J. Predicting and preventing post-ERCP pancreatitis. Rev Cur Gastroenterol Rep. 2002;4:112–9.

Byl B, Deviere J, Struelens MJ, et al. Antibiotic prophylaxis for infectious complications after therapeutic endoscopic retrograde cholangiopancreatography: a randomized, double-blind, placebo-controlled study. Clin Infect Dis. 1995;20:1236–40.

Demols A, Deviere J. New frontiers in the pharmacological prevention of post-ERCP pancreatitis: the cytokines. Pancreas. 2003;4:49–57.

Freeman ML. Adverse outcomes of endoscopic retrograde cholangiopancreatography: avoidance and management. Gastrointest Endosc Clin N Am. 2003;13:775–98.

Freeman ML, Nelson DB, Sherman S, Haber GB. Complications of endoscopic biliary sphincterotomy. N Engl J Med. 1996;335:909–18.

Ghazi A, Washington M. Endoscopic diagnosis and management of diseases of the pancreas and hepatobiliary tract. Curr Probl Surg. 1990;7:161–74.

Kullman E, Borch K, Lindstrom E, Ansehn S, Ilse I, Anderberg B. Bacteremia following diagnostic and therapeutic E.R.C.P. Gastrointest Endosc. 1992;38:444–9.

Lo AY, Washington M, Fischer MG. Splenic trauma following endoscopic retrograde cholangiopancreatography. Surg Endosc. 1994;8:692–3.

Low DE, Mioflikier AB, Kennedy JK, Stiver HG. Infectious complications of endoscopic retrograde cholangiopancreatography. Arch Intern Med. 1980;140:1076–7.

Pasricha P. Prevention of ERCP-induced pancreatitis: success at last. Gastroenterology. 1997;112:1415–7.

Skude G, Wehlin L, Maruyama T, Ariyama J. Hyperamylasemia after duodenoscopy and retrograde cholangiopancreatography. Gut. 1976;17:127–32.

Tarnasky PR, Cunningham JT, Hawes RH, et al. Transpapillary stenting of proximal biliary strictures: does biliary sphincterotomy reduce the risk of postprocedure pancreatitis? Gastrointest Endosc. 1997;45:46–51.

Part V
Laparoscopic Colectomy

31. Laparoscopic Ileocecectomy, Small Bowel Resection, and Strictureplasty for Crohn's Disease

Joanne Favuzza, D.O.
Conor P. Delaney, M.D., Ph.D.

A. Introduction

Crohn's disease is a chronic inflammatory bowel disease that can affect the entire digestive tract, most often the terminal ileum. Crohn's disease has steadily increased in incidence and prevalence in the USA over the last decade. The treatment of Crohn's disease consists of medical management primarily with the use of steroids and immunomodulating agents. Despite the advancements made over the years in the medical treatment for Crohn's disease, approximately 80% of patients will require surgical intervention during their lifetime. The most common surgery performed for Crohn's patients is an ileocolic resection for stricture or obstruction.

Laparoscopy has been shown to be a viable option in the literature for patients with benign and malignant colorectal disease. Two prospective randomized trials as well as numerous case-controlled studies have confirmed that laparoscopic techniques are a safe and acceptable option for Crohn's disease. The benefits of laparoscopic resection in Crohn's disease include decreased length of stay and reduced morbidity. These results are also associated with reduced use of nasogastric tubes, earlier resumption of diet, decreased ileus, and earlier return of bowel function. For Crohn's patients, typically a younger population requiring future surgical interventions, laparoscopy offers a smaller wound size with improved cosmesis and likely decreased adhesion formation and a rapid improvement of the quality of life after surgery.

N.T. Nguyen and C.E.H. Scott-Conner (eds.), *The SAGES Manual: Volume 2*   457
Advanced Laparoscopy and Endoscopy, DOI 10.1007/978-1-4614-2347-8_31,
© Springer Science+Business Media, LLC 2012

B. Indications for Surgery

The decision to operate on a patient with Crohn's disease is apparent when the presentation is perforation or massive bleeding (albeit both are unusual presentations). Aside from these emergent indications, the timing of surgery for Crohn's patients is more complicated and should be evaluated carefully on a case-by-case basis. Some important factors when attempting to determine the need for surgery include the patient's clinical course and disease location, complications, and number of relapses. Studies have shown that failure of conservative medical therapy and the presence of obstructive symptoms are reasonable indications. Complications from the disease, such as abscess or fistula, or medical therapy or evidence of dysplasia or cancer are also reasons for surgery.

C. Patient Position, Room Setup, Trocar Position

1. Place the patient in the supine position on a bean bag. Following intubation, insert an orogastric tube and a Foley catheter and place the legs in yellowfin stirrups. While a supine position may be used, in our experience the presence of ileo-sigmoid fistulas in some patients leads us to use a lithotomy position in all patients. Securely tuck the arms at the patient's side and aspirate the bean bag.

2. Place the primary monitor on the right side of the patient toward the patient's head. The secondary monitor is placed on the left side of the patient at the same level. The operating surgeon stands on the left side of the patient and the assistant on the patient's right. Once ports have been placed, the assistant moves to the patient's left side.

3. Gain access by using a modified Hassan approach. A vertical 1-cm infraumbilical incision is made. The fascia is grasped with two Kocher clamps and a 15 blade scalpel is used to open the fascia. A Kelly forcep is used to gain entrance into the peritoneum. A pursestring of 0 polyglyclic acid suture is used around the fascia and secured with a Rommel tourniquet. A 10 mm reusable port is inserted through this site and the abdomen is insufflated to 12 mmHg.

4. Insert a camera through the umbilical port and examine the liver, small bowel, and peritoneal surfaces.

5. Place a 5 mm port in the left lower quadrant about 2–3 cm medial and superior to the anterior superior iliac spine. Insert another 5 mm port in the left upper quadrant at least a hands breath superior to the lower quadrant port. A 5 mm right lower quadrant port may also be inserted on an as-needed basis.

D. Performing Laparoscopic-Assisted Ileocecectomy (Table 31.1)

1. Once the trocars are inserted, the assistant moves to the patient's left side. Tilt the table so that right side is up with a 15–20° tilt. Next, place the patient in slight Trendelenburg position.

2. Insert two atraumatic bowel clamps through the left sided ports and begin by reflecting the greater omentum over the transverse colon. Any small bowel located in the pelvis is reflected into the upper abdomen.

3. Reflect the terminal ileum cephalad to expose the plane between the ileal mesentery and the retroperitoneum. Use electrocautery to dissect the terminal ileum off the retroperitoneal structures. The dissection extends from the ileocecal junction towards the origin of the superior mesenteric artery, as far as the third part of the duodenum.

Table 31.1. Steps for laparoscopic-assisted ileocecectomy.

No. of step	Procedure
1	Port insertion
2	Slight Trendelenburg and rotation to left
3	Reflect omentum over stomach, if necessary take down adhesions
4	Take down fistulas to reduce phlegmon size
5	Drain abscesses, if present
6	Mobilize ileocolic pedicle (medial to lateral)
7	Mobilize hepatic flexure and lateral attachments
8	Mobilize cecum and small bowel mesentery
9	Confirm specimen mobilization
10	Midline or ostomy site extraction

4. The next steps involve mobilization of the ileocecal junction using a lateral to medial approach. Develop the plane between the retroperitoneum and the cecum using scissors and reflect the ascending colon medially and cephalad. Then, mobilize the remaining ascending colon from the paracolic gutter in a lateral to medial approach towards the hepatic flexure.

5. Now, return the patient to supine position by removing the Trendelenburg tilt and the assistant now grasps the transverse colon pushing it inferiorly while the surgeon grasps the distal ascending colon with medial and inferior traction. With the hepatic flexure under tension, divide the gastrocolic ligament.

6. Mobilize the transverse colon using a lateral to medial approach, bringing the entire right colon and its mesentery to the midline.

7. Once this is accomplished, evaluate the mobility of the specimen. The base of the ileal mesentery may have additional attachments that may need to be divided prior to removal of the specimen. Be particularly careful in this area to avoid extensive blood loss or a mesenteric hematoma because the mesentery may be thickened and friable in Crohn's patients.

8. Because of the inflammatory nature of the disease, many patients will have a large phlegmon, abscess, or fistula associated with their disease. In these cases, the pathology is dealt with until resection of the terminal ileum and cecum can be performed. Thus, the omentum is often mobilized off the phlegmon. An abscess may need drainage using a suction to minimize spillage. A fistula can be taken down sharply with scissors and cautery. Often most difficult is retroperitoneal inflammation and psoas abscess, and ureteral stents may selectively be required for these cases. Fistulas to the sigmoid colon may require combined laparoscopic sigmoid colectomy, and once the fistula tract has been taken down, this is performed by the standard technique in Chap. 32.

9. Once the entire right colon, small bowel, and their mesentery have been adequately mobilized, grasp the appendix or cecum and deflate the pneumoperitoneum.

10. Remove the umbilical port and extend the site into a 3–4 cm midline incision. Laparoscopic takedown of omentum, abscesses, and fistulas allows the specimen to be removed

through a small incision; however, the wound may require some extension for larger phlegmons. Determine an appropriate 2 cm margin on the distal small bowel and divide the small bowel mesentery extracorporally using 0 polygalactin ties for hemostasis. Divide the ascending colon mesentery with cautery and ligate vessels with 0 polygylcolate ties. Then, divide the small bowel and colon with a stapler, and perform a side-to-side anastomosis. Check the anastomosis for hemostasis and return it to abdomen.

11. The small bowel may be sequentially exteriorized and palpated through the midline incision up to the duodenojejunal flexure, to completely assess for Crohn's disease. Once this inspection is complete, close the fascia with interrupted figure of eight 1 polydioxanone sutures. Irrigate the wound and close it with 4/0 polyglycolate suture in a subcuticular fashion.

E. Performing Laparoscopic-Assisted Strictureplasty or Small Bowel Resection

Strictureplasty for Crohn's disease was a technique adopted by Katariya et al. applied to patients with small bowel strictures for intestinal length preservation and the avoidance of short bowel syndrome.

1. For patients with small bowel disease alone, a similar mobilization to ileocecectomy is performed, although the hepatic flexure is only mobilized selectively, and a small bowel resection performed in similar fashion.

2. Once the patient is positioned appropriately and the trocars are inserted similar to placement described above, the small bowel is carefully examined to confirm adequate mobilization. The terminal ileum and cecum are usually mobilized to ensure adequate mesenteric reach.

3. Strictured areas may be found laparoscopically and marked with a silk suture or the strictured segment may be grasped with an atraumatic bowel clamp and exteriorized through a vertical infraumbilical incision; however, we generally exteriorize and palpate the entire small bowel so that more subtle disease is not missed.

4. Identical to the open technique for strictureplasty, two common techniques are employed, generally Heinecke-Mikulicz for strictures less than 10 cm and Finney for strictures between 10 and 20 cm (Figs. 31.1 and 31.2). For a Heinecke-Mikulicz strictureplasty, make a longitudinal incision through the stricture, extending 3 cm onto normal bowel on either side. Then, close the bowel transversely using interrupted 3/0 absorbable sutures.

5. With a Finney strictureplasty, place the bowel in a U-shaped position and open the strictured area on the antimesenteric margin, and then close it in a side-to-side fashion.

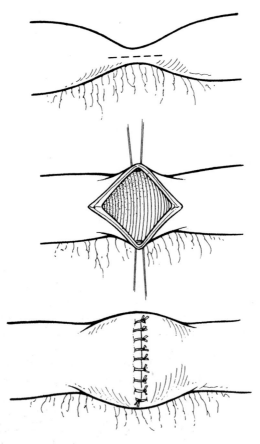

Fig. 31.1. For a short stricture, open the bowel longitudinally and close it transversely as shown.

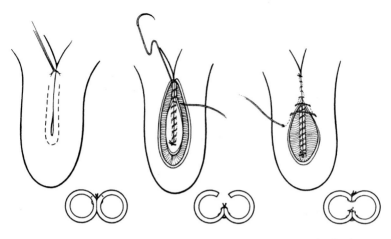

Fig. 31.2. Longer strictures may be manages by a Finney-type plastic closure, essentially a side-to-side anastomosis.

6. After performing the appropriate strictureplasty, return the bowel to the intra-abdominal compartment and close the wound in layers as above.

F. Reasons for Conversion

In some cases, the pathology may include difficult conditions, such as abscesses, masses, fistulae, or multiple strictures. More problematic are extensive adhesions from prior open surgery, and these may in some cases lead to conversion to an open procedure. The most common reason for conversion by Reissmann et al. was an inflammatory mass with an enterocutaneous fistula. In another study, the most common reasons for conversion were adhesions, followed by inflammation and size of inflammatory mass. The published conversion rates for laparoscopic surgery in Crohn's disease are 0-40% (Table 31.2). Patients who required conversion to open procedure have been compared to patients undergoing an open procedure with no significant differences in operative times, length of stay, outcomes, and morbidity as well as cost. Overall, the reasons for conversion in patients with Crohn's disease depend on the complexity of the disease but more particularly on the individual skill and experience, and comfort level of the operating surgeon.

Table 31.2. Laparoscopic-assisted resection for Crohn's disease.

Author	No. of patients	Major procedures	Conversion (%)	Reasons for conversion
Bauer et al.	18	Ileocolic resection	22	Large fixed mass, fistula
Kreissler-Haag et al.	20	Ileocolic, small bowel	0	None
Milsom et al.	9	Ileocolic resection	0	None
Schmidt et al.	113	Ileocecectomy, small bowel resection, strictureplasty	40	Adhesions, extent of disease, mass size, fistula, inability to assess anatomy
Duepree et al.	21	Ileocolic resection, small bowel, strictureplasty	4.8	Extent of disease
Reissman et al.	51	Ileocolic resection	14	Large mass, fistula, bleeding

Selected References

Alos R, Hinojosa J. Timing of surgery in Crohn's disease: a key issue in the management. World J Gastroenterol. 2008;14(36):5532–9.

Bauer J, Harris MT, Grumbach NM, Gorfine SR. Laparoscopic assisted intestinal resection for Crohn's disease. Dis Colon Rectum. 1995;38:712–5.

Bernell O, Lapidus A, Hellers G. Risk factors for surgery and recurrence in 907 patients with primary ileocaecal Crohn's disease. Br J Surg. 2000;87:1697–701.

Casillas S, Delaney CP. Laparoscopic surgery for inflammatory bowel disease. Dig Surg. 2005;22:135–42.

Delaney CP, Fazio VW. Crohn's disease of the small bowel. Surg Clin North Am. 2001;81(1):137–58.

Delaney CP, Kiran RP, Senagore AJ, O'Brien-Ermlich B, Church J, Hull TL, Remzi FH, Fazio VW. Quality of life improves within 30 days of surgery for Crohn's disease. J Am Coll Surg. 2003;196(5):714–21.

Duepree HJ, Senagore AJ, Delaney CP, Brady KM, Fazio VW. Advantages of laparoscopic resection for ileocecal Crohn's disease. Dis Colon Rectum. 2002;45(5):605–10.

Gardiner KR, Dasari BVM. Operative management of small bowel Crohn's disease. Surg Clin North Am. 2007;87:587–610.

Katariya RN, Sood S, Rao PG, et al. Strictureplasty for tubercular strictures of the gastrointestinal tract. Br J Surg. 1977;64:496–8.

Kiran RP, Delaney CP, Senagore AJ, O'Brien-Ermlich B, Mascha E, Thornton J, Fazio VW. Prospective assessment of Cleveland Global Quality of Life (CGQL) as a novel marker of quality of life and disease activity in Crohn's disease. Am J Gastroenterol. 2003;98(8):1783–9.

Kreissler-Haag D, Hildebrandt U, Pistorius G, et al. Laparoscopic surgery in Crohn' disease. Surg Endosc. 1994;8:1002 (Abstract).

Lee ECG, Papaioannou N. Minimal surgery for chronic obstruction in patients with extensive or universal Crohn's disease. Ann R Coll Surg Engl. 1982;64:229–33.

Ludwig KA, Milsom JW, Church JM, Fazio VW. Preliminary experience with laparoscopic intestinal surgery for Crohn's disease. Am J Surg. 1996;171:52–6.

Maartense S, Dunker MS, Slors JF, et al. Laparoscopic-assisted versus open ileocolic resection for Crohn's disease, a randomized trial. Ann Surg. 2006;243:143–9.

Milsom JW, Lavery IC, Bohm MB, Fazio VW. Laparoscopically assisted ileocecotomy in Crohn's disease. Surg Laparosc Endosc. 1993;3:77–80.

Milsom JW, Hammerhofer KA, Bohm B, Marcello P, Elson P, Fazio VW. Prospective, randomized trial comparing laparoscopic vs. conventional surgery for refractory ileocolic Crohn's disease. Dis Colon Rectum. 2001;44(1):1–9.

Naidu MN, Trang AC, Salky BA. Laparoscopy in Crohn's disease. Clin Colon Rectal Surg. 2007;20:329–35.

Pokala N, Delaney CP, Brady K, Senagore AJ. Elective laparoscopic surgery for benign internal enteric fistulae. Surg Endosc. 2005;19:222–5.

Reissman P, Salky BA, Edye M, Wexner SD. Laparoscopic surgery in Crohn's disease. Surg Endosc. 1996;10:1201–4.

Schmidt CM, Talamini MA, Kaufman HS, Lilliemoe KD, Learn P, Bayless T. Laparoscopic surgery for Crohn's disease: reasons for conversion. Ann Surg. 2001;233(6):733–9.

32. Laparoscopic Segmental Colectomy

Steven D. Wexner, M.D.
Marylise Boutros, M.D.

A. Indications

1. **Laparoscopic colon resection** may be considered whenever resection of a segment of colon is required. Rectal resection and total colectomy are discussed in later chapters. Laparoscopic segmental colectomy is most commonly performed for one of the following indications:
   a. Colon cancer
   b. Endoscopically unresectable polyps
   c. Diverticulitis
   d. Crohn's disease
   e. Volvulus
   f. Endometriosis
   g. Rectal prolapse

B. Patient Position and Room Setup

1. Position the patient supine on the operating table with both arms tucked, padded, and protected at the sides. Ensure that the patient is well secured to the table using an inflatable bean bag and/or padded foam and adhesive tape (across the chest).
2. Place the patient in a modified lithotomy position using Allen stirrups (Lloyd-Davies or other designs may be used). It is imperative that the thighs are at or lower than the level of the abdominal wall to obviate difficulty in maneuvering the lower

abdominal instruments. Regardless of the type of planned segmental resection, this position is preferred as it allows the greatest flexibility for the surgeon's position and enables intra-operative colonoscopy (if needed), as well as the introduction of a circular stapler through the anus for construction of a low anastomosis.

3. In general, the surgeon stands on the side of the patient opposite the pathology and site of dissection, with the first assistant standing across the table.

    a. Thus, for **right hemicolectomy or ileocolic resection**, the surgeon typically stands on the patient's left side. At times, it may be beneficial to stand between the patient's legs. Two monitors are placed at the right side of the patient (one by the head of the table and one more caudad).

    b. For **left colon resections** (including abdominoperineal resection), the surgeon usually stands on the patient's right side. During mobilization of the splenic flexure, it may be easier to stand between the patient's legs. Two monitors are placed at the left side of the patient (one by the foot of the table and one more cephalad).

4. **Trocar position and choice of laparoscope** are discussed with each individual procedure. In general, it is the authors' preference to use 10/12-mm trocars for all the ports so that a 10-mm camera and an endoscopic stapler can be inserted in any trocar. A 10-mm 30° laparoscope is preferred.

C. Special Instruments and Equipment

1. **Graspers**: It is important to choose graspers that have a firm grip on the bowel wall without causing any trauma to the serosa. There are several options available, including endoscopic babcocks (5 or 10 mm), atraumatic bowel graspers (5 or 10 mm), or padded bowel graspers (5 mm). It is not advisable to use any graspers with a rachet locking mechanism to manipulate the bowel during mobilization.

2. **Devices for vascular division**: There are several options for intracorporeal ligation of the ileocolic artery, inferior mesenteric artery or vein, and superior rectal artery. Although all are reliable methods, it is important to be aware of all methods

and have equipment available as backup if any vessel ligation failure were to occur.

- a. **Energy sources**: Electrothermal bipolar vessel sealers include LigaSure™ (Valleylab, Boulder, CO), available for 5- or 10-mm trocars, and EnSeal™ (Ethicon Endo-Surgery, Cincinnati, Ohio), available for 5-mm trocars. Use of a 5-mm instrument usually requires multiple fires.
- b. **Endoscopic staplers**: These must be used through a 10/12-mm trocar. A vascular (white) stapler cartridge is recommended.
- c. **Endoscopic clips**: 10-mm clips may be used to ligate any of the aforementioned vessels.

3. **Dissectors**: Cautery scissors (endoscopic scissors with cautery attached) can be used through a 5-mm trocar. Alternatively, 5-mm energy devices are suitable dissecting tools and can also be used to divide the colon mesentery. Two available types include ultrasonic shears (Harmonic™ Scalpel, Ethicon Endo-Surgery, Cinicinnati, Ohio) or electrothemal bipolar vessel sealers (LigaSure™ or EnSeal™).

4. **Wound protector**: This is used to protect the skin edges from contamination and to assist in wound retraction and extraction of the colon. An Alexis (Applied Medical, Rancho Santa Margarita, CA) or other similar self-expanding wound protector is ideal.

D. Approaches for Laparoscopic Segmental Colectomy

1. **Laparoscopic right hemicolectomy** can be performed by a lateral-to-medial, medial-to-lateral, or caudal-to-cephalic approach.
2. **Laparoscopic left hemicolectomy** can be performed by a lateral-to-medial or medial-to-lateral approach.
3. Each approach has its advantages. A lateral-to-medial approach approximates the open technique familiar to many surgeons. A medial-to-lateral approach prioritizes vessel isolation and division as the first step of the operation. A caudal-to-cephalic approach allows identification of the ureter early on in the operation.

4.   Familiarity with all approaches equips the surgeon with versatility to tackle unclear anatomy and unexpected intraoperative findings.

E. Performing the Laparoscopic-Assisted Ileocolic Resection or Right Hemicolectomy

1.   Perform a vertical supraumbilical incision within the site of the planned incision for specimen extraction to place the **camera port (10/12 mm)** using an open Hasson technique. In certain instances where an infraumbilical extraction may be possible (based on pathology and patient's body habitus), this site may be used.

2.   Insert a **30° laparoscope** through this trocar and establish pneumoperitoneum to 15-mm Hg with carbon dioxide.

3.   **Two other trocars are required**: Place one in the left lower quadrant and one in the left mid abdomen, both lateral to the rectus muscles.

4.   **Additional trocars** may be needed for retractors. These are generally placed in the right upper or lower quadrant (lateral to the rectus muscles). Occasionally, an additional trocar may be placed high in the left upper quadrant (this may be needed for division of the gastrocolic ligament by allowing simultaneous retraction of the greater omentum cephalad and the transverse colon caudad) (Fig 32.1).

5.   A thorough inspection of the liver and the peritoneal cavity is required for patients with cancer to exclude any metastatic disease.

6.   Position the patient in steep Trendelenburg with the left side of the table down.

7.   Gently bring the small bowel out of the pelvis and sweep it into the left upper quadrant.

1. Lateral-to-Medial Approach

8.   Identify the terminal ileum and base of cecum. Grasp the cecum with an endoscopic grasper and retract it toward the left upper quadrant (Fig. 32.2).

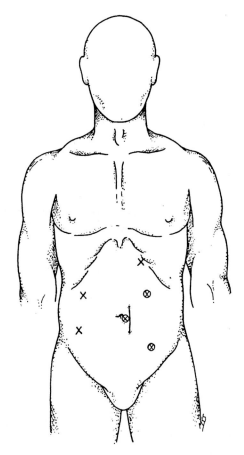

Fig. 32.1. Positions of trocars for laparoscopic ileocolic resection and right hemicolectomy. The small midline incision is made as an extension of the Hasson trocar site and is used for exteriorization of the specimen: ⊗, typical trocars; X, optional additional trocars.

9. Starting at the cecum, incise along the white line of Toldt with a 5-mm energy device or electrocautery scissors. Continue to mobilize the right colon superiorly to the level of the hepatic flexure.

10. Continually regrasp and manipulate the right colon as needed to maintain adequate superomedial traction. This facilitates medial dissection and exposes the ureter, Gerota's fascia, and duodenum. Once the duodenum is visualized, the extent of this dissection is complete.

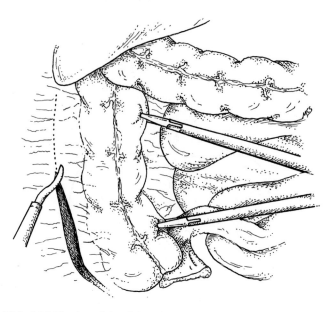

Fig. 32.2. Mobilization of the right colon. One or two graspers are used to pull the colon medially as the white line of Toldt is incised.

11. Reposition the patient in reverse Trendelenburg. Grasp the greater omentum and lift it cephalad. Begin to divide the gastro-colic ligament at the level of the middle colic artery, distal to the gastroepiploic vessels, heading toward the hepatic flexure. Inferior traction on the transverse colon allows the duodenum to be visualized.

12. Finally, grasp the hepatic flexure and retract it inferomedially. This allows identification of any remaining hepatocolic liga-ment that may be divided with a 5-mm energy device or electro-cautery scissors. When using electrocautery scissors, it is necessary to have ligaclips or endoclips available as bleeding may occur. Once the duodenum is clearly visualized and the right colon can easily (without tension) reach the extraction site, the extent of this dissection is complete.

13. Once the right colon has been completely mobilized as described, grasp the cecum with a locking forcep.

14. At the site of the initial trocar (camera port) in the supraumbili-cal position, make a 2- to 4-cm vertical incision in the skin and the fascia to allow extraction of the colon.

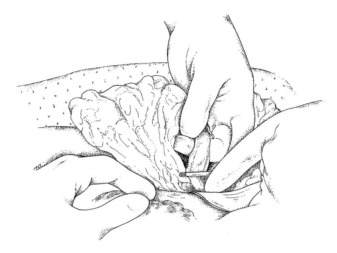

Fig. 32.3. Terminal ileum, cecum, ascending and proximal transverse colon eviscerated through the small incision. Extracorporeal resection and anastomosis are performed and the anastomosis is then returned to the abdominal cavity.

15. Allow the pneumoperitoneum to collapse and place a wound protector (usually, a small to medium size is required). An Alexis® or other similar self-expanding wound protector is ideal.

16. Deliver the cecum through the midline wound, and eviscerate the terminal ileum, cecum, and ascending and proximal transverse colon onto the abdominal wall (Fig. 32.3).

   a. The vascular ligation, bowel division, and anastomosis are performed as they would be during a laparotomy.

   b. The mesenteric defect may be closed in its entirety if it is feasible or it may be left open.

   c. Typically, a stapled functional end-to-end anastomosis is performed.

   d. When the anastomosis is complete, return it to the abdominal cavity, taking great care not to damage or tear the bowel or mesentery during this manipulation.

   e. Close the incision using interrupted absorbable sutures.

17. Reestablish pneumoperitoneum through one of the other trocar sites, and insert a laparoscope (at this point, a 5-mm 30° laparoscope may be used if only 5-mm trocars remain).

18. Inspect the bowel, anastomosis, and abdomen; irrigate and assure hemostasis.

19.   Close the fascia of all 10/12-mm trocar sites in the usual fashion.

2. Medial-to-Lateral Approach

20.   Using an endoscopic grasper (in the left lower quadrant trocar), apply right superolateral traction on the mesentery by elevating the cecum at the junction of the bowel and the mesentery. Identify the ileocolic artery.

21.   Isolate the ileocolic artery by scoring the mesentery and creating windows in the mesentery on each side of the artery. This vessel can be divided using electrothermal bipolar vessel sealing devices, an endoscopic stapler, or endoscopic clips. Typically, any of these devices are introduced through the left midabdominal trocar for an optimal angle. Prior to ligation, visualize the tissue on either side of the vessel and ensure that nothing else is incorporated in the ligation. After confirming satisfactory positioning, perform vessel ligation (Fig. 32.4).

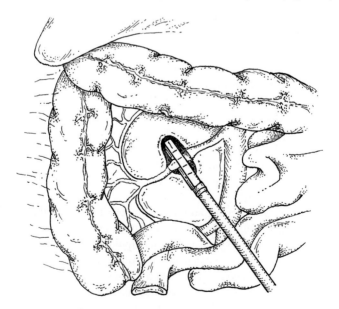

Fig. 32.4. Intracorporeal division of the ileocolic pedicle. The ileocolic artery is identified by superolateral traction of the mesentery and is ligated after creation of a mesenteric window on either side.

22. Divide the thin mesentery between the ileocolic and the middle colic artery.
23. Proceed to the lateral mobilization as described above (in lateral-to-medial approach: Steps 8–19).

3. Caudal-to-Cephalic Approach

24. Using an endoscopic grasper (in the left midabdominal trocar), elevate the terminal ileum superomedially.
25. Begin to dissect the ileal peritoneal attachments to the pelvic brim. Proceed in a cephalad direction, continually elevating the cecum and right colon off the retroperitoneum.
26. Continually regrasp and manipulate the right colon as needed to maintain adequate superomedial traction. This facilitates cephalad dissection and exposes the ureter, Gerota's fascia, and duodenum. Once the duodenum is visualized, the extent of this dissection is complete.
27. Proceed to mobilization of the transverse colon and hepatic flexure as described above (in lateral-to-medial approach: steps 11–19).

F. Performing the Laparoscopic-Assisted Left Hemicolectomy/Sigmoid Resection

1. Perform a vertical supraumbilical incision within the site of the planned incision for specimen extraction to place the **camera port (10/12 mm)** using an open Hasson technique. In certain instances where an infraumbilical extraction may be possible (based on pathology and patient's body habitus), this site may be used.
2. Insert a **30° laparoscope** through this trocar and establish pneumoperitoneum to 15-mm Hg with carbon dioxide.
3. **Two other trocars are required**: Place one trocar in the right upper quadrant and one in the right lower quadrant (will be used for endoscopic stapler), both lateral to the rectus muscle.
4. **Additional trocars**: A third trocar may be placed in the left lower quadrant to aid in mobilization of the splenic flexure

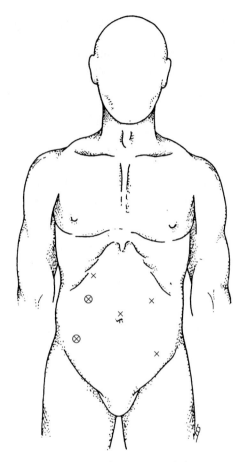

Fig. 32.5. Positions of trocars for laparoscopic left hemicolectomy and sigmoid resection. The small midline incision is made as an extension of the Hasson trocar site and is used for exteriorization of the specimen. ⊗, typical trocars; X, optional additional trocars.

(surgeon standing in between the legs using the right and left lower quadrant trocars). A left upper quadrant trocar placed lateral to the rectus muscle may be used for additional retraction. This site also provides an excellent vantage point for laparoscopic visualization of the anastomosis. A fifth trocar is sometimes placed high in the right upper quadrant if needed (Fig. 32.5).

5. A thorough inspection of the liver and the peritoneal cavity is required for patients with cancer to exclude any metastatic disease.

6. Place the patient in **steep Trendelenburg position** with the right side of the table down.

7. Gently bring the small bowel out of the pelvis and sweep it into the right upper quadrant.

1. Lateral-to-Medial Approach

8. Grasp the sigmoid colon with an endoscopic grasper and retract it medially to expose the white line of Toldt.

9. Using either a 5-mm energy device or cautery scissors, incise the peritoneum to mobilize the sigmoid and left colon to the level of the splenic flexure.

10. Continually regrasp and manipulate the left colon/sigmoid as needed to maintain adequate superomedial tract. This facilitates the dissection as it progresses medially to expose Gerota's fascia, ureter, and sacral promontory (Fig. 32.6).

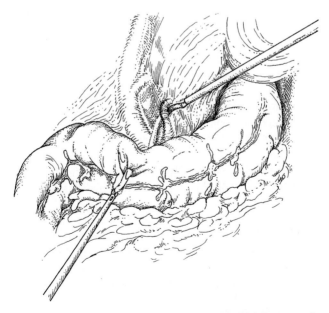

Fig. 32.6. Mobilization of the sigmoid colon to expose the left ureter as it crosses the pelvic brim. The iliac vessels are seen to the left of the ureter.

11. Next, reposition the patient in reverse Trendelenburg.

12. Mobilize the splenic flexure and distal transverse colon.

13. Grasp the greater omentum and lift it cephalad. Divide the gastrocolic omentum to the level of the middle colic artery.

14. Grasp the transverse colon with an endoscopic grasper and dissect the transverse colon and splenic flexure free of the retroperitoneum inferior to the spleen.

15. After complete mobilization, intracorporeally ligate the vascular pedicle.

   a. Medially isolate either the superior hemorrhoidal and the left colic arteries or the inferior mesenteric artery.

   b. Anterolateral retraction of the left colon facilitates this identification.

   c. **Isolate the vessels** by scoring the mesentery and creating windows in the mesentery on each side.

   d. These vessels can be divided using electrothermal bipolar vessel sealing devices, an endoscopic stapler, or endoscopic clips. Typically, any of these devices are introduced through the right lower quadrant trocar for an optimal angle.

   e. Prior to ligation, visualize the tissue on either side of the vessel and reconfirm the location of the ureter. **This is crucial** to ensure that nothing else is incorporated in the ligation. After confirming satisfactory positioning, perform vessel ligation.

   f. Continue dividing the mesentery heading cephalad and identify the inferior mesenteric vein. Isolate and divide the vein using electrothermal bipolar vessel sealers, clips, or an endoscopic stapler.

   g. Typically, only the above-named vessels are divided in this manner.

16. After isolating the smaller vessels in the sigmoid mesentery, control them with clips, electrothermal bipolar vessel sealers, or ultrasonic shears.

17. Choose the distal extent of resection and circumferentially expose the colonic or rectal wall. This may be performed using an energy source or a cautery-hook dissector, and at times curved dissector (such as Maryland forceps) may be useful to develop the plane between the bowel wall and the mesocolon. Bare colon or rectal wall should be demonstrated circumferentially.

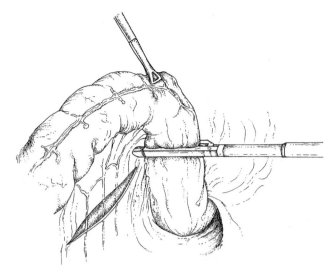

Fig. 32.7. The endoscopic linear stapler is used to divide the bowel at the distal resection margin.

18. Insert a 60-mm linear cutting stapler, encompass the bowel wall between the blades (making sure that laterally nothing else is incorporated into the blades), and fire the stapler (Fig. 32.7).

19. Once the left colon and sigmoid have been completely mobilized as described, grasp the proximal stapled colon end with a locking forcep.

20. At the site of the initial trocar (camera trocar) in the infraumbilical position, make a 2- to 4-cm vertical incision in the skin and the fascia to allow extraction of the colon. Alternatively, a small Pfannenstiel left lower quadrant or lower midline incision can be used.

21. Allow the pneumoperitoneum to collapse and place an Alexis® or other similar wound protector (usually, a small to medium size is required).

22. Deliver the colon through the midline wound, and eviscerate the left colon and sigmoid on the abdominal wall.

23. Perform the proximal resection extracorporeally in the conventional fashion. Place a purse-string suture and insert the circular stapling anvil into the proximal end of bowel. Secure the purse-string suture and replace the bowel into the abdominal cavity (Fig. 32.8).

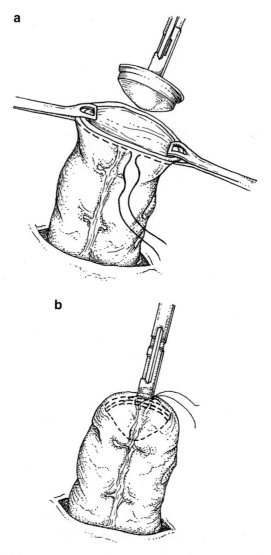

Fig. 32.8. (**a**) The anvil of the circular stapler is inserted in the proximal end of the bowel (which has been drawn out of the abdomen through a small incision). (**b**) The purse-string suture is tied. The bowel is then returned to the abdomen.

24.   In order to reestablish pneumoperitoneum, we recommend closing the fascia with two running absorbable sutures (one starting superiorly and one inferiorly) and leaving the ends untied in order to allow replacement of the Hasson trocar.

The sutures should be fastened to the trocar and should be long enough so that they can be tied at the end of the operation.

25. Grasp the anvil with a laparoscopic anvil-grasping clamp or alligator clamp. Assess the ability of the anvil to reach the planned anastomotic site. Further mobilization and/or vascular division may be needed, and should be performed if necessary.

26. Verify the correct orientation (i.e., no twist) for the proximal bowel.

27. Transanally insert a circular stapler and advance it to the distal staple line. Under direct laparoscopic visual control, extend the spike of the stapler through the distal staple line. Attach the anvil (Fig. 32.9).

28. Move the laparoscope to the right lower quadrant trocar to best visualize the anvil and stapler head coming together. Once satisfied, close, fire, and remove the stapler. Inspect the two donuts for completeness.

29. Test the anastomosis by placing an atraumatic clamp across the bowel proximal to the anastomosis. Use the suction irrigator, fill the pelvis with saline, and immerse the anastomosis. Insufflate the rectum with air using a bulb syringe, proctoscope, or flexible sigmoidoscope, and observe for air bubbles.

30. Irrigate the abdomen, obtain hemostasis, and close the trocar sites.

31. Remove the Hasson trocar and complete the closure of the small midline incision with the two sutures that were placed earlier on (in Step 24). Close the fascia of all 10/12-mm trocar sites in the usual fashion.

2. Medial-to-Lateral Approach

32. This approach starts with identification of the inferior mesenteric artery and its ligation.

33. Using an endoscopic grasper, retract the sigmoid colon superolaterally and identify the inferior mesenteric artery.

34. Proceed as described above (Steps 15c–g).

35. Proceed with lateral mobilization of the left colon and sigmoid as described above (Steps 8–14), followed by Steps 16–31 to complete the procedure.

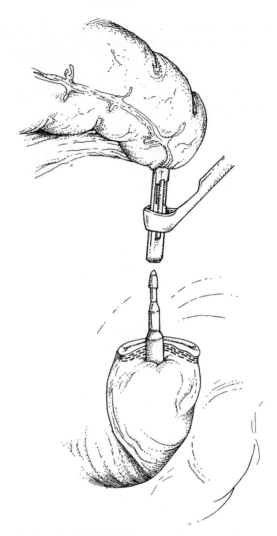

Fig. 32.9. The anvil is attached to the circular stapler (which has passed transanally); the stapler is closed and fired in the usual fashion.

G. Common Errors

1.   Trocar placement can facilitate or substantially hinder the operation. In order to ensure ease of instrument handling, place all trocars at least 1 hand span apart and at least 2 fingerbreadths

above and medial to the anterior superior iliac spine. Ensure that the trocars are not in the direct trajectory of the camera. In obese patients and patients with prior abdominal surgery, trocar insertion might be more complicated and time consuming; however, well-placed trocars will be of much assistance for the remainder of the case.

2. During lateral mobilization in right or left/sigmoid colectomy, a common error is to dissect too laterally on the abdominal wall resulting in retroperitoneal dissection and mobilization of the kidney. The dissection plane should be continually verified and brought medially as the colon is mobilized.

3. Traction and countertraction are of paramount importance in order to identify and dissect the correct planes. However, too much inadvertent traction causes serosal tears and splenic lacerations. Continually verify the site of endoscopic grasper application on the bowel to assess for such injuries.

4. One of the drawbacks of laparoscopy is loss of tactile feedback; thus, for endoscopically unresectable polyps, ensure that the colon is tattooed in all quadrants just distal to the lesion. Also, if the lesion could not be laparoscopically identified, availability of intraoperative endoscopy is important. In this case, carbon dioxide endoscopy is preferred because of its rapid absorption, which minimizes colonic distention and thus does not impede subsequent laparoscopic visualization. Finally, for such lesions, it is imperative that the resected colon is opened and examined for the desired lesion prior to fashioning the anastomosis.

H. Special Considerations

The following patient and disease factors increase the technical complexity of a laparoscopic colectomy. However, it has been demonstrated that laparoscopic segmental colectomy is safe and feasible, and renders good outcomes in each of these situations. It is important to anticipate the technical challenges that one may be faced with and to have careful operative planning.

1. **Obesity**
   a. Use of optical trocars (such as Visiport™) with a 0° laparoscope can be helpful for insertion of the first trocar

(camera trocar) under direct visualization in morbidly obese patients with thick subcutaneous tissue.

b.   Use of additional trocars and greater availability of instruments in the peritoneal cavity may assist in retracting the heavier, fatty mesentery and achieving adequate exposure.

c.   In many of these patients, the mesentery may be foreshortened; thus, intracoporeal vessel ligation may be necessary in order to exteriorize the colon through a small incision.

d.   Manipulation of the fatty mesentery is difficult in obese patients and obtaining hemostasis is often difficult. We recommend the use of energy devices (such as LigaSure™ or Harmonic scalpel™) for any dissection during laparoscopic colectomy in these patients.

2.   **Crohn's disease**

a.   In patients with Crohn's disease, it is imperative to "carefully inspect" the entire small bowel to find or exclude concomitant strictures, fistulae, or masses. Accomplish this maneuver by a "hand-over-hand" technique using two endoscopic graspers under direct vision.

b.   These patients often have fragile tissues and friable mesentery because of disease severity and immunosuppressants. We recommend the use of energy devices (such as LigaSure™ or Harmonic scalpel™) for any dissection during laparoscopic colectomy in these patients.

c.   Furthermore, the colon mesentery may be foreshortened. Ligation of the mesentery may be performed intracorporeally if a thin, less diseased area closer to the root of the mesentery can be identified. Alternatively, if the mesentery is too friable, extracorporeal vessel ligation may be necessary.

d.   In patients with recurrent disease or those with abscess, phlegmon, or fistula, the case complexity is further increased. Again, it is safe and feasible to perform laparoscopic colectomy in these cases; however, a judicious early threshold for conversion is important.

3.   **Reoperative surgery**

a.   Place the initial trocar away from areas of previous incisions. This may necessitate camera port placement off the midline. This can be done using an open Hasson technique with a muscle splitting approach or using an optical trocar.

b. Adhesiolysis should be performed in order to achieve appropriate exposure. Careful dissection is important in order to avoid bowel injuries. Use of meticulous sharp dissection is the preferred method of adhesiolysis, with limited use of energy devices as loops of bowel may be hidden by adhesive bands. Also, excessive traction on adhesions involving bowel should be avoided.

c. It is safe and feasible to perform laparoscopic colectomy in these cases; however, a judicious early threshold for conversion is important.

I. Complications

1. **Anastomotic leak**

    a. **Cause and prevention**: A well-vascularized, tension-free, circumferentially intact anastomosis is necessary to prevent anastomotic leakage. If any of the foregoing requirements are not present during a laparoscopic-assisted colectomy, then the anastomosis must be revised. It is often prudent, if not mandatory, to convert to a laparotomy at this point. Identification of ischemia may be difficult and the aid of intravenous fluorescein should be used. One ampule of fluorescein given intravenously followed by inspection with a Wood's lamp allows for identification of ischemic bowel. Resection proximally to viable colon alleviates this problem. Intraoperative testing of the anastomosis is mandatory as described earlier. Any leak requires, at minimum, reinforcement if not complete revision. The use of only a diverting stoma to protect such an anastomosis is inadequate.

    b. **Recognition and management**: Postoperative fevers, prolonged ileus, elevated leukocyte counts, and abdominal pain are all hallmarks of postoperative anastomotic leak. Aggressive detection and delineation often allow conservative therapy to be employed. Perform prompt radiologic evaluation of the anastomosis using a water-soluble contrast enema in concert with a computed tomography scan of the abdomen and pelvis. If a small leak or a leak associated with a localized abscess is identified, percutaneous drainage, antibiotics, bowel rest, and total parenteral nutrition often allow for spontaneous closure. If a large, free leak is identified, prompt surgical intervention with stoma creation is necessary.

2. **Anastomotic bleed**

   a. **Cause and prevention**: This complication can be reduced by careful intraoperative inspection of the staple line. In the case of a stapled side-to-side/functional end-to-end anastomosis, the incidence of this complication can be minimized by ensuring that the antimesenteric borders of each limb are used to construct the anastomosis. Also, before closing the enterotomy through which the linear stapler was fired, evert the edges of the bowel and inspect the staple line. Areas of bleeding can be controlled with sutures. In an end-to-end low colocolonic or colorectal anastomosis, we advocate intraoperative flexible endoscopy to assess the staple line. Endoscopic clips can be applied to the staple line if active bleeding is found. Routine intraoperative endoscopy after circular stapled distal anastomosis has been shown to reduce the combined incidence of bleeding and leak as compared to simple nonoptical air insufflation.

   b. **Recognition and management**: Most anastomotic bleeding identified postoperatively is minor and stops spontaneously. However, in rare instances, bleeding can be massive and may necessitate transfusion and intervention. Depending on the extent of the bleeding and the postoperative timing, bleeding can be managed surgically or endoscopically. Immediate postoperative massive bleeding is better managed by laparotomy, whereas anastomotic bleeding later in the postoperative period or of less severity is better initially diagnosed and managed endoscopically.

3. **Postoperative small bowel obstruction**

   a. **Cause and prevention**: Postoperative small bowel obstruction is almost universally caused by adhesion formation. Postoperative adhesions may be less common with the laparoscopic approach. However, internal hernias or trocar site hernias may still occur. Closing all trocar sites of 10 mm or greater should help minimize this problem. It is important to close both anterior and posterior fascia, as trocar site hernias through the posterior fascia have been reported.

b. **Recognition and management**: Abdominal distention, cessation, or no passage of flatus and the inability to tolerate oral intake associated with nausea or vomiting are all common signs and symptoms of small bowel obstruction. When these symptoms occur early in the postoperative course (3–10 days), it is often difficult to distinguish a bowel obstruction from a normal postoperative ileus. Initial management is similar in both cases with nasogastric tube decompression, intravenous fluids, and possibly nutritional support. This conservative management may continue in the absence of fevers, rising white blood counts, or peritonitis (which would indicate leak; see above). Consider evaluation of the trocar sites via CT scan in any patient who develops a bowel obstruction after a laparoscopic procedure. Failure to resolve mandates reexploration for lysis of adhesions and possible bowel resection. If possible, the addition of an antiadhesion product should be employed to prevent further postoperative adhesions.

Selected References

Braga M, Vignalli A, Gianotti L, et al. Laparoscopic versus open colorectal surgery: a randomized trial on short-term outcome. Ann Surg. 2002;236:759–67.

Clinical outcomes of surgical therapy study group. A comparison of laparoscopically assisted and open colectomy for colon cancer. N Engl J Med. 2004;350:2050–9.

Cohen SM, Wexner SD. Laparoscopic right hemicolectomy. In: Lezoche E, Paganini AM, Cuschieri A, editors. Minimally invasive surgery. Milan, Italy: Documento Editoriale; 1994. p. 23–6.

Duepree HJ, Senagore AJ, Delaney CP, Brady KM, Fazio VW. Advantages of laparoscopic resection for ileocecal Crohn's disease. Dis Colon Rectum. 2002;45:605–10.

Guillou PJ, Quirke P, Thorpe H, et al. Short-term endpoints of conventional versus laparoscopic-assisted surgery in patients with colorectal cancer MRC CLASICC trial: multicentre, randomised controlled trial. Lancet. 2005;365:1718.

Hamel CT, Hildebrandt U, Weiss EG, Feifelz G, Wexner SD. Laparoscopic surgery for inflammatory bowel disease. Surg Endosc. 2001;15:642–5.

Hewett PJ, Allardyce RA, Bagshaw PF, et al. Short-term outcomes of the Australasian randomized clinical study comparing laparoscopic and conventional open surgical treatments for colon cancer: the ALCCaS trial. Ann Surg. 2008;248:728–38.

Hong D, Lewis M, Tabet J, Anvari M. Prospective comparison of laparoscopic versus open resection for benign colorectal disease. Surg Laparosc Endosc Percutan Techniques. 2002;12:238–42.

Jacobs M, Verdeja JC, Goldstein MD. Minimally invasive colon resection (laparoscopic colectomy). Surg Laparosc Endosc. 1991;1:144–50.

Lacy AM, Garcia-Valdercasas JC, Delgado S, Grande L, et al. Postoperative complications of laparoscopic assisted colectomy. Surg Endosc. 1997;11:119–22.

Lacy AM, Garcia-Valdecassas JC, Delgado S, et al. Laparoscopy-assisted colectomy versus open colectomy for treatment of nonmetastatic colon cancer: a randomized trial. Lancet. 2002;359:2224–9.

Lascano CA, Kaidar-Person O, Szomstein S, et al. Challenges of laparoscopic colectomy in the obese patient: a review. Am J Surg. 2006;192:357–65.

Marcello P. Laparoscopy for inflammatory bowel disease: pushing the envelope. Clin Colon Rectal Surg. 2006;19(1):26–32.

Marcello PW, Milsom JW, Wong SK, et al. Laparoscopic restorative proctocolectomy: case-matched comparative study with open restorative proctocolectomy. Dis Colon Rectum. 2000;43:604–8.

Milsom JW, Hammerhofer KA, Bohm B, Marcello P, Elson P, Fazio VW. Prospective randomized trial comparing laparoscopic versus open conventional surgery for refractory ileocolic Crohn's disease. Dis Colon Rectum. 2001;44:1–8.

Neudecker J, Klein F, Bittner R, et al. Short-term outcomes from a prospective randomized trial comparing laparoscopic and open surgery for colorectal cancer. Br J Surg. 2009;96:1458–67.

Pietrabissa A, Moretto C, Carobbi A, Boggi U, Ghilli M, Mosca F. Hand assisted laparoscopic low anterior resection: initial experience with a new procedure. Surg Endosc. 2002;16:431–5.

Poulin EC, Schlachta CM, Seshardi PA, Cadeddu MO, Gregoire R, Mamazza J. Septic complications of elective laparoscopic colorectal resection. Surg Endosc. 2001;15:203–8.

Schwenk W, Haase O, Neudecker J, Muller JM (2005) Short term benefits for laparoscopic colorectal resection. Cochrane Database Syst Rev CD003145.

Targarona EM, Balague C, Marin J, et al. Energy sources for laparoscopic colectomy: a prospective randomized comparison of conventional electrosurgery, bipolar computer-controlled electrosurgery and ultrasonic dissection: operative outcome and costs analysis. Surg Innov. 2005;12(4):339–44.

Trebuchet G, Lechaux D, Lecalve JL. Laparoscopic left colon resection for diverticular disease. Surg Endosc. 2002;16:18–21.

Veldkamp R, Kuhry E, Hop WC, et al. Laparoscopic surgery versus open surgery for colon cancer: short-term outcomes of a randomised trial. Lancet Oncol. 2005;6:477–84.

Young-Fadok TM, Nelson H. Laparoscopic right colectomy: five step procedure. Dis Colon Rectum. 2000;43:267–71.

Zucker KA, Pitcher DE, Martin DT, Ford RS. Laparoscopic assisted colon resection. Surg Endosc. 1994;8:12–8.

33. Laparoscopic Low Anterior Resection

Christopher R. Oxner, M.D.
Alessio Pigazzi, M.D., Ph.D

A. Indications

1. Laparoscopic anterior resection is used for resection of the rectosigmoid or rectum for both benign and malignant conditions.
    a. Rectal polyps or tumours not amenable to endoscopic or transanal resection.
    b. Rectal cancer without sphincter invasion.
    c. Ulcerative colitis and Crohn's disease when appropriate or as part of other colonic procedures.

B. Preoperative Planning

1. Appropriate laboratory, cardiac and imaging evaluation as indicated. CT scanning and endoscopic ultrasound or pelvic MRI should be performed routinely in cases of rectal cancer.
2. Preoperative colon preparation is at the discretion of the surgeon; colostomy or ileostomy marking and antibiotic administration are recommended.

C. Patient Position and Room Set-Up

1. The preferred patient position is modified lithotomy. Place a large foam pad under the patient's back to prevent sliding. A strap is also placed across the patient's chest for further stability.

N.T. Nguyen and C.E.H. Scott-Conner (eds.), *The SAGES Manual: Volume 2*   489
Advanced Laparoscopy and Endoscopy, DOI 10.1007/978-1-4614-2347-8_33,
© Springer Science+Business Media, LLC 2012

The patient's arms are tucked and padded. The thighs remain in line with the operating table rather than flexed upward to allow wide instrument movement. Full access to the abdomen and perineum is required.

2. Prep the perineum sterile only if a transanal extraction and hand-sewn coloanal anastomosis are anticipated. The routine use of ureteral stents is not necessary.

3. The predominant table position is Trendelenburg with the left side up. However, a reverse Trendelenburg position may also be required during mobilization of the splenic flexure.

4. Set the room up with the surgeon and the assistant initially on the patient's right, opposite the pathology. Place the monitor on the patient's left, opposite to the surgeon and the assistant at eye level (Fig. 33.1.).

5. Recommended equipment (some items are optional):
   a. Energy-based vessel-sealing device.
   b. Atraumatic bowel graspers.
   c. Vascular clips.
   d. Wound protector for extraction.
   e. Linear and circular stapling devices.

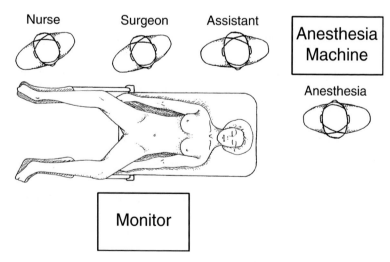

Fig. 33.1. OR set-up.

D. Performing the Laparoscopic (Low) Anterior Resection

1. **Port Placement** (Fig. 33.2.)—Establish pneumoperitoneum with the Verres needle or via a Hasson approach in the midline, where the scope will be inserted. Place this trocar halfway between the pubis and the xiphoid usually at or a few centimetres above the umbilicus (C). The minimum distance between trocars is roughly one medium-size palm. Place a 12-mm trocar halfway between port C and the anterior superior iliac spine. This site can be adjusted to coincide with preop-marked stoma site if within close proximity (P1). Place a 5-mm port 12–15 cm above P1 (P2) and a fourth port above and between P2 and the midline (P3). If needed, place another assistant port on the left between the periumbilical port (C) and the left ASIS (P4).

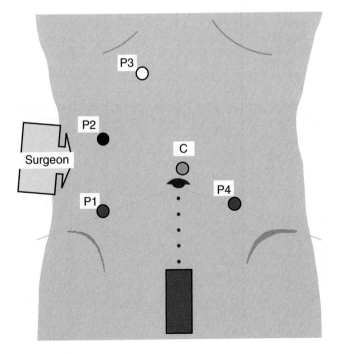

Fig. 33.2. Port placement.

2. **Mobilization of the Left Colon**—Our preferred technique for mobilization of the left colon is with a medial-to-lateral approach under the inferior mesenteric vein (IMV). Visualize the IMV by retracting the transverse colon and omentum cephalad and placing the small bowel in the right upper abdomen to get to the root of the mesentery. The jejunal attachments at the ligament of Trietz can be divided sharply to further delineate and get more length on that portion of the IMV, where the vein travels without a paired artery. Elevate, dissect and divide the IMV close to the pancreas (Figs. 33.3. and 33.4.). Then, carry the medial-to-lateral dissection to the lateral abdominal wall, sweeping down Toldt's fascia. Follow the IMV to the right in a caudal direction together with the left colic artery until the origin of the inferior mesenteric artery (IMA) is encountered. Alternatively, begin the mobilization under the superior haemorrhoidal artery at the level of the sacral promontory and divide the IMV after the IMA.

3. **Division of the Inferior Mesenteric Artery and Mobilization of the Splenic Flexure** (Fig. 33.5.)—After identifying the left ureter and gonadal vessels in the retroperitoneal plane, dissect the IMA free just distal to its origin. Create a window around the vessel and then divide it with a vascular stapler or an energy

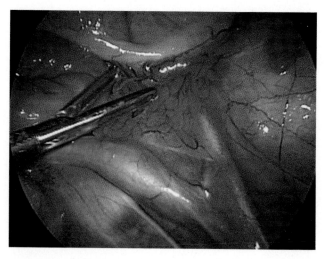

Fig. 33.3. Identification of IMV.

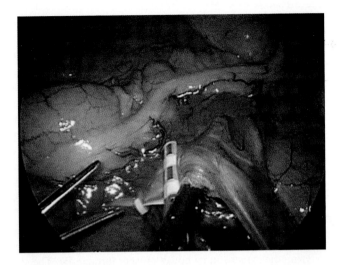

Fig. 33.4 Division of IMV.

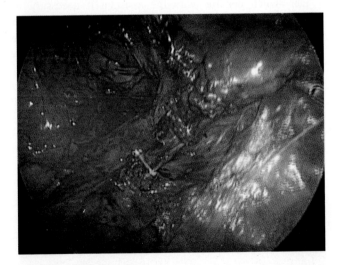

Fig. 33.5. Skeletonization of IMA and division of IMA.

device. Retract the colon medially and open the peritoneum along the white line of Toldt, freeing the descending and sigmoid colon. Next, take down the splenic flexure by opening the gastrocolic omentum just below the gastroepiploic vessels or dividing the avascular coloepiploic attachments next to the bowel wall. Divide the splenocolic ligament. An energy-based vessel-sealing device is recommended for these steps of the operation. Port P4 can be used as well to reach a high flexure from the left side of the abdomen.

4. Lastly, carefully divide the attachments of the body and tail of the pancreas to the colonic mesentery obtaining a full splenic flexure release. Divide the mesentery of the left colon, including the left colic artery, starting just proximal to the stump of the IMA and proceeding towards the colonic wall, usually at the point of anticipated division of the proximal bowel. Consider dividing the marginal artery at this time, particular if extraction of the specimen through the anus is anticipated, to avoid tearing the mesenteric vessels during the extraction manoeuvres.

5. **Mesorectal Dissection** (Figs. 33.6.–33.10.)—During the rectal dissection, the assistant can move to the patient's left manoeuvring the camera and a bowel grasper through P4. The surgeon will remain on the patient's right for most of the procedure but can switch position with the assistant if necessary. Steady cephalad retraction of the rectum out of the pelvis by the assistant is important for a proper dissection. Use electrocautery to enter the pre-sacral plane posterior to the superior rectal vessel. During this dissection, pay careful attention to identify and

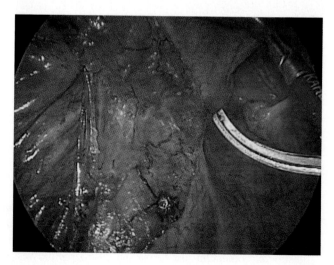

Fig. 33.6. Start of posterior TME (the ureter can be seen in the background).

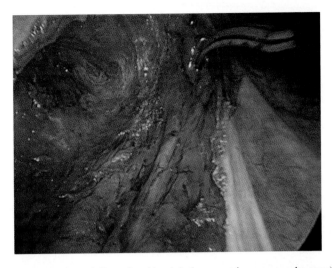

Fig. 33.7 Posterolateral dissection (the right hypogastric nerve can be seen).

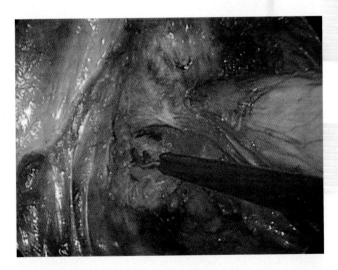

Fig. 33.8. Completion of the TME.

avoid injuring the hypogastric nerves travelling bilaterally from the sacral promontory to the side wall. Follow the posterior plane to below the level of the pathology, separating the pre-sacral fascia from the fascia propria of the rectum along what is called the "holy plane" of the mesorectum.

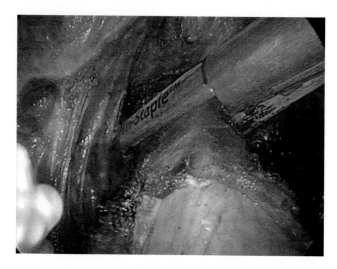

Fig. 33.9. Dividing the rectum.

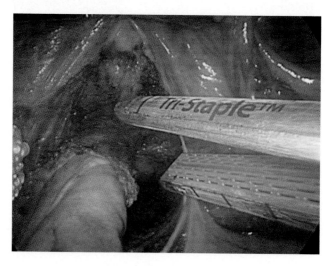

Fig. 33.10. Anastomosis with circular stapler.

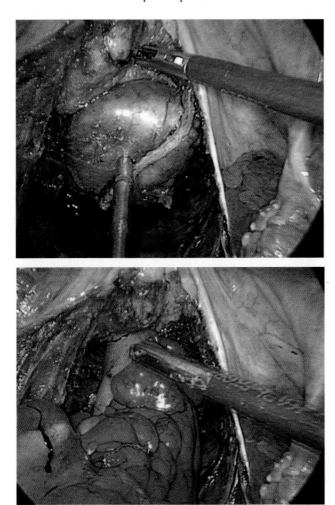

Fig. 33.10. (continued)

6. **The dissection continues laterally**, opening the peritoneal coverings along the side walls medial to the ureters. The middle rectal vessels may be divided with a vessel-sealing energy device. Open the peritoneal reflection anteriorly, proceeding along the rectovaginal space in women and Denonvillier's fascia in men. In large anterior neoplasms, the dissection may

proceed anterior to this fascia. Continue the dissection circumferentially below the level of pathology. In upper rectal cancers, a 5-cm margin with partial mesorectal excision is sufficient. In mid and low rectal cancers, a total mesorectal excision down to the level of the levators is warranted with the goal of achieving at least a 1-cm distal margin.

7. **Division and Re-anastomosis**—Perform a digital rectal examination under laparoscopic visualization to ensure an adequate distal margin. Next, prepare the rectum distal to the tumour by thinning the mesorectum with cautery or a vessel-sealing energy device. Our preferred approach is to utilize a reticulating linear stapler inserted through P1 in a right-to-left manner. A 45-mm cartridge is ideal, either a green load or the new Endo GIA with a Tristaple® purple load. Two or more firings may be necessary and it is important to maintain proper alignment of each successive cartridge to prevent crossing staple lines. In very low resection, no mesorectum is present around the rectum and no preparation of the fat is usually necessary. Deliver the specimen via a small Pfannenstiel incision and divide it. Secure the anvil with a purse string suture to the end of the proximal colon or to a colonic J-pouch. Perform the circular anastomosis under laparoscopic visualization making sure that the colon is not twisted or under tension. For very low rectal lesions, an intersphincteric resection can be chosen. In these cases, perform rectal division manually via a transanal approach at or near the dentate line followed by a hand-sewn coloanal anastomosis. Afterwards, mature a protective ileostomy, if indicated, according to patient conditions, level of the anastomosis, or intra-operative events.

E. Complications

1. **Bleeding**—Careful adherence to the natural planes when mobilizing the colon and mesorectal rectal dissection is important to prevent bleeding. Also, when taking the lateral stalks of the mesorectum, division of the middle colic may require bipolar cautery or clips. The risk of bleeding may be higher in patients previously treated with novel biologic chemotherapeutic agents.

2. **Anastomotic leak**—A tension-free, well-vascularized anastomosis is the primary requirement for proper healing. A post anastomotic air leak test can be beneficial in confirming that the anastomosis is circumferentially intact. The use of a protective ileostomy can help reduce the risk of symptomatic leak. Also, the surgeon should recognize when more mobilization of the colon or revision of the anastomosis is required.

Selected References

Agachan F, Joo JS, Weiss EG, et al. Intraoperative laparoscopic complications: are we getting better? Dis Colon Rectum. 1996;39:S14.

Bernstein MA, Dawson JW, Reissman PR, et al. Is complete laparoscopic colectomy superior to laparoscopic assisted colectomy? Am Surg. 1996;62:507–11.

Braga M, Vignalli A, Gianotti L, et al. Laparoscopic versus open colorectal surgery: a randomized trial on short-term outcome. Ann Surg. 2002;236:759–67.

Hong D, Lewis M, Tabet J, Anvari M. Prospective comparison of laparoscopic versus open resection for benign colorectal disease. Surg Laparosc Endosc. 2002;12:238–42.

Sackier JM and Chae FH. "Laparoscopic-Assisted Colon and Rectal Surgery", in *Colon and Rectal Surgery* Ed. By Corman, ML., (Philadelphia PA: Lippincott Williams & Wilkins, 2005), pp. 1225–1262.

34. Laparoscopic-Assisted Proctocolectomy and Ileal Pouch-Anal Anastomosis

Noelle L. Bertelson, M.D., F.A.C.S.
Tonia M. Young-Fadok, M.D., M.S., F.A.C.S., F.A.S.C.R.S.

A. Indications

Proctocolectomy with ileal pouch-anal anastomosis (IPAA) is most commonly indicated for patients with ulcerative colitis or familial adenomatous polyposis (FAP).

1. IPAA is indicated in the management of **ulcerative colitis** in the following settings: the disease is refractory to medical management; the patient is intolerant of medication side effects or cannot wean off steroids; growth retardation in pediatric patients: the patient wishes to avoid long-term immunosuppression; the patient has cancer or dysplasia; or the patient wishes to prevent cancer.

2. **FAP**, hereditary nonpolyposis colorectal cancer (HNPCC or Lynch Syndrome) with synchronous cancers involving the rectum, and ill-defined nonfamilial syndromes in which the colon is carpeted with polyps are also indications for cancer treatment or prophylaxis.

B. Contraindications

1. Proctocolectomy with IPAA is contraindicated in ulcerative colitis associated with severe malnutrition (low serum albumin or prealbumin, >10% weight loss), use of antitumor necrosis factor

N.T. Nguyen and C.E.H. Scott-Conner (eds.), *The SAGES Manual: Volume 2*   501
Advanced Laparoscopy and Endoscopy, DOI 10.1007/978-1-4614-2347-8_34,
© Springer Science+Business Media, LLC 2012

5. Type and screen is obtained.

6. A consultation with an ostomy nurse is important for education and marking of the planned ileostomy site, which improves patient satisfaction and capability in managing the ostomy postoperatively.

7. While bowel preparation is controversial in open cases, a decompressed colon is more easily manipulated laparoscopically and is utilized in our practice to minimize incision length.

8. Pre- and intraoperative use of a warming blanket assists in preventing hypothermia, which is associated with wound infection and poor coagulation.

9. A dose of IV steroids should be given preoperatively if the patient is on steroids currently or within the last year.
   a. If the patient is currently on steroids, methylprednisolone 10 mg greater than the current prednisone equivalent is administered.
   b. If the patient is not currently on steroids, methylprednisolone 20 mg is given.
   c. IV methylprednisolone is then tapered over 3 days back to the preoperative prednisone dose, which is then tapered by 5 mg per week until discontinued.

10. Preoperative intravenous antibiotics should be started within 60 min of incision.
    a. The first-line antibiotic choice is ertapenem 1 gm, which gives 24-h coverage.
    b. For penicillin allergic patients, ciprofloxacin 400 mg and metronidazole 500 mg are given.
    c. Antibiotics should not be continued past 24 h.

F. Positioning

1. Place the patient in the combined synchronous (modified lithotomy) position with legs in stirrups and thighs parallel to the abdominal wall (minimal hip flexion).

2. Tape medical-grade egg crate foam to the OR table over an underlying draw sheet and under the patient to prevent sliding.

3. Wrap the hands with foam, and tuck the arms using the draw sheet.

4. Place a warming blanket over the chest and secure it with an overlying regular blanket. Wrap cloth tape around both the blanket and the table.

5. Perform a "tilt test" with lateral tilt in both Trendelenburg and reverse Trendelenburg to ensure security in extreme positioning.

6. Place a Foley catheter in the bladder and an orogastric tube (to be removed at the end of the case).

G. Technique

1. Port Placement (Fig. 34.1)

a. Make a supraumbilical incision, open the fascia, and place a 12-mm blunt port under direct vision.

b. Place a 5-mm port in the left lower quadrant.

c. Place a 5-mm port in the suprapubic midline.

d. At the planned right lower quadrant ileostomy site, excise a disc of skin and subcutaneous fat down to the fascia, and place a 12-mm port through the site.

2. Left Colon Mobilization

a. We use a lateral-to-medial approach which allows preservation of the vessels, particularly the ileocolic artery, ease in finding the appropriate plane and protecting the ureters, and translation of the common way of performing open colectomy to laparoscopy.

b. Place the table in Trendelenburg with the left side tilted up.

c. Retract the sigmoid and descending colon medially, and incise the left lateral peritoneal reflection immediately medial to the white line of Toldt with cautery scissors, gently sweeping the retroperitoneum laterally.

d. Identify the left ureter, sweep it laterally, and protect it.

e. As dissection proceeds cephalad, identify the plane over Gerota's fascia to prevent undermining the left kidney.

f. Then, reposition the table in reverse Trendeleburg, still with the left side up.

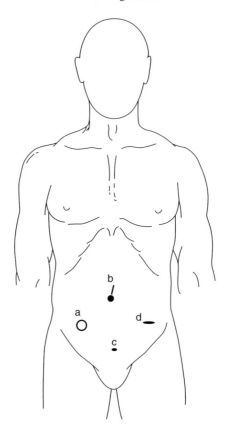

Fig. 34.1. Suggested port sites for laparoscopic proctocolectomy: (**a**) Ileostomy site with 12-mm trochar, (**b**) supraumbilical 12-mm Hasson trochar, (**c** and **d**) 5-mm trochar sites.

g.   Proceed with splenic flexure mobilization.

    i.   The omentum can be left on the colon or left attached to the stomach.

    ii.   The tissue at the flexure is thicker and no longer bloodless as the lateral dissection typically is; flexure mobilization is, thus, facilitated by switching from cautery scissors to use of a vessel sealing device.

    iii.   Direction of dissection:

        –   Dissection can proceed retrograde from descending to transverse in which the dissection of the proximal descending colon proceeds anterior to Gerota's fascia and then turns medially and superiorly to the flexure, entering the lesser sac from the lateral aspect.

–   Conversely, dissection can occur antegrade from transverse to descending in which the lesser sac is entered medially either by elevating the omentum and dissecting the omentum off the transverse colon or by incising the lesser omentum. This is then carried laterally around the flexure.

–   A combination of both directions of dissection may be used, particularly in the obese patient, leaving the omentum on the colon as planes are obscured by fat deposition.

3. Right Colon Mobilization

a.   Place the table in Trendelenburg with the right side elevated.
b.   Divide the peritoneal attachments of the inferior portion of the cecum and terminal ileum mesentery with cautery scissors (Fig. 34.2).
c.   Identify the right ureter.

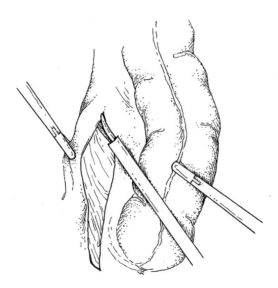

Fig. 34.2. With the patient in steep Trendelenberg with the left side up, the right colon is mobilized from lateral to medial.

d. Incise the white line of Toldt from inferior to superior, sweeping the retroperitoneum laterally with medial traction on the colon. Preserve Gerota's fascia posteriorly to avoid mobilizing the kidney on the right side.

e. Identify and protect the inferior vena cava and duodenum.

f. Place the patient in reverse Trendelenburg, and divide the hepatocolic ligaments with a vessel sealing device. Manage the omentum in the same manner as you have on the left side, i.e., either it with the colon or leave it with the patient.

4. Dissection of the Rectum

a. The table is placed in Trendelenburg with the left side slightly elevated.

b. Retract the left rectosigmoid mesentery anteriorly and to the right and out of the pelvis.

c. Identify the left ureter and protect it.

d. Note the subtle color change of the fat between the yellow mesorectum and white retroperitoneum and incise this line with cautery scissors.

e. Enter the presacral space and carry the dissection inferiorly, posteriorly, and laterally to the pelvic floor.

f. Visualize and protect the left hypogastric nerve.

g. Eliminate any side to side tilt in table position.

h. Identify the right ureter.

i. Incise the right pararectal peritoneum. Dissection proceeds posteriorly and laterally to join the previous dissection from the left.

j. Identify and protect the right hypogastric nerve.

k. Anterior dissection progresses with cephalad and posterior retraction of the rectum.

l. Protect the seminal vesicles and prostate in men, and the posterior vaginal wall in women.

m. If necessary, transfix the uterus or anterior peritoneal fold with a transabdominal suture and retract it anteriorly.

n. Sizers in the rectum and a sponge stick in the vagina may also assist in adequate visualization.

o. Complete the dissection to the level of the pelvic floor circumferentially and confirm this by digital rectal examination.

p. Transect the rectum at the level of the pelvic floor using an articulated laparoscopic stapler through the right lower quadrant 12-mm port.

q. Stapler size depends upon the size of the pelvis; a wide female pelvis may accommodate a 45- or 60-mm cartridge while a narrow male pelvis may require multiple firings of a 30-mm cartridge.

5. Transection of the Mesentery

a. In the setting of cancer or dysplasia, ligate the vascular pedicles at their bases to facilitate lymphadenectomy. Otherwise, take the mesentery where convenient. Sequentially divide the mesentery, commencing at the top of the presacral dissection using a vessel sealing device.

b. In a patient with a normal BMI, grasp the transected rectum with a locking grasper and exteriorize it through the planned ileostomy site after incising the fascia in a cruciate fashion, separating the rectus muscle fibers, and incising the posterior sheath. A 3–5-cm extension of the umbilical port site can also be used for extraction.

c. Alternatively, completely mobilize the colon and rectum, transect the rectum, and exteriorize the specimen via a periumbilical incision. Transect the mesentery.

d. In the obese patient or for a completely laparoscopic approach, transect the mesentery intracorporeally. In an obese patient, the transected mesentery will likely be too bulky to bring out through the ileostomy site. Rather, exteriorize it through a 3–5cm extension of the periumbilical incision.

e. Preserve the ileocolic pedicle to allow for subsequent choices of vessel division if pouch reach is an issue.

6. Pouch Creation

a. After exteriorization, transect the remaining right colon mesentery, preserving the ileocolic pedicle.

b. Transect the terminal ileum with a linear stapler.

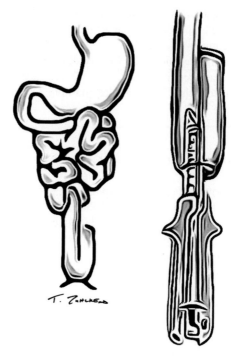

Fig. 34.3. The J pouch is created by firing a 100-mm GIA stapler twice through an apical enterotomy (Figure by Todd Zuhlke, MD).

c. Pull a point 15 cm from the transected end down to see if it reaches the pubis; if, after pulling down adjacent areas to find the best reach, the loop does not reach the pubis, a variety of mesenteric lengthening procedures can be attempted.

d. Create a 15-cm J-pouch by firing a 100-mm linear stapler twice through an apical enterotomy (Fig. 34.3).

e. Place a monofilament purse string around the enterotomy, and secure the anvil of a circular stapler in the apex of the pouch.

f. Suture the efferent limb of the pouch to the afferent limb to bury the staple line.

g. Return the pouch to the abdomen, irrigate the abdomen with saline and aspirate it, and close the extraction site with interrupted sutures such that the 12-mm port can be placed between two of the sutures left untied.

h. Reestablish pneumoperitoneum.

7. *Creation of the Ileal J-Pouch Anal Anastomosis*

a. Dilate the anus, and insert the circular stapler.

b. Bring the stapler spike out adjacent to (not through) the staple line, and remove the spike.

c. Trace the cut edge of the pouch mesentery to the duodenum to prevent twisting.

d. Dock the anvil on the stapler. Close and fire the stapler after confirming in female patients that the posterior vaginal wall is not trapped in the stapler.

e. After removing the stapler, examine the tissue rings for completeness, and send the distal ring for pathologic evaluation.

f. Place a 15 closed suction drain into the pelvis via the suprapubic port.

g. Run the small bowel retrograde from the pouch to a point approximately 30 cm proximal. Grasp this segment of small bowel and bring it out through the ileostomy site after removing the port, ensuring correct orientation by laparoscopic visualization.

h. Remove the remaining ports under direct vision to assure hemostasis.

i. Close the fascia at the midline extraction site (if one was used) or the periumbilical 12-mm port site, and approximate the skin incisions with subcuticular monofilament 3–0 suture.

j. Mature the ileostomy in a loop fashion with 3–0 monofilament suture.

k. Place a 24 French red rubber catheter into the pouch transanally.

8. *Single-Incision Proctocolectomy and IPAA*

a. The ileostomy site is the single-incision site of access.

b. The site is moved more cephalad and medially than traditional marking to allow access to all four quadrants, leaving sufficient space between the site and the umbilicus to permit placement of an ostomy appliance.

c. The same order of steps is performed.

d. The specimen is exteriorized via the stoma site.

e. No additional transabdominal drain is placed in the presacral space, but a drain is placed into the pouch transanally to keep the pouch decompressed.

9. Postoperative Management

a. The orogastric tube is removed at the end of the operation.

b. Scheduled IV ketorolac and oral acetaminophen are given for baseline pain management, as long as there is no contraindication.

c. Patient-controlled analgesia (PCA) is used for breakthrough pain.

d. A total of 24 h of antibiotics are given, with ertapenem given as a single dose preoperatively or ciprofloxacin and metronidazole given for two additional doses postoperatively.

e. Clear liquids are given on postoperative day (POD) 0 or 1, and if the patient tolerates 500 ml of liquids or has ileostomy output the diet is advanced to low residue with thickening snacks.

f. The PCA and foley are removed when the patient tolerates solid food.

g. Ostomy care teaching starts on POD 1, and home health services are recommended to assist with ostomy management after discharge.

h. Once the patient tolerates 2,000 ml of oral intake and ileostomy output is 1,000 ml or less, the patient is discharged.

i. Loperamide 2–4 mg 30 min prior to meals and bedtime is recommended to keep ileostomy output under 1,000 ml and to prevent dehydration.

10. Complications

a. Intraoperative complications
   i. Bleeding
   ii. Ureteral injury
   iii. Hypogastric nerve injury
b. Postoperative complications
   i. Postoperative ileus
   ii. High ileostomy output
   iii. Small bowel obstruction
   iv. Wound infection, possibly reduced in laparoscopic versus open
   v. Urinary tract infection
   vi. Pouch leak

    vii.   Urinary retention

    viii. Sexual dysfunction (impotence or retrograde ejaculation in men)

  c. Long-term complications

    i.   Pouchitis

    ii. Pouch dysfunction

    iii. Small bowel obstruction, possibly decreased relative to open

11. Results

a. Discharge occurs in 3–5 days, which is fewer days when compared to open.

b. Four to six bowel movements per day and zero to two at night are to be expected.

c. Patients are generally satisfied with IPAA: they no longer have symptoms of colitis, nor medication side effects, or in the case of FAP they no longer carry the elevated colon cancer risk.

Selected References

Ahmed Ali U. Keus F. Heikens JT. Bemelman WA. Berdah SV. Gooszen HG. van Laarhoven CJ (2009) Open versus laparoscopic (assisted) ileo pouch anal anastomosis for ulcerative colitis and familial adenomatous polyposis. Cochrane Database Systematic Reviews CD006267.

Bemelman WA. Laparoscopic ileoanal pouch surgery. Brit J Surg. 2010;97:2–3.

Chung TP, Fleshman JW, Birnbaum EH, Hunt SR, Dietz DW, Read TE, Mutch MG. Laparoscopic vs. open total abdominal colectomy for severe colitis: impact on recovery and subsequent completion restorative proctectomy. Dis Colon Rectum. 2009;52: 4–10.

Indar AA, Efron JE, Young-Fadok TM. Laparoscopic ileal pouch-anal anastomosis reduces abdominal and pelvic adhesions. Surg Endosc. 2009;23:174–7.

Lawes DA, Young-Fadok TM. Minimally invasive proctocolectomy and ileal pouch-anal anastomosis. In: Frantzides CT, Carlson MA, editors. Atlas of minimally invasive surgery. Philadelphia, PA: Saunders Elsevier; 2009. p. 139–46.

Polle SW, Dunker MS, Slors JF, Sprangers MA, Cuesta MA, Gouma DJ, Bemelman WA. Body image, cosmesis, quality of life, and functional outcome of hand-assisted laparoscopic versus open restorative proctocolectomy: long-term results of a randomized trial. Surg Endosc. 2007;21:1301–7.

Vivas D, Khaikin M, Wexner SD. Laparoscopic proctocolectomy and Brooke ileostomy. In: Asbun HJ, Young-Fadok TM, editors. American college of surgeons multimedia atlas of surgery; colorectal surgery volume. Chicago: American College of Surgeons; 2008. p. 111–6.

Young-Fadok TM, Nunoo-Mensah JW. Laparoscopic proctocolectomy and ileal pouch-anal anastomosis (IPAA). In: Asbun HJ, Young-Fadok TM, editors. American college of surgeons multimedia atlas of surgery; colorectal surgery volume. Chicago: American College of Surgeons; 2008. p. 117–29.

35. Laparoscopy for Crohn's Colitis

Assar A. Rather, M.D.
Eric G. Weiss, M.D.

A. Introduction

Crohn's Disease (CD) is estimated to affect more than half a million people in North America with an incidence ranging from 3.1 to 14.6 cases per 100,000 person-years. The most common form of CD is ileocolic disease (50%). Crohn's colitis is relatively less common and is reported in 30–52% of patients with Crohn's Disease. Typical features of Crohn's Disease, such as thickened mesentery, enteric fistulae, inflammatory masses, abscesses, or multiple "skip" areas of intestinal involvement, have deterred many surgeons from offering laparoscopic resections to their patients. Furthermore, a large percentage of patients with Crohn's Disease have a history of previous abdominal surgery, often for prior Crohn's Disease, making laparoscopy potentially more complex and time consuming. The first case of a laparoscopic ileo-colectomy for CD was in the early 1990s and demonstrated the initial feasibility and low morbidity of the procedure. Since then, multiple studies have shown the benefits of laparoscopic surgery for ileocolic Crohn's Disease.

In recent years, technical advances and increased surgeon experience with minimally invasive surgery (MIS) techniques, including both laparoscopic-assisted and hand-assisted laparoscopic surgery (HALS), have led to MIS being increasingly performed in patients with all forms of Crohn's Disease including Crohn's colitis. A number of reports have been published describing the advantages of laparoscopic colectomy in Crohn's colitis which include reduced operative blood loss, quicker return of bowel function, and shorter hospital stay with reasonable operative times and conversion rates.

N.T. Nguyen and C.E.H. Scott-Conner (eds.), *The SAGES Manual: Volume 2*   515
Advanced Laparoscopy and Endoscopy, DOI 10.1007/978-1-4614-2347-8_35,
© Springer Science+Business Media, LLC 2012

Laparoscopic colectomy has been used for essentially all situations for which a colon resection might otherwise be done via laparotomy. Specific indications for the surgical management of Crohn's colitis include:

1. Failure of medical management
2. Dysplasia
3. Cancer
4. Fistulas and intra-abdominal abscesses
5. Stricture and obstruction
6. Proctitis with or without perineal disease
7. Toxic colitis
8. Lower GI bleed
9. Perforation
10. Extraintestinal manifestations
11. Growth retardation

MIS resections for Crohn's colitis can be divided into two categories.

1. **Total/Subtotal Colectomy with or Without Anastomosis**
   Total abdominal colectomy with ileorectal anastomosis
   Total abdominal colectomy with end ileostomy
   Total proctocolectomy with end ileostomy
   Subtotal colectomy with ileosigmoid or ileodescending anastomosis
   Subtotal colectomy with end ileostomy
2. **Segmental Colectomy**
   Right colectomy
   Left colectomy
   Sigmoid colectomy

B. Patient Positioning and Room Setup

1. Position the patient supine on the operating room table with both arms tucked at the patient's sides. The arms must be appropriately padded and protected on the sides to prevent ulnar nerve injuries and brachial plexus injuries. A moldable beanbag may be placed under the patient's torso on the operating room table to further secure the patient. Alternative taping of the

patient's chest by "wrapping tape around the patient and the OR table" can be utilized. This helps to keep the patient's body from sliding during the steep changes in position often required for laparoscopic colectomy.

2. Place the patient in a modified lithotomy position using Allen stirrups (Allen Medical system), Lloyd Davis, or other designs. Position the patient so that the pelvis is just above the break at the lower end of operating table and there is adequate access to the anus for stapled anastomosis, intraoperative endoscopy, and/or perineal dissection if required. Place the legs in a 20° to 25° abducted position, with the thighs at a lower level than that of the abdominal wall (in order to obviate difficulty in maneuvering instruments via the lower abdominal quadrant ports). This position enables intraop endoscopy if needed as well as the introduction of the circular stapler through the anus for the construction of anastomosis.

3. The surgeon generally stands on the side of the operating room table opposite the site of pathology but may stand between the legs for a variety of reasons, including mobilization of either colonic flexure. The first assistant should stand opposite the surgeon or on the same side of the pathology. The second assistant (camera person) should stand next to the surgeon when the surgeon stands alongside the patient or next to the first assistant so that the operating team views the monitors from the same vantage point, which facilitates guidance of the laparoscope.

The trocar positions, extraction incisions, and the choice of laparoscope are discussed with each individual procedure.

C. Total/Subtotal Colectomy

1. **Trocar position and choice of a laparoscope**

    a. The first trocar is typically placed in the supraumblical region; however, in certain cases, an infraumbilical initial trocar may be utilized. This is typically done when a vertical midline extraction in the lower abdomen is possible (based on patients' body habitus and pathology) this site may be used.

    b. It is recommended that the initial trocar is placed via an open technique particularly for reoperative surgery, but

Veress needle and optical trocars may be used based on the surgeon's experience and practice.

c.   A 30° angled laparoscope is used in all procedures. A flexible, deflectable-tip laparoscope may also be used at the surgeon's discretion.

d.   In general, four operating trocars are placed—one in each quadrant lateral to the rectus sheath. The exact number and the location depend on the patient's body habitus, previous incisions if any, and planned stoma sites. Modifications of the trocar sites can also allow one to hide a site in, for example, the proposed right lower quadrant ostomy site or to the left of midline in the anticipated site of pfannenstiel incision for HALS.

e.   If a HALS approach is being used, the incision for the hand-assist device is one ½ size larger than the surgeon's glove size. The surgeon then uses his nondominant hand for palpation and retraction while the dominant hand is reserved for manipulation of laparoscopic instruments. The limitations of laparoscopic surgery, such as loss of direct tactile sensation, diminished depth perception, and retrieval of organs, are compensated by the insertion of a hand into the laparoscopic field. The hand can be used for blunt dissection, palpation of lesions or blood vessels, organ retraction, hemorrhage control, and knot tying. This is particularly helpful in Crohn's patients with thickened mesentery, and when the colon is excessively fragile as in fulminant colitis.

f.   The sizes of trocars vary based on the instruments used for dissection, vessel ligation, bowel transection, and surgical technique (HALS vs. laparoscopic assisted). Clearly, there is more versatility with 10–12-mm ports as compared to 5-mm ports, but it is rarely required to have all the ports of larger sizes. This is particularly true with the 5-mm vessel sealing devices, 5-mm laparoscopes, and other instrumentation now available.

The dissection can begin on either side, beginning in the right or left iliac fossa.

2.   **Mobilization of Right Colon**
Both medial-to-lateral and lateral-to-medial approaches have been described and the choice depends on surgeons' experience

and preference. We describe our preferred lateral-to-medial approach first.

a. Position the patient in steep Trendelenburg position with the left side of the table down. This facilitates displacement of small bowel loops from right lower quadrant. The assistant retracts the ascending colon medially using an atraumatic bowel grasper. In patients with friable bowel, the mesentery or epiploical appendices of the colon can be grasped instead to minimize trauma to the bowel wall.

b. Begin dissection along the white line of Toldt. Dissection can be performed with a variety of instruments, including the Harmonic Scalpel, Ligasure, or electrocautery using scissors or hooks (Ethicon Endo-Surgery).

c. If a hand port device is utilized, retract the colon medially through the hand port site and use the upper abdominal cannula sites for the dissecting instrument.

d. Continuous regrasping and manipulating of the right colon for medial dissection expose the ureter, Gerota's fascia, and duodenum. Recognize complete dissection of all attachments by clear identification of Gerota's fascia overlying the right kidney and the duodenal sweep.

e. Carry the dissection cephalad toward the hepatic flexure, exposing the third portion of the duodenum with dissection of the small bowel mesentery to that level and then to the transverse colon. Next, grasp the hepatic flexure and divide the hepaticocolic ligament. Regardless of the device being used for dissection, one should have readily available endoscopic clip appliers and endoloops as bleeding may occur. Careful medial traction at the hepatic flexure avoids tearing the middle colic vein near the superior mesenteric vein (Fig. 35.1).

3. **Mobilization of Transverse Colon**

a. Place the patient in reverse Trendelenburg position during this portion of the procedure.

b. Separate the gastrocolic omentum from the superior surface of the transverse colon. Grasp the colon with one atraumatic grasper and the omentum with the other, and dissect the avascular plane, separating the two structures. Alternatively, the omentum may remain attached to the colon and omentum divided distal to the gastroepiploic with great

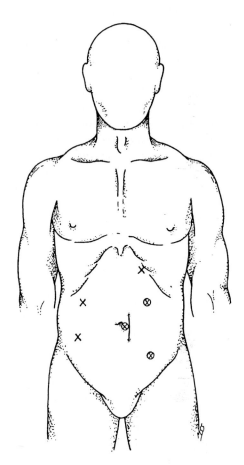

Fig. 35.1. Mobilization of right colon.

attention vessels at the surgeon's discretion. Perform this
phase of the dissection because of the extreme mobility of
this segment and the tendency of the omentum to hang over
the operative field. Carefully identify and preserve the
gastroepiploic vessels.

c. Applying constant traction and countertraction on the
omentum in cephalad direction and transverse colon in
caudal direction exposes the lesser sac.

d. Once in the lesser sac, lyse any adhesions from the stomach
to transverse mesocolon and completely separate the

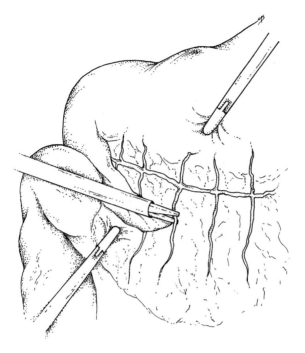

Fig. 35.2. Mobilization of transverse colon.

omentum from the transverse colon until the splenic flexure is reached. In order to facilitate complete mobilization, the surgeon may need to change position and move to right side or in between the patient's legs (Fig. 35.2).

4. **Mobilization of Left Colon**

   a. Place the patient in steep Trendelenburg position with right side of the table down and perform mobilization on the left side along the white line of Toldt in a manner similar to that on the right side starting at the left pelvic brim.

   b. Identify and preserve the left ureter and the gonadal vessels. Again, complete dissection of all attachments and clear identification of Gerota's fascia overlying the left kidney completely mobilize the left mesocolon.

   c. Next, mobilize the splenic flexure and the distal transverse colon. The dissection is made easier if the surgeon stands between the patient's legs and uses left lower quadrant port site. It is important that the dissection remains within a few millimeters of the colon as the flexure is taken down to avoid injury to the spleen. This is an avascular plane, and staying in this plane minimizes the bleeding from large omental vessels and avoids unnecessary traction on the spleen.

5. **Transection of the Mesenteric Vessels**

   a. After complete mobilization of the colon, ligate the vessels intracorporeally. The assistant (or the surgeon if using the hand port) grasps the colon or the mesentery adjacent to the colon and retracts the mesentery upward toward the anterior abdominal wall. Anterolateral retraction of the colon facilitates this identification of major vascular trunks. Isolate the vessels by scoring the mesentery on both sides of the vessel and creating windows in the mesentery on each side. These vessels are typically divided by using a vessel-sealing device or endoscopic linear stapler with a (white or gray) vascular cartridge.

   b. In the medial-to-lateral approach, the major vascular pedicles are identified and divided first before the lateral mobilization of the colon. Identify the ileocolic pedicle as the first vessels cross over the duodenal sweep. The assistant then grasps the pedicle and elevates the vessels and mesentery. Score the mesentery just inferior and underneath the pedicle near its origin from the superior mesenteric vessels. Develop a plane underneath the ileocolic pedicle until the duodenum is identified and this structure is swept posteriorly. Then, isolate the pedicle from surrounding structures. Trace the ileocolic pedicle distally to the cecum before division to correctly distinguish it from the superior mesenteric artery and vein. Once identification is confirmed, ligate and divide the pedicle as described above.

   c. Once the pedicle is divided, perform the medial-to-lateral dissection bluntly, making sure that the right ureter, gonadal vessels, and duodenum are free from mesocolon.

6. **Completion of Dissection and Anastomosis**

   a. Continue dissection cephalad around the hepatic flexure until the middle colic vessels are identified. Score the transverse mesocolon and isolate the middle colic vessels. By incising the mesocolon to the left of the left colic branch of the middle colic vessel, a free space usually emerges into the lesser sac. This expedites freeing of the pedicle. The main trunk of middle colic vessels is short and difficult to visualize and hence it may be prudent to target the branches of the middle colic vessels.

b. Mobilize the right colon, hepatic flexure, transverse colon, and splenic flexure as described above. The procedure then shifts to the left colon. The assistant elevates the inferior mesenteric pedicle and the surgeon makes an incision along the right peritoneal fold of the recto sigmoid mesentery beginning at the sacral promontory. The incision parallels the course of the inferior mesenteric pedicle and should be opened widely.

c. Using blunt dissection, sweep the inferior mesenteric artery and vein ventrally away from the preaortic hypogastric nerve plexus.

d. As dissection is continued medially beneath the inferior mesenteric artery and vein, identify and sweep the left ureter and gonadal vessels posteriorly. If the ureter cannot be readily and easily identified at this point in the dissection, incise the lateral attachments of the sigmoid colon, and mobilize the sigmoid colon from left to right. Identify the gonadal vessels and left ureter laterally and dissect them free of the mesentery.

e. Once the origin of the inferior mesenteric artery is identified, incise the peritoneum anteriorly over this pedicle and across the inferior mesenteric vein.

f. Then, use blunt dissection under the pedicle to create a window lateral to the inferior mesenteric artery and vein below the left colic vessels. A high ligation of the pedicle is not necessary for benign disease. Ligate and divide the inferior mesenteric pedicle as described above.

g. Once the pedicle is divided, the left colon mesentery then opens. Mobilize the left colon mesentery from medial to lateral in a similar manner as was done for the right colon.

h. Identify the distal end of resection and circumferentially expose the colonic or rectal wall. Transect the bowel using a 60-mm endostapler. Place a Babcock clamp on the proximal staple line to help in specimen extraction.

i. Extend the skin incision in the midline or, in case of hand-assisted laparoscopy, use the Pfannenstiel hand port incision for specimen extraction after protecting the wound with an Alexis wound protector (Applied Medical, Rancho Santa Margarita, CA).

j. It is imperative to run the small bowel from the Ligament of Trietz to the terminal ileum to ensure that there is no involvement of Crohn's disease in the small bowel. This can be accomplished either intracorporeally by a "hand-over-hand technique" or extracorporeally once the specimen is extracted. If there is no small bowel disease in the terminal ileum, transect the small bowel close to cecum. Again, this can be performed intracorporeally with 45 or 60-mm endoscopic stapler or extracorporeally through the extraction site.

k. If an ileorectal anastomosis is to be constructed, introduce the anvil of a circular stapler into the ileum and secure it with a purse-string suture. Return the ileum to the peritoneal cavity, and reestablish pneumoperitoneum.

l. Pass a circular stapler transanally, and move the camera to the right iliac fossa; fire the stapler. As with conventional surgery, verify the integrity of the anastomosis for leakage by air testing. Immerse the anastomosis in saline, proximally occlude the bowel with an atraumatic clamp, and instill air transanally via either a syringe or flexible sigmoidoscope. There may be advantages to testing via intraoperative endoscopy.

7. **Proctectomy**

a. Perform proctectomy with the patient in steep Trendelenburg position to allow for gravity retraction of the small bowel from the pelvis. Anterior retraction of the uterus can be achieved by suspending it with a suture through the abdominal wall.

b. After dividing the superior hemorrhoidal artery, mobilize the rectum by dissecting the presacral plane in the loose areolar tissue plane. Once the presacral space is entered posterior to the rectosigmoid junction at the sacral promontory in the avascular plane, carry dissection distally to the levator muscles. Identify and preserve the ureters as they cross the pelvic brim to enter the bladder.

c. Carry the dissection laterally and subsequently anteriorly staying on the rectal side of the Denonvillier's Fascia. Separate the rectum from vagina in females and prostrate/seminal vesicles in males.

d. Once the rectum is completely mobilized up to the level of levators, the perineal phase commences. This involves removal of anorectum with preservation of external sphincter. It is accomplished as in open surgery and the dissection is carried proximally in a circumferential manner to the level of levator ani muscle, where the dissection meets with the mobilized rectum from above.

e. The entire colon can be removed through the perineal incision. Then, place a moist sponge to temporarily seal the wound and reinstate pneumoperitoneum.

D. Segmental Colectomy

1. **Right Colectomy**

a. Place the first trocar (10–12-mm Hasson) in the supraumblical region at the site of planned incision for specimen extraction. Two additional trocars are placed in the left upper and left lower quadrant lateral to the rectus muscles at least a hand's breadth apart. Additional trocars may be used at surgeon's discretion for retraction and they are generally placed in the right upper or right lower quadrants (again, lateral to the rectus muscle). Alternatively, a subxiphoid port may be used for additional retraction.

b. Place the patient in steep Trendelenberg position with the left side of the table down.

c. Mobilization is performed in a manner similar to that described under right colon mobilization in total colectomy section.

d. Vascular ligation may be performed intracorporeally or extracorporeally. Intracorporeal vessel ligation in Crohn's Disease can be difficult and treacherous depending on the thickness of the mesentery.

e. Once the right colon is fully mobilized from the right iliac fossa to the Falciform Ligament, a fascial incision in the midline is made extending from the initial trocar periumbilically. A wound protector facilitates extraction but is not mandatory in a noncancer operation.

f. The mobilized colon, including the terminal ileum, cecum, ascending colon, hepatic flexure, and proximal transverse colon, is extracorporealized via the midline wound.

g.   Typically, a stapled functional end-to-end anastomosis is performed. When the anastomosis is complete, return it to the abdominal cavity, taking great care not to damage or tear the bowel or mesentery during this manipulation. One can reestablish pneumoperitoneum by occluding the wound protector or closing the extraction site and insufflating through one of the other port sites. Inspect the bowel, anastomosis, and abdomen; irrigate and assure hemostasis.

2.   **Left Colectomy or Sigmoid Colon Resection**

a.   Introduce the first trocar (10–12-mm Hasson) in the supraumbilical region. Next, place two 10–12-mm trocars in the right upper and lower quadrants, lateral to the rectus muscle.

b.   Place the patient in steep Trendelenburg position with the right side of the table down. Additional trocars may be used at the surgeon's discretion for retraction and they are generally placed in the left upper or left lower quadrants (again, lateral to the rectus muscle). This site also provides an excellent vantage point for laparoscopic visualization of the anastomosis.

c.   Mobilization is performed in a manner similar to that described under left colon mobilization in total colectomy section starting at the pelvic brim. Splenic flexure is mobilized more often than not in order to have a tension-free anastomosis.

d.   After complete mobilization, ligate the vascular pedicle intracorporeally. This dissection at the origin of the IMA involves a risk of injury to the left sympathetic trunk situated on the left border of the IMA. A meticulous dissection of the artery helps to avoid this risk because only the vessel will be divided, and not the surrounding tissues. The inferior mesenteric vein (IMV) is identified to the left of the IMA or in case of difficulty, higher, just to the left of the ligament of Treitz. The vein is divided below the inferior border of the pancreas or above the left colic vein.

e.   After vascular ligation, identify the distal extent of resection and circumferentially expose the colonic or rectal wall. Transect the bowel with a 45- or 60-mm linear cutting endoscopic stapler.

f.   Make a fascial incision in the midline and extrude the specimen after using a wound protector. A pfannenstiel or

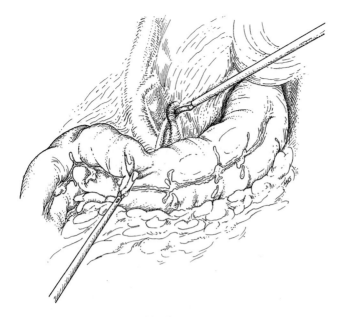

Fig. 35.3. Mobilization of sigmoid colon.

transverse incision in the left lower abdomen may occasionally be used for improved cosmesis. Anastomotic technique is the same as described for ileorectal anastomosis (Fig. 35.3).

E. Avoiding, Recognizing, and Managing Complications

1. Bowel Trauma/Anastomotic Leak

a. Cause and Prevention

Inadvertent enterotomy usually occurs due to excessive trauma to the bowel during retraction. This problem can be avoided by using atraumatic graspers, retracting the colon by the epiploica whenever possible being cognizant of the amount of force being placed on the instruments.

Avoiding the use of the "locking mechanisms" may also help. The use of energy devices or cautery may also result in thermal injury and delayed enterotomy. Ensuring that the entire tip of the dissecting instrument is always within the full field of view minimizes the complication. Careful manipulation of laparoscopic instruments especially during introduction also helps in avoiding traumatic injury and ideally should be performed under direct vision. Sometimes, bowel may be excessive friable secondary to fulminant colitis; inability to retract without tearing may preclude a laparoscopic approach. In such a situation, hand port is very helpful.

A well-vascularized, tension-free, circumferentially intact anastomosis is necessary to prevent anastamotic leakage. If any of the foregoing requirements are not present during a laparoscopic-assisted colectomy, then the anastomosis must be revised or the conditions improved by further mobilization and/or vascular division to achieve it. It is often prudent, if not mandatory, to convert to a laparotomy at this point. Identification of ischemia may be difficult and the aid of intravenous fluorescein may be used, as would intraoperative endoscopy to view the mucosa, as that is the most vulnerable to blood flow insufficiency. One ampoule of fluorescein given intravenously followed by inspection with a Wood's Lamp allows for identification of ischemic bowel. Resection proximally to viable colon corrects this problem. Intraoperative testing of the anastomosis is mandatory as described earlier. Any leak requires, at minimum, reinforcement if not complete revision. The use of only a diverting stoma to protect such an anastomosis may also be required.

b. Recognition and Management

Postoperative fevers, prolonged ileus, elevated leukocyte counts, and abdominal pain are all hallmarks of postoperative anastomotic leak. Aggressive detection and delineation often allows conservative therapy to be employed. The time course for the signs and symptoms of a leak or enterotomy may be much earlier than one is accustomed to seeing for patients undergoing laparotomy. This is due to rapid return of bowel function and lack of ileus that can occur with laparoscopic surgery. Any patient who has undergone laparoscopy and is not behaving as the typical patient in the early postoperative period should require the surgeon to assume the worst. This requires aggressive and prompt evaluation and action. This may require prompt radiologic evaluation of the anastomosis using a water-soluble contrast enema (perhaps, in concert with a computed tomography [CT] scan of the abdomen and pelvis). Alternatively returning to the OR for the reexploration may be most efficacious. If a small leak or a leak associated with a localized abscess is identified, percutaneous drainage, antibiotics, bowel rest, and total parenteral nutrition often allow for spontaneous closure. If a large, free leak is identified, prompt laparotomy with stoma creation is necessary.

2. Ureteric Injury

a. Cause and Prevention

This is most commonly caused by either misidentification or non-identification and then division or incorporation while dissecting or ligating structures. In addition, this can be caused by inadvertent energy transfer from vessel-sealing devices or electrocautery, or inclusion in the stapling devices or blades of energy devices during transection of the mesenteric pedicle. Clear identification of the ureter by careful observation of the steps enumerated in the chapter minimizes the chances of such an injury. The addition of lighted ureteric stents may be a useful adjunct in laparoscopic surgery to safeguard ureteric integrity. If the ureters are not adequately seen conversion to laparotomy so that identification prior to vascular or bowel division is mandatory.

b. Recognition and Management

Recognition during surgery often mandates conversion to open procedure for repair. The complication can manifest in post-op period by postoperative fever, ileus, or excessive drainage from pelvic drains that is high in creatinine.

3. Port Site Hernias

Intestinal obstruction from port site hernias is an uncommon complication after laparoscopic surgery. Various factors that have been implicated are large trocar size, incomplete closure of fascia at the trocar site, midline trocars, stretching the port site for organ retrieval, obesity, poor nutrition, and surgical site infections. Most of these hernias occur in sites, where the trocar diameter is more than 10 mm. Prevention of trocar site hernias includes closing of all port sites more than 10 mm at the fascial level. Many authors have recommended the deflation of pneumoperitoneum prior to port removal so that omentum and intestines are not drawn into the fascial defect. Other techniques to prevent herniation include use of fascial closure devices and nonbladed trocars.

4. Bleeding

Even with the most careful dissection and meticulous hemostasis, bleeding may be occasionally encountered, especially when dealing with thickened mesentery as is usually the case in Crohn's Disease. Failure of energy sources while achieving hemostasis is the usual culprit, and in those situations mechanical methods of hemostasis, like endoscopic clips, pretied vessel loops, and endoscopic staplers, may be used.

Selected References

Loftus Jr EV. Clinical epidemiology of inflammatory bowel disease: incidence, prevalence, and environmental influences. Gastroenterology. 2004;126:1504–17.

Lapidus A. Crohn's disease in Stockholm County during 1990–2001: an epidemiological update. World J Gastroenterol. 2006;12(1):75–81.

Loftus CG, Loftus Jr EV, Harmsen WS, et al. Update on the incidence and prevalence of Crohn's disease and ulcerative colitis in Olmsted County, Minnesota, 1940–2000. Inflamm Bowel Dis. 2007;13(3):254–61.

Henriksen M, Jahnsen J, Lygren I, et al. Clinical course in Crohn's disease: results of a five-year population-based follow-up study (the IBSEN study). Scand J Gastroenterol. 2007;42(5):602–10.

Milsom JW, Lavery IC, Bohm B, et al. Laparoscopically assisted ileocolectomy in Crohn's disease. Surge Laparosc Endosc. 1993;3:77–80.

Tan JJY, Tjandra JJ. Laparoscopic surgery for Crohn's disease: a metaanalysis. Dis Colon Rectum. 2007;50:576–85.

Holubar SD, Dozois EJ, Privitera A, et al. Minimally invasive colectomy for Crohn's colitis: a single institution experience. Inflamm Bowel Dis. 2010;16:1940–6.

Moreira ADL, Stocchi L, Remzi FH, et al. Laparoscopic surgery for patients with Crohn's colitis: a case-matched study. J Gastrointest Surg. 2007;11:1529–33.

Umanskiy K, Malhotra G, Chase A, et al. Laparoscopic colectomy for crohn's colitis. A large prospective comparative study. J Gastrointest Surg. 2010;14:658–63.

Li VK, Wexner SD, Pulido N, et al. Use of routine intraoperative endoscopy in elective laparoscopic colorectal surgery: can it further avoid anastomotic failure? Surg Endosc. 2009;23(11):2459–65.

36. Single-Site Laparoscopic Colectomy

Joseph C. Carmichael, M.D.
Michael J. Stamos, M.D.

A. Indications

Single-site laparoscopic colectomy can be utilized in almost any situation in which colectomy is indicated. It may also be used in procedures requiring proctectomy, but that is beyond the scope of this chapter.

1. Diverticular disease
   a. Complicated diverticulitis, including abscess, fistula, bleeding, or obstruction
   b. Recurrent acute diverticulitis
2. Colon cancer
3. Colon polyps that are not resectable endoscopically
4. Inflammatory bowel disease
   a. Segmental colectomy for Crohn's disease
      i. Indicated in patients with stricture, fistula, or uncontrolled segmental colitis
   b. Total colectomy for Crohn's disease
      ii. Indicated in patients with fulminant colitis
   c. Total colectomy with ileostomy for ulcerative colitis (UC): This would be considered the first step in a three-stage treatment process. The second step would be completion proctectomy with creation of ileal pouch-anal anastomosis and diverting ileostomy. The third step would be closure of the ileostomy. It is also possible to treat UC in a two-stage process. The first step in a two-stage plan would be total proctocolectomy with ileal pouch anal anastomosis and diverting ileostomy. The second step in a

N.T. Nguyen and C.E.H. Scott-Conner (eds.), *The SAGES Manual: Volume 2*   531
Advanced Laparoscopy and Endoscopy, DOI 10.1007/978-1-4614-2347-8_36,
© Springer Science+Business Media, LLC 2012

two-stage plan would be ileostomy closure. Finally, it is possible to treat ulcerative colitis with a single-stage approach that would be total proctocolectomy with ileal pouch-anal anastomosis or total proctocolectomy with end ileostomy. The complex process of choosing between one-stage, two-stage, and three-stage approaches to the treatment of UC is beyond the scope of this chapter; however, general indications for surgery in ulcerative colitis are as follows:

   i.   Fulminant disease unresponsive to maximal medical management
   ii.   Chronic disease refractory to medical therapy
   iii.   Complications related to adverse effects of chronic medical therapy
   iv.   Hemorrhage
   v.   High-grade dysplasia, dysplasia-associated lesion or mass (DALM)
   vi.   Malignancy
   vii.   Growth retardation in children

B. Contraindications to Single-Site Colectomy

1. Locally advanced tumors requiring multivisceral or abdominal wall resection.
2. The presence of a large phlegmon, such as may be found in perforated diverticulitis or Crohn's disease.
3. Large bowel obstruction: If the colon is significantly dilated and cannot be decompressed via colonic stent, then it may be impossible to establish a large enough working space with pneumoperitoneum to perform laparoscopic surgery.
4. Previous surgery is NOT a specific contraindication for this approach. Often, the adhesions from previous surgery are not significant enough to preclude a minimally invasive approach. In addition, scars from previous skin incisions may be used as a site for insertion of the trocars.

C. Definition of Single Site

1. Single-site surgery is a form of minimally invasive surgery defined as surgery through a small incision at one location. In the case of colectomy, the incision is usually located at the umbilicus, but may be located anywhere on the abdomen.
2. References to single-site surgery may be found under many names in the academic literature. The following acronyms all refer to this topic:
   a. LaparoEndoscopic Single-Site (LESS) surgery
   b. No VIsible Scar (NVIS) surgery
   c. Embryonic Natural Orifice Transumbilical Endoscopic Surgery (E-NOTES)
   d. Single-Incision Laparoscopic Colectomy (SILC)
   e. Single-Port Laparoscopic Surgery (SPLS)

D. Single-Incision Access Devices Available

Single-incision surgery frequently involves a special access device to be used at the surgical incision. There are several of these devices that are commercially available. All of them offer a way to insufflate CO_2 into the abdomen, a camera port, and at least two working ports. Some of the devices have an integrated wound protector for specimen extraction and others do not. The following are a few of the devices available.

1. SILS™ Port Multiple Instrument Access Port (Covidien, Mansfield, MA, USA)
2. GelPoint® Advanced Access Platform (Applied Medical, Rancho Santa Margarita, CA)
3. TriPort and QuadPort (Advanced Surgical Concepts Ltd., Wicklow, Ireland)

E. Operating Without a Single-Incision Access Device

Some surgeons have described single-site surgery techniques that avoid using the single-incision access device. There is a cost advantage to these techniques, but they can be more technically challenging. Two of these techniques are listed.

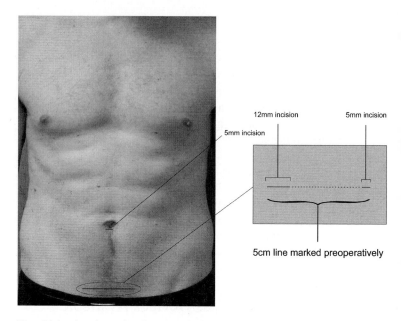

Fig. 36.1. A schematic diagram of the No Visible Scar (NVIS) surgery is depicted. This is a three-trocar procedure in which the two lower trocars are inserted through separate puncture sites. At the end of the procedure, the skin and fascia between the trocar sites are opened to create a site large enough for specimen extraction.

1. **Low-profile multiport approach**: In this approach, a skin incision is made and multiple trocars pierce the fascia at different points through the single skin incision. It is important to adequately separate the fascial incision sites so that pneumoperitoneum may be maintained. This has been described previously for the NVIS approach and is depicted in Fig. 36.1.

2. **Alexis® wound retractor (Applied Medical, Rancho Santa Margarita, CA) and surgical glove**: In this technique, an incision is made through the skin and fascia. A wound protector is inserted. A surgical glove is placed over the wound protector and trocars are inserted through the glove fingers. The abdomen is insufflated through the trocars. It can be difficult to keep the trocars inserted in the surgical glove fingers and authors have described various strategies to accomplish this task.

F. Patient Position and Room Setup

1. Right Colectomy
   a. Position the patient supine on the operating room table.
   b. Tuck the left arm and extend the right arm. Place sequential compression devices on the patient's legs.
   c. Fix a gel pad in place over the shoulders to prevent sliding when the patient is in steep Trendelenburg position. Similarly, place a securing strap across the thighs and chest to prevent patient movement when the right side of the table is elevated.
   d. Insert a foley catheter.
   e. Place patient warming devices (Bair Hugger® blanket) over the chest and legs.
   f. Check patient security to the table before draping by moving the table to maximum Trendelenburg and lateral positions.
   g. Place two laparoscopic monitors on the patient's right side, one by the right leg and one by the right shoulder. The surgeon and assistant stand on the patient's left. Use additional monitors if needed.

2. Left Colectomy
   a. Place the patient in a low lithotomy position with Allen® Surgical Stirrups (Allen Medical Systems, Acton, MA). Put sequential compression devices on the patient's legs.
   b. The stirrups need to be low, with a hip angle of <10°, ensuring minimal external collision between the thighs and laparoscopic instruments. The proper leg positioning is depicted in Fig. 36.2.
   c. Tuck the right arm and extend the left arm.
   d. Place gel pads, securing straps, Foley catheter, and warming devices as previously described. Check that the patient is securely positioned by moving the table into steep Trendelenburg position before draping as noted above.
   e. Place two laparoscopic monitors on the patient's left side, one by the shoulder and one by the hip. The surgeon and assistant stand on the patient's right. Use additional monitors if needed.

3. Total Colectomy
   a. Set up as for left colectomy, except both arms are tucked. Laparoscopic monitors need to be in place on both sides of the patient.

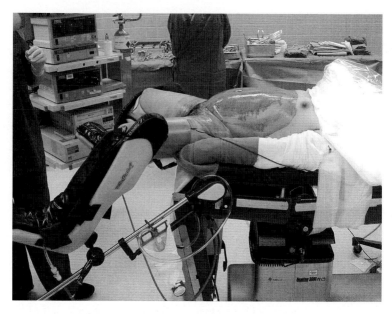

Fig. 36.2. The proper leg positioning should have less than 10° of hip flexion.

G. Minimizing the Effects of Loss of Triangulation

1. Loss of triangulation is a basic problem in single-site surgery procedures in which both instruments and the camera come from the same direction. This leads to a loss of perspective, difficulty with tissue retraction, and external collisions between the instrument handles. There are several ways to overcome these problems.

2. **Angled laparoscopic instruments**: There are now multiple laparoscopic graspers and dissectors that flex 0–80° in the instrument shaft. This assists with the problems of tissue retraction and external collisions. The problem with these instruments is that they can be cumbersome and more difficult to control (nonintuitive ergonomics). They also add considerably to the expense.

3. **Long laparoscopes**: Laparoscopes with a longer (45 cm) shaft help minimize external collisions.

4. **Flexible-tip laparoscopes**: Laparoscopes with a flexible tip improve perspective and minimize external collisions as the laparoscopic handle is moved away from the operative instrument handles. Additionally, the angulation of the lens helps considerably to restore triangulation. Angled (30 and 45°) lens help with this problem to a lesser degree.

5. **Integrated laparoscope without a separate light cord**: Integrated laparoscopes that have no separate light cord are less likely to cause external collisions.

6. **Low-profile and variable-length ports**: Instrument ports with a low-profile external component and variable lengths are less likely to have external collisions (most useful when a multiport device is not utilized).

7. **NVIS Colectomy**: In this technique, the single port site is a low-transverse incision on the abdomen. An additional trocar is placed through the umbilicus. This restores some triangulation, but maintains the cosmetic results of a single-site surgery (see Fig. 36.3).

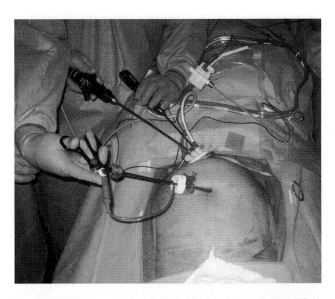

Fig. 36.3. In this NVIS approach, a multiport is placed through a low Pfannenstiel incision. The additional umbilical port site is used to improve triangulation. Also, note that a flexible-tip laparoscope with integrated cord is utilized to help minimize external collisions and improve triangulation.

H. Technique: Right Colectomy

1. After the abdomen is prepped and draped, make a 2.5-cm vertical periumbilical incision. Open the fascia vertically and insert a single-incision access device (see Fig. 36.4).
2. Alternatively, the NVIS approach may improve triangulation. In this approach, two trocars (one 5 mm and one 10 mm) are placed via a low-transverse Pfannenstiel incision, one trocar at each end of a planned incision (see Fig. 36.1). A third 5-mm port is placed through the umbilicus. This NVIS approach restores triangulation, but requires the operator to perform an intracorporeal anastomosis prior to specimen extraction.
3. Use a 5-mm 30° laparoscope or a 5-mm deflectable-tip laparoscope (Olympus, Tokyo, Japan) (see Fig. 36.5).
4. Use two long atraumatic straight laparoscopic graspers.
5. Place the patient in a Trendelenburg position with the right side elevated.

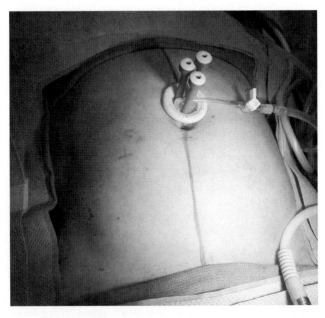

Fig. 36.4. An SILS port has been placed for a right hemicolectomy. Note that the ports are of low profile and staggered to minimize external collisions.

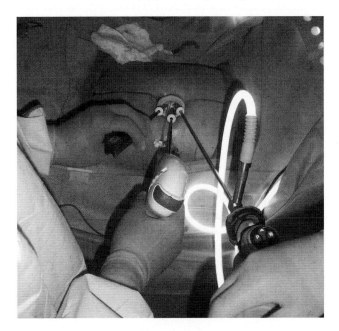

Fig. 36.5. In this intraoperative photo of a right hemicolectomy, a long laparo-scope lens (45 cm) is utilized to minimize external collisions.

6. Medial-to-lateral mesenteric mobilization begins with elevation of the mesentery at the base of the cecum toward the right lower quadrant so that the ileocolic pedicle is visible.

7. Open the peritoneum at the base of the pedicle and begin mobilization by elevating the mesentery off the retroperitoneum.

8. Identify the duodenum and divide the ileocolic pedicle with a 5 mm LigaSure™ (Covidien, Mansfield, MA, USA) or Enseal® (Ethicon Endo-Surgery Inc, Cincinnati, Ohio, USA) energy device.

9. The right ureter is not routinely identified prior to vascular division.

10. Extend the retroperitoneal mobilization to the right abdominal sidewall and superiorly to the hepatic flexure.

11. Mobilize the base of the cecum and terminal ileum to connect with the previous retroperitoneal dissection via an inferior-to-superior approach or lateral–medial approach.

12. Mobilize the ascending colon along the white line of Toldt.

13. Place the patient in slight reverse Trendelenburg position and mobilize the hepatic flexure and transverse colon. Identify the proximal portion of the duodenum here and further expose the second and third portions of the duodenum.

14. Place a grasper on the terminal ileum. Remove the single-access device and enlarge the fascial and skin incisions as needed to allow for specimen removal.

15. Insert an Alexis® wound retractor (Applied Medical, Rancho Santa Margarita, CA) (see Fig. 36.6) and pull the terminal ileum into the field.

16. Divide the terminal ileum with a linear stapler. Divide the remaining mesentery at that site and place a stay stitch on the ileum staple line. Allow the ileum to drop into the abdomen and exteriorize the colon. Divide it at the planned distal line of transection with a linear stapler. Next, exteriorize the ileum and create a side-to-side anastomosis.

17. Return the bowel to the abdomen and close the wound in layers.

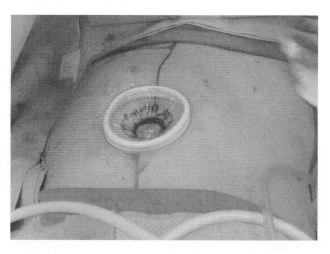

Fig. 36.6. The SILS port has been removed and a wound protector has been inserted in anticipation of specimen extraction.

I. Technique: Left Colectomy

1. After the abdomen is prepped and draped, make a 2.5-cm vertical periumbilical incision. Open the fascia vertically and insert a single-incision access device.

2. Alternatively, the NVIS approach may improve triangulation. In this approach, a multiport device may be placed via a low-transverse Pfannenstiel incision. A second 5-mm port is placed through the umbilicus (see Fig. 36.3).

3. Place three 5-mm trocars in the multiport devices and umbilical trocar if utilized and establish pneumoperitoneum.

4. Use a 5-mm 30° laparoscope or a 5-mm deflectable-tip laparoscope (Olympus, Tokyo, Japan).

5. Use two long atraumatic straight laparoscopic graspers.

6. Place the patient in a Trendelenburg position with the left side elevated.

7. Begin a medial-to-lateral mesenteric mobilization by grasping and elevating the sigmoid colon, tenting up the inferior mesenteric artery.

8. Open the peritoneum at the base of the sigmoid mesentery and elevate the mesentery off the retroperitoneum.

9. Identify the left ureter.

10. Divide the vascular pedicle with a 5 mm LigaSure™ (Covidien, Mansfield, MA, USA) or Enseal® (Ethicon Endo-Surgery Inc, Cincinnati, Ohio, USA) energy device.

11. Continue the retroperitoneal medial-to-lateral mobilization laterally, and then cranially and caudally. The extent of mobilization depends on the individual anatomy and pathology.

12. Mobilize the descending colon along the line of Toldt and mobilize the splenic flexure. Divide the inferior mesenteric vein at the base of the pancreas if increased mobilization is needed.

13. Divide the mesentery of the proximal rectum at the planned location of distal margin in a tangential direction. Use a linear endostapler to divide the rectum.

14. Place an atraumatic grasper on the proximal bowel staple line and exteriorize it via the sleeve of the multiport device or Alexis® wound retractor.

15. Divide the proximal residual mesentery and proximal colon. Pass the specimen off the table.

16. Place a purse-string suture of 2–0 Prolene and insert the circular stapler anvil into the proximal colon. Reinsufflate the abdomen after replacing the multiport device cap and complete the anastomosis. Perform a standard leak test, and inspect the donuts, to confirm anastomotic integrity. Close the wound in layers.

J. Technique: Total Colectomy

1. After the abdomen is prepped and draped, make a 2.5-cm incision at the planned ileostomy site in the right lower quadrant. Open the fascia vertically and insert a single-incision access device.

2. Place three 5-mm trocars in the port and establish pneumoperitoneum.

3. Use a 5-mm 30° laparoscope or a 5-mm deflectable-tip laparoscope (Olympus, Tokyo, Japan).

4. Use two long atraumatic straight laparoscopic graspers.

5. Place the patient in a Trendelenburg position with the right side elevated.

6. Mobilize the right colon using medial-to-lateral mesenteric mobilization, and divide the ileocolic vascular pedicle as described above.

7. Place the patient in slight reverse Trendelenburg position and mobilize the hepatic flexure and transverse colon. Identify the proximal duodenum and expose the second and third portions of the duodenum.

8. Elevate the greater omentum off the transverse colon and enter the lesser sac. Divide the transverse colon mesentery and mobilize the splenic flexure.

9. Return the patient to Trendelenburg position and elevate the sigmoid colon, and identify and divide the inferior mesenteric artery pedicle (after identifying the left ureter) as described above.

10. Divide the mesentery to the transverse colon. Next, divide the mesentery of the upper rectum transect with a linear endostapler.

11. Place a grasper on the distal colon. Remove the single-access device and enlarge the fascial and skin incisions, if necessary, to allow for specimen removal.

12. Insert an Alexis® wound retractor and pull the ileum and colon into the field.
13. Divide the terminal ileum with a GIA stapler.
14. If necessary, close the fascia slightly with absorbable suture to avoid parastomal hernia.
15. Mature the ileostomy in the standard Brooke fashion.

K. Complications

1. Wound infection
2. Hernia
3. Venous thromboembolism
4. Anastomotic leak
5. Surgical bleeding

Selected References

Adair J, Gromski MA, Lim RB, et al. Single-incision laparoscopic right colectomy: experience with 17 consecutive cases and comparison with muliport laparoscopic right colectomy. Dis Colon Rectum. 2010;53:1549–54.

Geisler DP, Kirat HT, Remzi FH. Single-port laparoscopic total proctocolectomy with ileal pouch-anal anastomosis: initial operative experience. Surg Endosc. 2011;25(7): 2175–8.

Hong TH, You YK, Lee KH. Transumbilical single-port laparoscopic cholecystectomy. Surg Endosc. 2009;23:1393–7.

Leblanc F, Makhija R, Champagne MD, Delaney CP. Single incision laparoscopic total colectomy and proctocolectomy for benign disease—initial experience. Colorectal Dis. 2011;13(11):1290–3.

Remzi FH, Kirat HT, Geisler DP. Laparoscopic single-port colectomy for sigmoid cancer. Tech Coloproctol. 2010;14:253–5.

Tung VS, Buchberg B, Masoomi H, Reavis K, Nguyen NT, Mills S, Stamos MJ. No Visible Scar (NVIS) colectomy: a new approach to minimal access surgery to the colon. Surg Innov. 2011;18(1):79–85.

Waters JA, Guzman MJ, Fajardo AD, et al. Single-port laparoscopic right hemicolectomy: a safe alternative to conventional laparoscopy. Dis Colon Rectum. 2010;53: 1467–72.

Wong MTC, Ng KH, Ho KS, et al. Single-incision laparoscopic surgery for right hemicolectomy: our initial experience with 10 cases. Tech Coloproctol. 2010;14:225–8.

37. Colonoscopic Stenting: Indications and Technique

Joseph L. Frenkel, M.D.
Elsa B. Valsdottir, M.D.
Anthony P. D'Andrea, M.S.
John H. Marks, M.D.

A. Indications

Indications for colorectal stenting include a variety of disorders which cause large bowel obstruction (LBO) both partial and complete. The majority of LBOs are caused by lesions in the descending and sigmoid colon and the rectosigmoid junction (75%). Because the proximal colon has a wider lumen and contains liquid stool, it is less commonly the site of bowel obstruction. Although initially reported in 1991 as an option for patients who presented with stage IV colorectal cancer, the indications for colonic stents have expanded considerably to include the management of both benign and malignant diseases at all stages. **The causes of LBO include the following.**

1. **Colorectal cancer** is the main cause of LBO. These cancers can present in several forms.
   a. A primary tumor alone
   b. Colorectal tumors that present in the setting of metastatic disease
   c. Locally recurrent disease after a prior resection (e.g., anastomotic, regional)
2. **Extrinsic compression** from other malignancies can cause LBO. These patients may have a lower clinical success rate with colonic stenting as there are often multiple sites of obstruction. This can lead to technical difficulties with the procedure as well.
   a. **Gynecologic malignancies** (e.g., ovarian cancer) are often multifocal with obstruction at several levels.

N.T. Nguyen and C.E.H. Scott-Conner (eds.), *The SAGES Manual: Volume 2*   545
Advanced Laparoscopy and Endoscopy, DOI 10.1007/978-1-4614-2347-8_37,
© Springer Science+Business Media, LLC 2012

  b. **Gastric carcinoma** can lead to colonic obstruction as well, particularly in the transverse colon. This is more frequently seen in the Asian population, where there is a higher incidence of this disease.

  c. **Carcinomatosis** from various etiologies can cause direct compression of the bowel lumen and result in LBO.

 3. **Benign conditions** can cause severe colorectal strictures resulting in chronic LBOs in very select instances. Initial stenting of these lesions may be performed, so bowel preparation can be performed followed by surgical intervention.

  a. Diverticulitis

  b. Crohn's colitis

  c. Anastomotic stricture

  d. Colonic ischemia

  e. Radiation injury

B. Patients with LBO Present

Patients with LBO present with variable severity and acuity. Several factors are common.

 1. In chronically obstructed patients, a recent change in bowel habits is noted. The patient may note narrow stools, constipation leading to laxative dependence, or present with frank obstipation.

 2. In the more acutely obstructed patient, signs and symptoms of obstruction are present. These include:

  a. Nausea

  b. Vomiting, with feculent emesis in some circumstances

  c. Severe, crampy abdominal pain

  d. Anorexia and inanition

  e. Abdominal distension

C. Initial Evaluation of LBO

 1. Plain abdominal X-rays can show proximal colonic and small intestinal dilatation.

 2. CT scan is essential in this situation, and in many cases can give you both the location of obstruction as well as potential causes.

It evaluates for perforation. If the obstruction is from extrinsic compression, it may give you an idea of the source of the primary tumor. If a cancer, it assists with staging.

3: Diagnostic endoscopy and biopsy can be performed. This confirms the presence of an obstructing lesion.

    a. The inability to pass the lesion with a standard colonoscope is a confirmatory characteristic of LBO.

    b. No visible lesion on endoscopy raises the possibility of acute colonic pseudo-obstruction (Ogilvie's Syndrome), extrinsic compression, or submucosal masses.

D. There Are Several Classic Surgical Options for an Acutely Presenting LBO

1. **Three-stage procedures** can be performed in those presenting emergently and with significant medical comorbidities. This option is reserved for only the extremely ill patients because it leaves the pathology in place.

    a. Proximal colostomy is the initial procedure. Avoiding formal resection of the site of obstruction can expedite the procedure and may be performed by those not experienced in what can be a complicated colorectal procedure.

    b. Resection of the obstructing lesion is the second stage.

    c. Colostomy reversal is then undertaken after evaluating the anastomosis for leak with enema studies or endoscopy.

2. **Two-stage procedures** decrease the risk because there is one fewer major abdominal procedure involved while still offering some protection against anastomotic leak. It does remove the offending pathology. It is currently considered the procedure of choice for high-risk patients.

    a. The initial resection of the obstructing lesion is performed with the formation of an end colostomy (Hartman's procedure) OR

    b. Resection can be performed with immediate anastomosis and proximal loop colostomy or ileostomy, and then

    c. Stoma reversal is undertaken at a later date.

3. **One-stage procedures** can be undertaken only in select instances. Anastomotic leak in an already medically compromised individual

is a significant concern. Selection for this option should, therefore, be based on parameters, such as age, ASA grade, extent of disease, and the patient's clinical condition. There is also increased risk of infection complications due to performing surgery with unprepared bowel (e.g., wound infections). Options include:

a.   Resection with primary anastomosis (with or without on-table lavage).

b.   Subtotal colectomy with ileorectal anastomosis.

E. Benefits of Colorectal Stenting for LBO

1.   For the acutely obstructed patient, stenting transitions an emergent situation into a nonemergent one.

    a.   Emergent colorectal surgery is a high-risk undertaking and has been shown to be an independent predictor of morbidity and mortality. The risks of emergent major abdominal interventions in this patient population increase with age, ASA class, and cancer stage. Mortality rates can be as high as 30% in emergent interventions, but are as low as 1–5% in the elective setting.

    b.   Stenting can be used as a temporizing measure in complex cases, so evaluation of the etiology of the lesion can be adequately performed with eventual resection by a surgeon with colorectal expertise.

2.   Stenting decreases the need for stoma formation by facilitating bowel preparation.

    a.   Patients with LBO are often poor candidates for surgical resection with primary anastomosis. They can be elderly patients with multiple comorbidities or present with significant malnourishment. If they are candidates for surgery, the majority would need diversion of some form at their initial operation. If stenting can successfully allow for adequate bowel preparation, one may be able to consider resection with primary anastomosis.

    b.   Up to two-third of patients who end up with a stoma in emergent situations never have their stomas reversed, and this is particularly true in the above-mentioned patient population.

    c.   Stoma formation reduces patient's quality of life and increases psychological stress significantly.

3. Stenting continues to be used as a palliative option for patients with advanced disease.

    a. Forty percent of patients with cancer and LBO present with metastatic disease or locally advanced fixed tumors. The surgeon is, therefore, put in the position of bringing a high-risk patient to the operating room with increased morbidity and mortality rates and little chance for cure.

    b. In the properly selected patient, there is evidence that patients who receive stents as palliation in stage IV cancer have equal survival times to those who undergo surgical procedures. Ultimately, patients succumb to their metastatic disease burden and not to reobstruction at the primary tumor site.

    c. Although stents have a very high clinical success rate in relieving colorectal obstructions, they cannot control bleeding. Control of clinically significant amounts of bleeding requires other interventions (e.g., surgery).

4. Colorectal stenting postpones major abdominal surgery in patients with obstructing colorectal lesions.

    a. LBO puts the surgeon in the situation of bringing patients to the operating room for major operative interventions when they may have significant cardiac or pulmonary comorbidities.

    b. Major surgery in the acute situation frequently requires intensive care unit admissions, long hospitalizations, and long recovery times.

    c. Patients may present with LBO and what is considered to be a hostile abdomen (e.g., multiple prior surgeries, adhesions).

    d. Stoma care will be necessary depending on the procedure type.

F. Contraindications to Colorectal Stenting

1. Perforation is an absolute contraindication.
2. Septic signs, such as fever or elevated white blood cell count.
3. Closed loop obstruction.
4. Complete obstruction

    a. No flow of contrast through the lesion is possible in these instances.

        b.   This is a strong predictor of technical failure and nearly always requires surgical management.

    5.   Obstruction of the cecum and lower rectum

        a.   Stenting of the lower rectum needs to be considered carefully. Stents may cause pain and tenesmus. In addition, because stents cannot always be retrieved, the presence of a stent may impair future attempts at resection. In these instances, the level of resection may be significantly lower in the pelvis than originally necessary and may impact future bowel function (e.g., turning a resection with a low colorectal anastomosis in to a coloanal anastomosis to resect beneath the stent or even worse turning a low anterior resection into an abdominoperineal resection).

    6.   Severe cecal dilation and concern for perforation with instillation of air through a colonoscope during the procedure.

G. Preoperative Evaluation

    1.   Full history and physical exam.

    2.   Patients should be medically optimized if they present acutely.

        a.   Nasogastric decompression may be necessary for abdominal distension and vomiting.

        b.   Fluid resuscitation is usually necessary, as patients have been unable to tolerate a diet.

        c.   Laboratory workup should be performed to evaluate the degree of electrolyte abnormalities and look for signs of sepsis.

    3.   Abdominal films and CT of the abdomen and pelvis, as described above.

    4.   Contrast enema is performed to assess the length and location of the obstructing lesion(s).

        a.   Pre-procedural evaluation with gastrograffin enema is particularly useful in cases of extrinsic compression (e.g., carcinomatosis, ovarian cancer) since they frequently have multiple areas of obstruction and may require more than one stent.

        b.   The decision to perform contrast enema is based on CT findings.

5. Endoscopy with biopsy can be performed within 12 h of presentation in the acutely presenting patient for diagnostic purposes, but in the chronically obstructed patient this is likely to have already been performed.

a. An enema may be administered first per rectum to attempt to clean residual stool beneath obstruction.

H. Available Colorectal Stents

1. **Covered vs. uncovered stents**
    a. Uncovered stents have a lower rate of migration but a higher rate of tumor ingrowth.
    b. Covered stents have a higher rate of migration but prevent tumor ingrowth.
2. **Stent size**
    a. There are a variety of stent sizes available. Generally speaking, the stent should be approximately 8 cm longer than the stricture, with at least a 3–4-cm margin on either side of the lesion. Stents shorten to varying degrees after deployment, so good overlap is essential.
    b. Stents are self-expanding and conform to the bowel lumen.
3. **Stent types**
    There are a number of commercially available stent systems. Please refer to company Web sites for specific information about available stents. There are some additional things to consider when choosing a stent.
    a. Stents are recapturable to varying degrees. You can begin deployment of a stent and resheath it if you are not happy with placement.
    b. Some systems require larger working channels in endoscopes than others. While some require a therapeutic colonoscope with a large working channel (e.g., 4.2 mm), many can be deployed through standard endoscopes (3.7-mm channel).
    c. Some stents are constructed with flares at their ends to prevent migration.

I. Technique

The technique of colorectal stenting has many variations, but we present the two most common methods. Stents can be deployed by using a combination of fluoroscopic and endoscopic guidance, which we find to be the most beneficial. It is particularly helpful for lesions in the right colon, as it can be very challenging or impossible to pass a guide wire through an obstruction at this site without endoscopic assistance and visualization. In addition, when using an endoscope to place stents, one can perform biopsies simultaneously if necessary. Stents may also be deployed with fluoroscopic guidance alone in the interventional suite.

1. **Patient preparation**
   a. In a nonacute setting with a partially obstructing lesion, full bowel preparation may be necessary. Otherwise, an enema per rectum on the morning of the procedure is adequate.
   b. Administer conscious sedation and place the patient in the lateral decubitus position.
   c. If using fluoroscopy, turn the patient supine as necessary to provide a better anatomic view of the lesion or stent.
2. **Description of the procedure**—combined endoscopic and fluoroscopic technique
   a. Use a therapeutic colonoscope with 4.2-mm working channel if available. This allows delivery of most stent systems through the colonoscope itself, as opposed to entering the system adjacent to the colonoscope. Many stent systems can now be employed through a standard colonoscope with a 3.7-mm channel as well. This is a particularly important point in stenting more proximal lesions. One can also attempt using a stricture scope initially if it seems possible to traverse the lesion with this scope as opposed to a standard adult colonoscope.
   b. Advance a .035″ guide wire through tumor or stricture (Fig. 37.1).
      i. The ability to advance a guide wire through the stricture is of critical importance. Technical success cannot be achieved without this vital step. One may instill contrast via a catheter into the bowel with fluoroscopy to help identify a lumen in the obstructive lesion if it is not easily apparent endoscopically (Fig. 37.2).

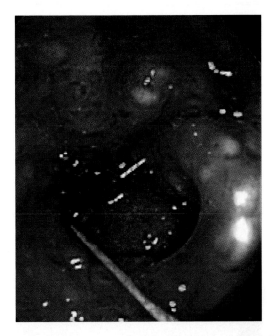

Fig. 37.1. Guide wire advancement through colonic anastomotic stricture.

        ii.   Time can be saved by preloading the guide wire though a catheter. Otherwise, feed a catheter over the guide wire after you successfully traverse the lesion.

   c.   Administer contrast through catheter.

        i.   This demonstrates the length of the stricture, its position, and degree of patency fluoroscopically.

        ii.   Due to instillation of air in addition to the contrast, one can usually visualize the stricture as well as the surrounding bowel, which is dilated with air and outlined with contrast (as in a double-contrast barium enema study).

   d.   Advance a stiff guide wire through the catheter, as the stiff wire facilitates stent delivery. The wire should be passed as far as can easily be accomplished proximal to the lesion (up to 20 cm) to be sure that it does not migrate distally during further manipulation of the colonoscope or stent system.

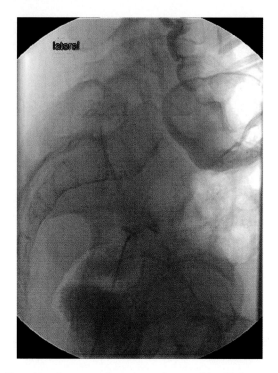

Fig. 37.2. Insertion of contrast through a catheter to identify lumen.

e. Advance the stent system over the stiff guide wire under
    fluoroscopic and endoscopic guidance.
    i.   Radio-opaque markers are present at either end of the
         stent. The marker on the tip of the stent system should
         be placed past lesion with fluoroscopic guidance to
         confirm adequate proximal placement.
    ii. Careful attention must be paid to the proximal tip to
         be certain that it is not at an angulation in the bowel
         or in a diverticulum to avoid perforation.
f. Stent delivery is performed with endoscopic and
    fluoroscopic guidance. The stent is deployed by withdrawal
    of the delivery system over sheath (Fig. 37.3).
    i.   It is an excellent idea to place metallic clips endo-
         scopically distal to the site of obstruction for a clear
         point of reference that is easily visualized with
         fluoroscopy.

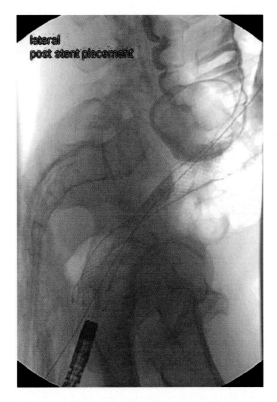

Fig. 37.3. Deployment of stent with both endoscopic and fluoroscopic guidance.

       ii.   Deployment of the stent itself can be inspected fluoroscopically so that repositioning maneuvers might be performed prior to full deployment.

      iii. One can visualize the distal end of the stent deployment endoscopically with the colonoscope in place (Fig. 37.4). This can help avoid a "watermelon seed" effect in which stents with too little distal overlap can be pulled proximally and "squirt out" of the obstruction.

  g. Instillation of contrast via a catheter placed proximal to the stent may be performed if there is concern that the entire lesion has not been covered.

  h. If the stent system cannot be advanced through the endoscope, it may not be possible to leave the colonoscope

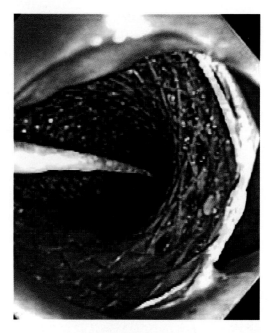

Fig. 37.4.   Endoscopic view of stent after deployment (distal end).

in place while advancing the stent system alongside the scope per anus. In this instance:

   i.   Advance the guide wire with both endoscopic and fluoroscopic guidance.

   ii.   Remove the colonoscope.

   iii.   Place the stent system over the wire with fluoroscopic guidance alone, using the radio-opaque markers as a guide to proper positioning.

   iv.   Replace the colonoscope to evaluate distal positioning.

   v.   Deploy the stent with both endoscopic and fluoroscopic guidance.

3.   Stent placement can be performed with fluoroscopic guidance alone.

   a.   The obstruction is located with fluoroscopy and water-soluble contrast enema.

   b.   The stricture is passed with a guide wire using fluoroscopic guidance and a catheter is advanced above the lesion.

A stiff guide wire is advanced through the catheter and the catheter is removed.

c. The stent system is inserted per anus over the stiff guide wire.

d. Radiologic markers are placed proximally and distally to the lesion.

e. The stent is deployed with fluoroscopic guidance alone.

J. Post-procedure Evaluation

1. Plain abdominal films should be performed to check and document stent position and to rule out perforation.
2. Water-soluble contrast enema may be used to confirm the stent position and efficacy in decompression.
3. Additional abdominal films 24 h later can be used in select circumstances to check for proper deployment, placement, and early delayed complications if questions exist.

K. Technical Issues

Success of stent placement is generally reported at greater than 90%.

1. Immediate failures
   a. Inability to pass the guide wire through the obstruction
   b. Inability to reach a more proximal lesion without looping the colonoscope
   c. Technical difficulty with stent deployment
      i. Proximal lesions may have issues with full stent expansion.
      ii. Failure of proper stent deployment may necessitate urgent surgery.
2. Better outcomes are seen with shorter stenoses. The reason for this may be more angulation with longer lesions.
3. Longer patency times are seen when stents are placed for more distal obstructions.
4. Multiple stents can be placed simultaneously in an overlapping fashion. This is normally indicated when there is a long area of

stenosis or if the stent was misplaced proximally or distally to the lesion.

5. For patients presenting with carcinomatosis, the immobility of the bowel caused by the peritoneal tumor deposits may lead to difficulty with colonoscopic advancement to the site of interest.

L. Complications

1. **Perforation** can be observed at the time of stent placement or shortly after. Perforation rates are reported to be up to 5%. This is the single most serious complication.
   a. **Causes**
      i. There is a high association with perforation and the use of balloon catheters to predilate the obstruction.
      ii. An overzealous guide wire exploration can cause a perforation.
      iii. Manipulation of the anchoring wires at the ends of the stents can cause perforation in rare instances.
   b. **Management**
      i. The treatment of acute perforation is emergent surgical intervention with colostomy in most instances.
      ii. Subtotal colectomy may be performed in select instances with the right surgical candidate.
      iii. Conservative management has been reported in patients with advanced disease, but is very risky and leads to poor outcomes (including death).
2. **Clinical reobstruction** from ingrowth or overgrowth can occur more often with uncovered stents. Ingrowth refers to tumor growth through the mesh of the stent itself, and overgrowth refers to tumor growing around the ends of the stent.
   a. Workup for reobstruction after stent placement includes abdominal plain films, water-soluble contrast enema, and endoscopic evaluation.
   b. Options for management include placement of an additional stent over the original stent (which is left in situ), intraluminal laser ablation of the ingrowth (theoretically), or ultimately a diverting stoma or resection.

3. **Stent migration**, which as stated above, is more frequent with covered stents.
    a. This can occur in particular after adjuvant therapies for colorectal tumors and may require colonoscopic stent retrieval. If there has been significant reduction in tumor size, placement of another stent may not be necessary.
    b. Occasionally, patients may pass the stent per anus.
4. Less common adverse outcomes and symptoms.
    a. **Pain and tenesmus** are usually the results of stent placement in lower rectal lesions (<6 cm from the anal verge).
    b. **Rectal bleeding** can occur but is usually self-limited and managed medically.
    c. Increased **bowel frequency**, diarrhea, and incontinence have been reported. However, it is unclear whether this is related to stent placement or the underlying disease process.
5. **Silent bowel perforation** has been seen in specimens after secondary procedures. The cause of this may be erosion of the stent or anchoring wires through the bowel wall. This finding has raised concerns about the oncologic aspects of the procedure and possible tumor dissemination. Water-soluble contrast enema can be used to evaluate for delayed perforation if there is clinical suspicion.
6. **Stent impaction** with stool is not uncommon. This needs to be kept in mind as an aggressive bowel regimen after stent placement can be preventative.

M. Post-procedure Options

Clinical success of colonoscopic decompression with stenting is usually defined as flatus or stool within 48 h of stent placement.

1. **Definitive management**: Patients can be discharged home after 24 h of observation for palliative indications or if no immediate secondary procedure is planned. Stenting may be considered as definitive therapy for those with advanced disease. These patients may be followed with clinical exam and abdominal films at intervals depending on the circumstances (Fig. 37.5).

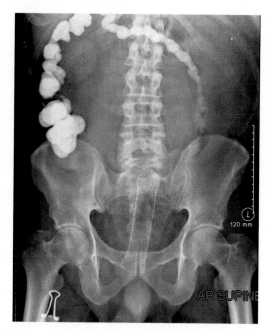

Fig. 37.5. Follow-up imaging showing full expansion of stent.

    a.   For patients with benign conditions, stent removal may be all that is eventually necessary. In this instance, use of a covered stent is preferable (Fig. 37.6).

2.   A second option is to have patients remain in the hospital in preparation for a necessary **secondary procedure**.

    a.   Cardiac evaluation and risk stratification can be performed.

    b.   Hyperalimentation can be administered to the malnourished patient.

    c.   Full bowel preparation can be undertaken now that the obstruction has been temporarily relieved.

    d.   Total colonoscopy can be performed if not already done recently to reevaluate the obstruction and look for synchronous lesions proximally.

    e.   Staging workup can be completed if not already done, including:

        i.   CEA level

        ii.   CT imaging

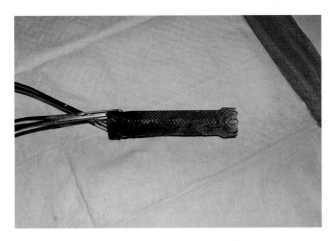

Fig. 37.6. Successful removal of covered stent after placement for anastomotic stricture.

       iii.   MRI (if indicated): MRI is not contraindicated after most stents are placed.

    f.   Laparoscopy or laparotomy can be performed in 7–14 days for nonmetastatic disease.

    i.   In particular, bowel decompression with colonic stenting assists with a laparoscopic approach by resolving proximal bowel dilation. The stent can be removed in situ with the colon or rectum through an extraction site as is done with standard laparoscopic resections.

3. **Delayed surgical procedure**

    a.   Alternatively, surgery can be delayed for 4–6 weeks at the discretion of the physician. This may depend on the extent of disease, comorbidities, and nutritional status.

    b.   A bowel regimen is helpful to prevent reobstruction in the interim.

Selected References

Cheung H, Chung C, Tsang W, Wong J, Yau K, Li M. Endolaparoscopic approach vs conventional open surgery in the treatment of obstructing left-sided colon cancer: a randomized controlled trial. Arch Surg. 2009;144(12):1127–32.

Davies RJ, D'Sa IB, Lucarotti ME, Fowler AL, Tottle A, Birch P, Cook TA. Bowel function following insertion of self-expanding metallic stents for palliation of colorectal cancer. Colorectal Dis. 2005;7(3):251–3.

Dronamraju S, Ramamurthy S, Kelly S, Hayat M. Role of self-expanding metallic stents in the management of malignant obstruction of the proximal colon. Dis Colon Rectum. 2009;52(9):1657–61.

Faragher I, Chaitowitz I, Stupart D. Long-term results of palliative stenting or surgery for incurable obstructing colon cancer. Colorectal Dis. 2008;10(7):668–72.

Johnson R, Marsh R, Corson J, Seymour K. A comparison of two methods of palliation of large bowel obstruction due to irremovable colon cancer. Ann R Coll Surg Engl. 2004;86(2):99–103.

Jung M, Park S, Jeon S, et al. Factors associated with the long-term outcome of a self-expandable colon stent used for palliation of malignant colorectal obstruction. Surg Endosc. 2010;24(3):525–30.

Keswani R, Azar R, Edmundowicz S, et al. Stenting for malignant colonic obstruction: a comparison of efficacy and complications in colonic versus extracolonic malignancy. Gastrointest Endosc. 2009;69(3 Pt 2):675–80.

Pirlet I, Slim K, Kwiatkowski F, Michot F, Millat B. Emergency preoperative stenting versus surgery for acute left-sided malignant colonic obstruction: a multicenter randomized controlled trial. Surg Endosc. 2011;25(6):1814–21.

Shin S, Kim T, Kim B, Lee Y, Song S, Kim W. Clinical application of self-expandable metallic stent for treatment of colorectal obstruction caused by extrinsic invasive tumors. Dis Colon Rectum. 2008;51(5):578–83.

Stipa F, Pigazzi A, Bascone B, et al. Management of obstructive colorectal cancer with endoscopic stenting followed by single-stage surgery: open or laparoscopic resection? Surg Endosc. 2008;22(6):1477–81.

Trompetas V. Emergency management of malignant acute left-sided colonic obstruction. Ann R Coll Surg Engl. 2008;90(3):181–6.

Part VI

Other Adjunct Minimally Invasive Procedures for Gastrointestinal Surgeons

38. Hand-Assisted Laparoscopic Live Donor Nephrectomy[*]

Kent W. Kercher, M.D., F.A.C.S.

A. Indications, Contraindications, and Preoperative Evaluation

1. Laparoscopic donor nephrectomy is indicated in patients who meet the criteria for live organ donation to an intended recipient for kidney transplantation. Live kidney donors are, by definition, healthy individuals with two normal kidneys and no medical contraindications to unilateral nephrectomy. Relative contraindications to live kidney donation include hypertension, diabetes, intrinsic renal disease, malignancy, or other significant medical comorbidities. Kidney donors must be approved for live organ donation through a rigorous selection process that focuses on minimizing risk for the organ donor. This process includes medical and psychological screening and formal approval by a live donor selection committee.

2. For live donor nephrectomy, hand-assisted laparoscopy has the potential to decrease operative and warm ischemia times, and may provide an additional margin of comfort and safety when compared to a totally laparoscopic approach. These advantages appear to be conferred without an increase in morbidity or overall cost.

3. CT angiogram of the abdomen and pelvis with 3-dimensional image reconstruction is used to assess renal anatomy and to rule out other intra-abdominal or retroperitoneal processes that could

---

[*]This chapter was contributed by Aloke K. Mandal, M.D., Ph.D., and Michael J. Conlin, M.D., in the previous edition.

N.T. Nguyen and C.E.H. Scott-Conner (eds.), *The SAGES Manual: Volume 2 Advanced Laparoscopy and Endoscopy*, DOI 10.1007/978-1-4614-2347-8_38, © Springer Science+Business Media, LLC 2012

contraindicate laparoscopic nephrectomy. CT angiography allows for delineation of arterial, venous, and ureteral anatomy and provides information regarding the number and caliber of renal vessels as well as kidney size and volume. If there is concern that renal size or function is asymmetric on angiography, then nuclear renogram can determine the degree to which each kidney contributes to overall renal function.

4. In the large majority (approximately 80%) of cases, the left kidney is selected for organ donation. This relates to the fact that the left renal vein is anatomically longer than the right renal vein, making implantation into the recipient technically easier. Relative contraindications to the use of the left kidney include (1) multiple left renal arteries or veins; (2) a small accessory lower pole artery potentially supplying the left ureter; (3) a small right kidney and/or disproportionately low split renal function of the right kidney; (4) an indeterminate cystic lesion or stone in the right kidney; (5) an extrarenal lesion on the right side requiring concomitant evaluation or treatment; and (6) an extrarenal lesion or anatomic variation on the left that could increase operative risk to the donor. In essence, if there is any significant discrepancy in size or function, the donor should be left with the "better" of the two kidneys.

B. Patient Position and Room Setup

1. Following induction of general anesthesia, insert a Foley catheter to monitor urine output during the case. Place the patient in a true lateral decubitus position on a bean bag. Flex the table, with the break in the table just above the umbilicus. Insert an axillary roll and place the arms outstretched on an arm board, with pillows between them. Place sequential compression devices on both legs. Secure and pad all extremities.

2. Widely prep and drape the entire abdomen and ipsilateral flank in the usual sterile fashion.

3. The surgeon and first assistant stand facing the patient's abdomen (Fig. 38.1).

4. Place two monitors at the head of the table on either side of the patient.

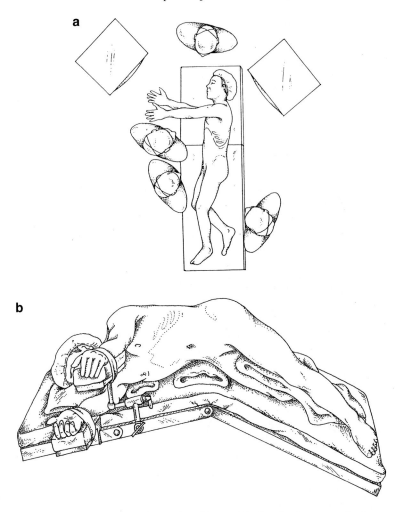

Fig. 38.1. Room setup and lateral patient positioning for laparoscopic donor nephrectomy. (**a**) Room setup allows the surgeon and assistant to stand facing the patient. The scrub nurse and instrument table are on the opposite side of the patient. (**b**) Placing the patient in the true lateral position takes advantage of gravity in allowing for medial rotation of adjacent viscera (spleen, pancreas, and colon). Note that the operating table is flexed, and all extremities are secured and padded.

C. Equipment

1. Hand-assist device
2. Two 12-mm ports (left nephrectomy): One additional 5-mm port needed for right nephrectomy (liver retractor)
3. 10-mm 30° laparoscope
4. Monopolar cautery (hook and scissors)
5. Ultrasonic dissector (harmonic scalpel)
6. Vascular load (2.0 mm) endo-GIA stapler
7. Endoscopic clip applier (10 mm)
8. 10-mm right-angle dissector (used for vascular dissection—renal artery, renal vein, and lumbar veins)

D. Trocar Position and Location of Hand-Assist Device: Left Donor Nephrectomy

1. Insert the hand-assist device through a 6.5–7-cm midline periumbilical incision (Fig. 38.2). Establish pneumoperitoneum by placing a trocar into the hand-assist port. Wrap the surgeon's

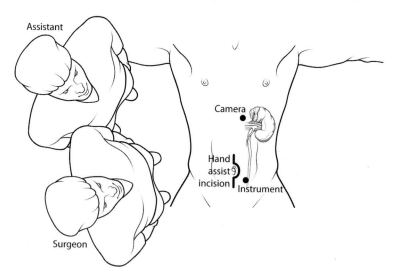

Fig. 38.2. Port placement and surgeon/assistant position for hand-assisted laparoscopic left nephrectomy (printed with permission of Carolinas Healthcare System).

left wrist and forearm with Ioban drape to facilitate passage through hand-assist device. The surgeon's left hand is placed intraperitoneal through the device. Use of K-Y jelly facilitates ease of passage of hand through the device.

2. Insert two 12-mm ports using the guidance of the intra-abdominal hand. Place the superior (camera) port in the midclavicular line at the left costal margin. Place the inferior port at the left rectus border, four fingerbreadths medial to the iliac crest. This is the surgeon's right-hand working port.

E. Performing Laparoscopic Left Donor Nephrectomy

1. A complete medial visceral rotation (colon, spleen, tail of pancreas, and greater curvature of the stomach) is required for full exposure of the left kidney.

2. First, mobilize the splenic flexure of the colon using sharp and blunt dissection, and judicious use of electrocautery. Mobilize the entire left colon medially along the avascular plane (white line of Toldt). Use your left hand for blunt dissection and retraction.

3. Divide the splenorenal ligament with cautery or harmonic scalpel. Gravity allows for the spleen to fall medially, exposing the tail of the pancreas and the splenic vessels.

4. Carefully mobilize the pancreatic tail away from Gerota's fascia.

5. Take care to mobilize the greater curvature of the stomach and short gastric vessels superior to the upper pole of the spleen.

6. Open Gerota's fascia sharply just lateral to the aorta and several centimeters caudal to the lower pole of the left kidney. Bluntly elevate the left ureter and gonadal vein up away from the psoas muscle. Carefully protect the blood supply to the ureter by leaving the entire mesoureter intact.

7. Retract the kidney medially and divide the posterior renal attachments with electrocautery. The entire kidney must be mobilized out of the retroperitoneum.

8. Elevate the gonadal vein and ureter. Follow the left gonadal vein cephalad to the left renal vein.

Expose the left renal and adrenal veins. Circumferentially dissect the adrenal vein using a right-angle dissector, clip it proximally and distally with two to three clips on each side, and sharply divide it.

9. Dissect the adrenal gland away from the upper pole of the kidney using the ultrasonic shears. Take care to avoid injury to any adjacent upper pole renal vessels.

10. After confirming adequate hydration, administer mannitol (12.5–25 gm IV) before the hilar vascular dissection.

11. Rotate the kidney medially and dissect, clip, and divide the lumbar veins (usually one to three in number).

12. Circumferentially dissect the renal artery down to its origin from the aorta.

13. Dissect the renal vein well below the adrenal vein entry point, and medial to the point at which the renal vein crosses the aorta.

14. Dissect the distal ureter down to the pelvic brim and beyond the iliac bifurcation. Divide the gonadal vein at this level with clips or a vascular stapler.

15. Once the recipient team is prepared in the adjacent operating room, administer lasix (10 mg IV). A brisk diuresis should ensue.

16. Control the distal ureter with two to three clips and then sharply divide it just proximal to the clips. Confirm urine output from the cut ureter prior to vascular division.

17. Elevate the kidney with your left hand, and divide the renal artery, followed by the renal vein, using two separate loads of a vascular endo-GIA stapler. Divide the artery flush with the aorta and the vein well below the adrenal vein entry point in order to ensure maximal vessel length.

18. Rapidly extract the kidney through the hand-assist port and place on ice.

19. Inspect the operative field to rule out staple-line bleeding. Inspect the colon mesentery and close any mesenteric defects to prevent internal herniation of bowel. Close the ports and hand-assist incision in standard fashion.

F. Trocar Position and Location of Hand-Assist Device: Right Donor Nephrectomy

1. Place the patient in the true lateral position as described for left nephrectomy.

2. Port setup for right donor nephrectomy (Fig. 38.3) is a mirror image of the left, except that an additional 5-mm port is needed

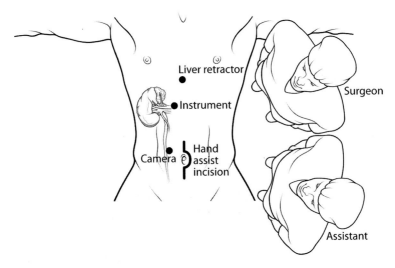

Fig. 38.3. Port placement and surgeon/assistant position for hand-assisted laparoscopic right nephrectomy (printed with permission of Carolinas Healthcare System).

for liver retraction. This port is placed in a subxiphoid position just to the patient's right of the falciform ligament.

3. Pass your left hand intraperitoneally through the hand-assist device.

4. Use the superior (12 mm) port for the right-hand working instrument.

5. Use the inferior (12 mm) port for the laparoscope.

G. Performing Laparoscopic Right Donor Nephrectomy

1. Medially mobilize the hepatic flexure and the right colon away from Gerota's fascia.

2. A Kocher maneuver is usually required to mobilize the duodenum away from the vena cava and to provide access to the right renal vein.

3. Open Gerota's fascia just below the lower pole of the kidney and along the lateral edge of the vena cava. Bluntly elevate the right ureter and gonadal vein up away from the psoas muscle.

4. Control the gonadal vein with clips and divide just proximal to its entry into the IVC.

5. Divide the posterolateral/retroperitoneal renal attachments and mobilize the kidney from lateral to medial.

6. Elevate the kidney and open Gerota's fascia along the lateral border of the IVC, from the lower pole of the kidney up to the interface between the kidney and the inferior pole of the right adrenal gland. This maneuver exposes the anterior aspect of the right renal vein.

7. Divide the attachments between the upper pole of the kidney and the adrenal gland with the harmonic scalpel.

8. Rotate the kidney medially and identify and circumferentially dissect the renal artery from a posterior approach. Take care to avoid injuring the underlying renal vein and IVC while dissecting the artery with a right-angle clamp.

9. Once the renal artery and vein are circumferentially dissected, the distal ureteral and gonadal dissection and division are carried out as described for left nephrectomy.

10. For vascular transection and kidney extraction, bring the endo-GIA stapler in through the inferior 12-mm port and move the camera to the superior port. Place your right hand through the hand-assist device and operate the stapler with your left hand. This orientation allows for the renal vein to be divided flush with the vena cava in order to maximize vein length.

H. Complications

1. **Hemorrhage**

    a. Cause and prevention: Laparoscopic nephrectomy requires dissection and division of the adrenal vein, renal artery, and renal vein. Meticulous hemostasis must be maintained throughout the case in order to provide for maximal donor safety. Major bleeding is rare, but can be substantial if there is a stapler malfunction during division of the hilar vessels. Vascular staplers should be loaded by an experienced scrub technician. The surgeon must obtain clear visualization prior to stapler firing and avoid stapling across previously placed titanium clips (typically located on the adrenal and lumbar veins).

b. Recognition and management: Bleeding is easily recognized by monitoring the operative field during and at the conclusion of the case. Minor bleeding can be controlled with local pressure using the intraperitoneal hand or with the use of clips for small vessels. Major hemorrhage should prompt conversion to open.

2. **Injury to adjacent organs (colon, spleen, pancreas, stomach)**

a. Cause and prevention: Capsular splenic tears are the most common injury during medial visceral rotation. Injury can be avoided by applying only gentle traction on the spleen during division of the splenorenal ligament. Injury to the pancreas and splenic vessels occurs when the plane of dissection is too close to the pancreas. Injury can be avoided by staying immediately adjacent to Gerota's fascia during medial visceral rotation. Hollow viscus injuries usually are the result of direct thermal injury. Maintaining complete visualization of the operative field during dissection is important to avoid these types of injuries. Care must be taken to avoid contact between energy sources and the bowel.

b. Recognition and management: Injury to adjacent organs is ideally recognized intraoperatively and repaired in the standard fashion. Most splenic bleeding is minor and can be managed by taking tension off of the spenic capsule (by completing division of the splenorenal ligament) or by application of topical hemostatic agents and use of local tamponade with the intraperitoneal hand. Injury to the pancreas may manifest postoperatively in the form of pancreatitis, pseudocyst, or subphrenic fluid collections. Management is generally conservative but may require percutaneous drainage. Bowel injury may present in a delayed fashion and can be characterized by signs of sepsis. A high index of suspicion for delayed bowel injury should prompt further radiographic investigation and/or reexploration.

3. Colon mesenteric defects resulting in internal hernia and small bowel obstruction

a. Cause and prevention: Windows in the left colon mesentery can occur during mobilization of the colon away from Gerota's fascia. Mesenteric defects are more likely to occur in thin patients with very little retroperitoneal fat. In these patients in particular, care must be taken to meticulously dissect the mesentery off of Gerota's fascia using sharp and blunt dissection, often facilitated by the surgeon's intra-abdominal hand.

b.　Recognition and management: The colon mesentery should be inspected at the conclusion of the case. Holes in the mesentery should be closed by reapproximating the edges of the defect with running suture or titanium clips. Defects that are left open can predispose to internal herniation of small bowel and subsequent bowel obstruction.

Selected References

Flowers JL, Jacobs S, Cho E, et al. Comparison of open and laparoscopic live donor nephrectomy. Ann Surg. 1997;226(4):483–9. discussion 489–490.

Philosophe B, Kuo PC, Schweitzer EJ, et al. Laparoscopic versus open donor nephrectomy: comparing ureteral complications in the recipients and improving the laparoscopic technique. Transplantation. 1999;68(4):497–502.

Kercher KW, Heniford BT, Mathews BD, Hayes D, Eskind LB, Smith TI, Lincourt AE, Irby PB, Teigland CM. Laparoscopic vs open nephrectomy in 210 consecutive patients: outcomes, cost, and changes in practice patterns. Surg Endosc. 2003a;17: 1889–95.

Jacobs SC, Cho E, Liao P, Bartlett ST. Laparoscopic donor nephrectomy: the University of Maryland 6-year experience. J Urol. 2004;171(1):47–51.

Ratner LE, Montgomery RA, Maley WR, et al. Laparoscopic live donor nephrectomy: the recipient. Transplantation. 2000;69(11):2319–23.

Keller JE, Dolce CJ, Griffin D, Norton HJ, Heniford BT, Kercher KW. Maximizing the donor pool: use of right kidneys and kidneys with multiple arteries for live donor transplantation. Surg Endosc. 2009;23(10):2327–31.

Ruiz-Deya G, Cheng S, Palmer E, Thomas R, Slakey D. Open donor, laparoscopic donor and hand assisted laparoscopic donor nephrectomy: a comparison of outcomes. J Urol. 2001;166(4):1270–3. discussion 1273–1274.

Slakey DP, Wood JC, Hender D, Thomas R, Cheng S. Laparoscopic living donor nephrectomy: advantages of the hand-assisted method. Transplantation. 1999;68(4): 581–3.

Kercher KW, Dahl D, Harland R, Blute R, Gallagher K, Litwin D. Hand-assisted laparoscopic donor nephrectomy minimizes warm ischemia. Urology. 2001;58(2): 152–6.

Lindstrom P, Haggman M, Wadstrom J. Hand-assisted laparoscopic surgery (HALS) for live donor nephrectomy is more time- and cost-effective than standard laparoscopic nephrectomy. Surg Endosc. 2002;16(3):422–5.

Dolce CJ, Keller JE, Walters KC, Griffin D, Norton HJ, Heniford BT, Kercher KW. Laparoscopic versus open live donor nephrectomy: outcomes alalysis of 266 consecutive patients. Surg Endosc. 2009;23(7):1564–8.

Kercher KW, Joels CS, Matthews BD, Lincourt AE, Smith TI, Heniford BT. Hand-assisted surgery improves outcomes for laparoscopic nephrectomy. Am Surg. 2003b;69(12): 1061–6.

39. Adolescent Bariatric Surgery

Marc P. Michalsky, M.D.
Steven Teich, M.D.

A. Introduction

The prevalence of obesity among children and adolescents is rapidly increasing and poses one of the most serious major healthcare challenges of the twenty-first century. Along with a reported threefold rise in childhood obesity in the last several decades, the pediatric population has seen a corresponding increase in serious obesity-related comorbid diseases, such as hypertension, type 2 diabetes mellitus, dyslipidemia, cardiovascular derangement, and obstructive sleep apnea (OSA) to name a few. The recognition of the establishment of such disease patterns in patients as young as 5 years of age has recently helped to focus the medical community on the increasing need for clinical and translational research focused on effective prevention and treatment strategies in an effort to reverse the current epidemic.

Recent data from the Centers for Disease Control and Prevention (CDC) indicate that 32% of children in the USA have a body mass index (BMI) for age ≥85th percentile (compared to historic reference values which define normal weight in children to be BMI for age >5th and <85th percentile), with approximately 17% being defined as obese (≥95th percentile). Although data from the latest National Health and Nutrition Examination Survey (NHANES) shows some leveling off of the persistent rise in childhood obesity, with the exception of males in the highest weight group, recent estimates suggest that as many as 4% of American children suffer from extreme obesity (BMI ≥99th), outnumbering those affected by childhood cancer, HIV, diabetes mellitus, and cystic fibrosis combined. Even more worrisome, an increasing body of evidence has demonstrated a high propensity for severely obese adolescents to become severely obese adults. The ramifications of such trends cannot be fully

N.T. Nguyen and C.E.H. Scott-Conner (eds.), *The SAGES Manual: Volume 2*   577
Advanced Laparoscopy and Endoscopy, DOI 10.1007/978-1-4614-2347-8_39,
© Springer Science+Business Media, LLC 2012

appreciated without the comprehensive consideration of the impact (both on the individual patient and overall healthcare system) of the progression of multiple obesity-related diseases as this population ages.

B. Childhood Obesity and Comorbid Disease

Although the majority of literature regarding obesity-related comorbid disease is focused on adults, recent data highlights the establishment of obesity-related chronic illnesses in children as young as 5 years of age. Seventy-five percent of obese adults and 25–50% of extremely obese adults become obese *during adulthood*, and thus do not suffer the same cumulative physiological effects (i.e., "pound years," Fig. 39.1) and associated comorbid disease risks compared to individuals who develop severe obesity early in life (i.e., juvenile-onset obesity). Given the rapidly rising prevalence of obesity in childhood, the lifetime burden of disease risk in these individuals is of major concern. An increasing body of literature has highlighted the broad spectrum of disease processes that are being increasingly recognized in the severely obese pediatric and adolescent population with almost every organ system being negatively affected. Common comorbid diseases seen among severely obese adolescents appear strikingly similar to those among severely obese adult populations and include sleep-disordered breathing, hypertension, nonalcoholic fatty liver disease (NAFLD), cardiovascular abnormalities, impaired glucose tolerance, type 2 diabetes mellitus, polycystic ovary syndrome, and psychological disorders to name a few.

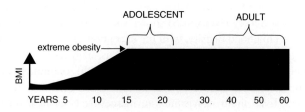

Fig. 39.1. Morbidly obese adolescents are considered "early" in the longitudinal spectrum of juvenile-onset obesity and have a shorter duration of obesity-related burden (i.e., "*pound years*") compared to adults (reprinted with permission from Michalsky MP, Garcia V, Adolescent Bariatric Surgery. Handbook of Obesity Surgery Current Concepts and Therapy of Morbid Obesity and Related Disease, edited by Mervyn Deitel, Michel Gagner, John B. Dixon, Jacques Himpens, Atul K. Madan, FD-Communications, Inc., Toronto, Canada, 2010).

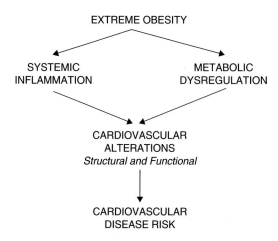

Fig. 39.2. Extreme obesity is mechanistically linked to chronic inflammation and metabolic derangement, leading to increased risk of cardiovascular disease.

Despite increasing recognition of obesity-related diseases in the child-hood and adolescent population, debate exists regarding the mechanism(s) responsible for the development and progression of individual disease processes. Recently, however, emerging evidence has suggested that obesity is associated with a state of chronic inflammation, which may subsequently serve to potentiate several mechanisms culminating in impaired insulin-glucose metabolism and hypertension culminating in increased cardiovascular disease risk and premature death (Fig. 39.2). This association is strikingly apparent in the adult population when considering the link between obesity and "metabolic syndrome" (i.e., hyperinsulinemia, glucose intolerance, hypertension, dyslipidemia, and central adiposity), albeit a less stable diagnostic entity in the pediatric population. Recent evidence from both human and animal studies has suggested that obesity-related inflammation and oxidative stress may cause a disruption in the endothelial production of nitric oxide (NO), which is important in the homeostatic mechanism(s) responsible for vascular performance. In addition, numerous reports have cited an association between diminished endothelial NO bioavailability and many forms of obesity-related comorbid diseases, including atherosclerosis, hypercholesterolemia, diabetes mellitus, and hypertension. Thus, it appears that the phenomenon of early inflammation and/or stress-induced endothelial cell dysfunction may be a common and unifying feature in the development and progression of obesity-related comorbid disease.

1. Cardiovascular Disease

Although the major complications from obesity-related cardiovascular disease (i.e., atherosclerosis, myocardial infarction, heart failure, peripheral vascular disease, and stroke) are not typically apparent until later in life, the pathophysiologic processes that lead to the development and progression of cardiovascular disease begin during childhood as a consequence of juvenile-onset obesity. Even though large vessel disease and myocardial fibrosis are rarely reported in the severely obese adolescent population, structural and functional cardiovascular abnormalities, including left ventricular hypertrophy, diminished diastolic performance, and cardiac work load, have been observed in adolescents undergoing bariatric surgery and have been shown to demonstrate at least partial improvement following surgical weight loss.

2. Nonalcoholic Fatty Liver Disease

NAFLD is a disease spectrum that ranges in severity from uncomplicated steatosis to nonalcoholic steatohepatitis (NASH) and has been shown to have a prevalence as high as 80% in the obese pediatric population. Although current trends predict an increasing incidence of liver-related deaths, recent reports demonstrate a reversal of disease following reduction in excess body weight.

3. Glucose Impairment

The link between childhood obesity and the development of impaired glucose metabolism is quite striking with recent reports of basal hyper-insulinemia in as much as 80% of obese children studied, with 1-6% demonstrating type 2 diabetes mellitus. As illustrated in Fig. 39.2., disturbances of mechanisms responsible for glucose regulation appear to be mechanistically linked to a state of chronic inflammation as evidenced by numerous reports demonstrating the link among obesity, insulin resistance as determined by homeostatic model assessment (HOMA-IR), and elevated serum levels of C-reactive protein (CRP). Although the specific mechanisms are debated, recent evidence has highlighted the role of insulin resistance and proatherogenic pathways leading to endovascular dysfunction and obesity-related cardiovascular disease. As with other forms of obesity-related comorbid diseases during childhood, an increasing body of evidence has shown improvement and/or complete reversal of metabolic dysregulation following surgical weight loss.

4. Obstructive Sleep Apnea

Sleep-disordered breathing is strongly associated with childhood as well as adult obesity. In addition to potential social and demographic ramifications as a consequence of chronic fatigue, OSA can result in hypertension as well as cardiac dysfunction and an associated increased risk of sudden death if left untreated. Evidence shows that significant improvement and abrogation of associated risks from OSA are seen as a result of even modest reduction of excess body weight (i.e., 10%) in the affected pediatric population.

5. Psychological Disorders

Relatively little is known regarding the potential impact of childhood obesity, and more specifically severe childhood obesity, on the complex developmental changes involved in the transition from childhood to adulthood. Current consensus suggests that such individuals experience significant difficulties during this important transition period as evidenced by a number of recent studies demonstrating an association between childhood obesity and depression. As with other obesity-related comorbid diseases, several recent reports have suggested that childhood obesity, in individuals as young as 5 years of age, is a risk factor for depression during adulthood.

C. The Argument for Early Intervention

Although the focus of ongoing academic debate, supporters of early intervention (i.e., adolescent bariatric surgery) cite the current literature demonstrating the beneficial effect(s) of early weight loss on the development and progression of multiple obesity-related comorbid conditions. In a recent report by Inge et al., evaluation of adolescents undergoing bariatric surgery shows reversal of type 2 diabetes, with associated improvement in fasting serum glucose and insulin levels, as well as improved hypertension. In addition, Ippish et al., in a recent study examining baseline cardiac geometry and functional characteristics using transthoracic echocardiography, clearly demonstrated improved cardiac structure and function after surgically induced weight loss. Combined with numerous reports demonstrating improvement in dyslipidemia, OSA, and hypertension, a hypothesis highlighting a potential window of opportunity for comorbid disease reversal has emerged. As discussed earlier and illustrated in Fig. 39.1., it is currently believed, although not yet proven, that intervention earlier in life (i.e., during the adolescent time period) may take advantage of the potential for greater cellular plasticity and associated organ remodeling seen in younger individuals resulting in an overall diminished state of cumulative disease burden (i.e., pound years). While clinical data comparing the longitudinal consequences of surgical weight loss with regards to the natural history of comorbid disease are presently lacking, such end points are the focus of a large multi-institutional observational study sponsored by the National Institutes of Health (NIH), Teen-Longitudinal Assessment of Bariatric Surgery (LABS) (www.Teen-LABS.org). The results of this study will hopefully lead to improved insight with regards to the surgical treatment and outcomes in this important population.

D. Surgical Trends and Outcomes

In contrast to the previous decade, where population-based adolescent bariatric surgery varied little (between 1996 and 2000), recently there has been a dramatic increase in the utilization of bariatric surgical procedures as a primary treatment modality for severe childhood obesity. In parallel to the increased number of operations being performed, there has been a recent proliferation of pediatric tertiary care centers offering comprehensive multidisciplinary care for the obese population. In a recent survey (2007) of 180 pediatric hospitals by the National Association of Children's Hospital's and Related Institutions (NACHRI), designed to characterize the existing pediatric obesity programs in the USA, 50% ($n = 80$) of responding institutions reported having an organized childhood obesity program, with 26% having a multidisciplinary team (consisting of a physician, dietician, physical activity specialist, and psychologist) and 19% offering bariatric surgery. Interestingly, however, results showed that approximately 30% of these designated disease-specific programs became operational only within a 3-year time period preceding administration of the survey. Although effective mechanisms to track longitudinal changes in the number of institutions offering this type of comprehensive care are not well developed, it is widely believed that the development of centers designed to treat childhood obesity, including the establishment of adolescent-specific bariatric surgical programs, continues to rise.

Multiple recent reports in favor of adolescent bariatric surgery cite postoperative complication rates that appear to be the same or better when compared to parallel adult cohorts and/or historic data. In addition to the concept of cumulative disease burden as a manifestation of obesity duration and as a variable in support of "early" surgical intervention, recent results raise the question of optimal timing based on the overall spectrum of preoperative body mass. Assessment of 61 adolescents who underwent RYGB at a single pediatric center demonstrated that though patients demonstrated an improvement or reversal of cardiovascular risk factors with a mean reduction of BMI of approximately 37% overall only 17% of patients achieved a BMI consistent with a nonobese state (i.e., $BMI < 30$ kg/m^2 or $BMI < 85$th percentile for age). Although further longitudinal research is needed, these results suggest the existence of an inverse relationship between the severity of preoperative body mass and the probability of achieving a nonobese state during the postoperative time period. This observation is similar to multiple reports in the adult bariatric population and supports the contention that delaying weight loss surgery until an adolescent is super-obese ($BMI > 50$ kg/m^2) may preclude complete reversal of obesity and amelioration of associated comorbid diseases and increase the probability of weight regain in the long-term postoperative time period.

E. Weight Loss Procedures

While there is literature reporting the use of various weight loss procedures in the adolescent population including RYGB, adjustable gastric band, sleeve gastrectomy, and biliopancreatic diversion, there is no clear consensus on which procedure(s) is the most effective or appropriate in the adolescent population. As mentioned earlier, current reports examining the use of various bariatric procedures in the adolescent population demonstrate safety and efficacy profiles that are similar to those seen in the adult population. Additional multi-institutional studies will be required before a consensus is likely to be achieved.

F. Adolescent Guidelines

The appropriate BMI threshold for the consideration of adolescent bariatric surgery has previously been a source of heated controversy. However, as discussed earlier, current data suggests that intervening at a higher BMI may result in a lower propensity to achieve a nonobese state during the postoperative period (i.e., BMI < 30 kg/m^2 or BMI < 85th percentile for age). Although no final consensus exists and initial recommendations for the pediatric community call for a higher threshold from that used in the adult population (as a result of the 1991 NIH consensus conference on the use of bariatric surgery in adults), current recommendations call for the application of bariatric surgical procedures in adolescent patients who have a BMI ≥ 35 kg/m^2 with serious comorbidities (i.e., type 2 diabetes, OSA, pseudotumor cerebri, etc.) or BMI ≥ 40 kg/m^2 with no identified obesity-related comorbidities.

In an effort to model to programmatic development for the administration of unified bariatric care in the adolescent population, similar to the organizational quality assurance oversight framework recently developed in the adult bariatric community through national organizations, such as the American College of Surgeons and American Society of Metabolic and Bariatric Surgery (ASMBS), guidelines for adolescent bariatric surgical centers of excellence designation are currently under development. In general, adolescent bariatric weight loss centers need to have adolescent-centered resources and associated specialists with expertise specifically geared toward this population. The multidisciplinary team should consist of specialists with expertise in adolescent obesity evaluation and behavioral health, an adolescent trained registered dietician, and an adolescent exercise physiologist and/or physical trainer. Access to pediatric subspecialists through well-established consulting relationships should include pulmonary medicine, endocrinology, cardiology, and orthopedics. In addition, programs should have a multidisciplinary review process to discuss and review both preoperative surgical candidates as well as patients that have already undergone surgical intervention in an effort to foster individual structured treatment plans for each adolescent.

The optimal timing of adolescent bariatric surgery has not been settled. Adolescent bariatric surgery should not occur until physiological maturation is generally complete and sexual maturation is at Tanner stage III–IV. Overweight children generally have accelerated onset of puberty and are likely to have advanced bone age compared to age-matched normal-weight children. Radiographs of the hand and wrist can be used to accurately determine skeletal maturation (i.e., the attainment of adult stature and assessment of epiphyseal plate status). As new less invasive technologies for the treatment of adolescent obesity are developed (e.g., endoluminal device systems, vagal nerve stimulation, and gastric stimulation), the guidelines for surgical weight loss therapies for severely obese adolescents will most likely continue to evolve.

G. Ethical Considerations

The consideration of adolescent bariatric surgery carries significant ethical burdens that are likely to evolve, along with the advances in the clinical applications of such surgical modalities that must be addressed by individual surgeons and institutions providing such care. The decision to provide bariatric services and/or to proceed with a bariatric procedure on an individual basis requires recognition of the associated ethic as it pertains to all stakeholders (i.e., the patient, parents, pediatric physicians, healthcare institution, and society in general). Although a comprehensive discussion regarding such ethical issues is beyond the scope of this chapter, there are several overall guidelines that warrant recognition to serve as a foundation for additional in-depth consideration.

The decision to proceed with a bariatric surgical procedures should be made after a comprehensive assessment has determined that (1) an individual patient is unlikely to achieve amelioration of his or her associated comorbid disease using nonsurgical methods, (2) the patient has an acceptable surgical risk/benefit profile, (3) the patient and family have received extensive educational material and preoperative counseling regarding bariatric surgery, (4) informed consent has been obtained, and (5) the adolescent bariatric team has established a reliable system for the administration of short-and long-term care. In addition, it is important for the surgeon to engage the family on an open dialogue regarding the innovative aspects of adolescent bariatric surgery, including a clear discussion regarding the degree of uncertainty with respect to some longitudinal outcomes. Finally, tertiary care facilities offering bariatric surgery for the adolescent population should be encouraged to participate in clinical research endeavors in an effort to obtain valuable data which will be used to optimize clinical care.

H. Summary

Childhood obesity poses a serious healthcare issue of epidemic proportions both in the USA and globally, and has resulted in a growing population of children and adolescents with obesity-related diseases that were previously only considered in relation to the obese adult population. As has been observed in the obese adult population, surgical weight loss procedures appear to be the most effective means of achieving durable weight loss that results in the amelioration and/or resolution of the majority of the obesity-related comorbidities. The adolescent undergoing weight loss surgery requires lifelong follow-up and may benefit from the partnership of pediatric and adolescent specialists with adult bariatric centers. The uncertainty about long-term outcomes of weight loss surgery in adolescents supports the need for continued prospective multi-institutional studies designed to evaluate the longitudinal outcomes of this therapy.

Selected References

Brandt ML, Harmon CM, Helmrath MA, Inge TH, McKay SV, Michalsky MP. Morbid obesity in pediatric diabetes mellitus: surgical options and outcomes. Nat Rev Endocrinol. 2010;6(11):637–45.

Garcia V, DeMaria E. Adolescent bariatric surgery treatment delayed, treatment denied, a crisis invented. Obes Surg. 2006;16(1):1–4.

Inge TH, Miyano G, Bean J, et al. Reversal of type 2 diabetes mellitus and improvements in cardiovascular risk factors after surgical weight loss in adolescents. Pediatrics. 2009;123(1):214–22.

Ippisch H, Inge T, Daniels S, et al. Reversibility of cardiac abnormalities in morbidly obese adolescents. J Am Coll Cardiol. 2008;51:1342.

Michalsky M, Reichard K, Inge T, et al. ASMBS pediatric committee best practice guidelines. Surg Obes Relat Dis. 2012;8:1–7.

Teich S, Michalsky MP. Chronic diseases in childhood obesity: risks and benifits of early intervention. Ohio April 2–3, 2009. Semin Pediatr Srug 2009;18(3):125.

Varela E, Hinojosa M, Nguyen N. Perioperative outcomes of bariatric surgery in adolescents compared with adults at academic medical centers. Surg Obes Relat Dis. 2007;3:537–40.

Index

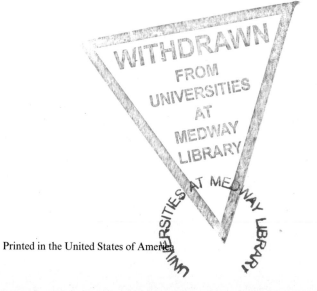